S0-CRQ-224

MedStudy®

RHEUMATOLOGY

SECTION EDITOR

Lisabeth V. Scalzi, MD, MS
Associate Professor of Pediatrics and
 Internal Medicine
Division of Rheumatology
Penn State Hershey Children's Hospital
Milton S. Hershey Medical Center
Hershey, PA

MEDICAL EDITOR

Jonathan S. Caudill, MD
Oxford, MS

REVIEWER

Randy Q. Cron, MD, PhD
Professor of Pediatrics & Medicine
Arthritis Foundation, Alabama Chapter,
 Endowed Chair
Director, Division of Pediatric Rheumatology
Children's Hospital of Alabama/
 University of Alabama at Birmingham
Birmingham, AL

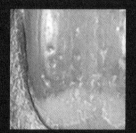

Table of Contents

RHEUMATOLOGY

GUIDELINES AND REVIEW ARTICLES AVAILABLE
ON THE MEDSTUDY HUB AT: medstudy.com/hub

JUVENILE IDIOPATHIC ARTHRITIS

PREVIEW | REVIEW

- Which cytokines are believed to mediate JIA?
- Name and describe the fever seen in sJIA.
- Name 2 poor prognostic indicators for sJIA.
- Describe the rash of sJIA.
- What is macrophage activation syndrome (MAS)?
- Which cell type engulfs other cell types (hemophagocytosis) in MAS?
- Which joint is frequently involved in JIA but is often silent, requiring diagnosis by MRI?
- In which eye chamber is uveitis due to JIA found?
- In oJIA, the presence of a positive ANA increases the risk of developing what eye finding?
- In poJIA, what does the presence of RF and anti-CCP antibodies indicate?
- What criteria are required to make the diagnosis of psJIA?
- In psJIA, can the arthritis precede the psoriasis by years?
- Arthritis of which joints is unique to psJIA?
- What is ERA?
- Which biologics can be used for JIA?

TERMINOLOGY / OCCURRENCE

Juvenile idiopathic arthritis (JIA) is the most common rheumatic disease diagnosed in children, affecting about 300,000 children in the United States. Incidence (new cases) per year varies by location and is ~ 10/100,000. Prevalence of JIA in North America is ~ 1/1,000 children.

The International League of Associations for Rheumatology (ILAR) renamed and replaced the terms juvenile rheumatoid arthritis and juvenile chronic arthritis with the new nomenclature, juvenile idiopathic arthritis. The ILAR JIA criteria have been endorsed by the World Health Organization and widely accepted in the U.S. and the international community.

JIA is defined as follows:

- Occurring before the age of 16 years
- Persistent synovitis in ≥ 1 joints
- Synovitis for at least 6 weeks

All other potential diagnoses must be excluded (e.g., infection and malignancy).

JIA TYPES

Overview

The ILAR classification system identifies 7 JIA categories:

1) **Systemic** (sJIA): arthritis + fever + systemic finding, including rash, hepatomegaly, splenomegaly, lymphadenopathy, or serositis
2) **Oligoarthritis** (oJIA): no more than 4 joints affected during the 1st 6 months of disease; 2 subcategories:
   - Persistent oligoarthritis (affecting ≤ 4 joints for the duration of the disease)
   - Extended arthritis (affecting ≥ 5 joints after the first 6 months of disease)
3) **Polyarthritis rheumatoid factor negative** (poJIA RF−): affecting ≥ 5 joints during the 1st 6 months of disease and RF−
4) **Polyarthritis RF positive** (poJIA RF+): affecting ≥ 5 joints during 1st 6 months of disease and RF+
5) **Psoriatic** arthritis (psJIA)
6) **Enthesitis-related arthropathies** (ERAs)
7) **Undifferentiated** (uJIA)

Keep going back to Table 20-1 on page 20-2 as you read through the following. It puts it all together and makes it easy to compare and contrast findings of these different subtypes.

The etiologies of these autoimmune disorders differ based on the subtypes. Genetic predispositions and environmental exposures that increase an individual's risk also likely differ based on subtype. Some HLA alleles appear to be important, and many believe that some microbial antigens are responsible as well.

JIA is thought to be initiated by presentation of antigens to T lymphocytes by antigen-presenting cells (e.g., macrophages, B cells, dendritic cells). This T-cell activation causes production of T and B lymphocytes. Cytokines are then released, including tumor necrosis factor alpha (TNF-α), interleukin-1 (IL-1), and interleukin-6 (IL-6), which cause release of other mediators such as prostaglandins, complements, proteases, and others. *[handwritten: TNFα IL1 IL6]*

Synovial fluid white blood cell counts, comprised mostly of lymphocytes, are usually between 2,000 and 30,000 cells/mL but can be as high as 100,000 cells/mL in some patients. The inflamed synovium is infiltrated with lymphocytes and plasma cells. Pannus formation occurs, which is growth of the synovium into the articular cartilage.

Clues for diagnosis of JIA:

- Morning stiffness that improves with movement later in the morning.
- Changes in walking, running, climbing, or willingness to play, especially in the morning hours. Sometimes described by the parents as the child walking like an old man/woman.

- Voluntary guarding of an inflamed joint.
- Leg length discrepancies.
- Return of need for assistance with dressing, eating, bathing, and using the toilet.
- Loss of developmental milestones.

Radiologic studies are nonspecific early in the course but can be helpful if you notice certain things. For example: If the JIA involves the fingers, it is characteristic to see widening of the midportion of the affected phalanges from periosteal new bone formation, although it takes months to years of active inflammation for these changes to appear. Unlike adult rheumatoid arthritis (RA), erosions are rarely seen early in the course of the disease, with the occasional exception of the temporomandibular joint, which can present with erosive changes.

Systemic JIA

Overview

By definition, sJIA (formerly called Still disease) requires the occurrence of daily fever, arthritis, and other systemic findings (Table 20-1). sJIA occurs in about 10–20% of those with JIA. This type affects boys and girls equally. Peak age is 2 years, and it trails off into adulthood. The key is finding 1 or 2 fever spikes on a daily basis, which returns to normal without any antipyretics; this is called a quotidian fever. Usually, the fever is in the evening and can be associated with severe myalgia and arthralgia. However, the fever is only present in this pattern in 30% of children at disease onset.

When the fever is gone, the child appears better and may have no significant symptoms. Poor prognostic indicators with sJIA include persistent, active disease 1 year after onset and diagnosis before 4 years of age.

Things to look for (in addition to fever and arthritis) with sJIA:

- Rash is migratory with macular, pink-to-salmon coloring and discrete borders with or without central clearing, usually coinciding with the fever. You see the rash on the trunk, thighs, and axillae. Mild irritation, such as rubbing or scratching (Koebner phenomenon), may cause the rash to appear. Occasionally, the rash is very pruritic. Biopsy shows only nonspecific lymphocytic infiltration, so this is not a recommended diagnostic test.
- Synovitis may or may not appear initially, but the diagnosis is more difficult—until the joint involvement has declared itself. Arthritis can occur as oligoarticular (~ 25–30%) or polyarticular (70–75%) involvement. The amount of arthritis predicts the long-term outcome.
- Severe myalgias may be present. Creatine phosphokinase (CPK) is usually normal, but the aldolase can be quite elevated.
- Pericarditis and myocarditis.
- Pleuritis.
- Lymphadenopathy.
- Hepatosplenomegaly.
- Abdominal pain.
- Weight loss and fatigue.

Table 20-1: JIA Subtypes						
	Oligoarticular	**Polyarticular RF–**	**Polyarticular RF+**	**Systemic**	**ERA**	**Psoriatic**
Peak age of onset	1–3 years	Dual peaks (1–3 years, then 9–14 years)	Teenage	2 years	Teenage	Dual peaks (2–3 years, then mean age of 10 years)
Sex	F > M	F > M	F > M	Equal	M > F	*F > M
ANA+	Majority	Majority	Rare	Rare	Rare	Majority of younger age
RF+	No	No	Yes	No	No	No
HLA-B27+	No	No	No	No	Majority	Majority of older age
Uveitis	Silent	Silent	Rare	Rare	Typically, acute	Silent
Enthesitis	No	No	No	No	Yes	Older age
Dactylitis	Rare	No	No	No	Yes	Yes
Fevers	No	No	No	High-spiking	Rare	No

By definition, children with unclassified JIA meet criteria for none of the categories listed in the table or for two or more of the categories.

*Among psoriatics with an older age of onset, the male:female ratio is close to 1, and the incidence of positive ANA is lower.

Adapted from Stoll ML and Cron RQ. *Pediatr Rheumatol Online J.* 2014 Apr 23;12:13.

Laboratory findings in sJIA can be very abnormal, with occasional leukemoid reaction (> 40,000 WBC/μL), thrombocytosis (occasionally >1 million cells/μL), and high C-reactive protein (CRP) and erythrocyte sedimentation rate (ESR) values. Ferritin levels are often elevated (normal < 200 ng/mL). Ferritin levels that are very elevated (e.g., > 5,000–100,000 ng/mL or higher) raise suspicion of macrophage activation syndrome, as described next. RF is negative, and the antinuclear antibody (ANA) is rarely positive.

Macrophage Activation Syndrome

Children severely affected by sJIA can develop a life-threatening condition called macrophage activation syndrome (MAS), also known as acquired hemophagocytic syndrome. Although MAS can be caused by infections (e.g., Epstein-Barr virus [EBV], parvovirus B19, and varicella) and drugs (e.g., sulfa drugs, NSAIDs), the usual cause in these patients is uncontrolled sJIA.

Characteristics of MAS:

- Persistent fever
- Hepatosplenomegaly
- Markedly high ferritin
- Cytopenias (affecting at least 2 of the 3 cell lines)
- Liver dysfunction marked by elevated liver function tests (LFTs), coagulopathy, low fibrinogen, and/or elevated triglycerides
- Neurologic dysfunction

Prompt diagnosis is possible with frequent laboratory (1–2× a week) and clinical (every 1–2 weeks) monitoring during active systemic disease. ESR can drop precipitously due to the low fibrinogen. Hemophagocytosis by macrophages/histiocytes is evident on bone marrow biopsy, although not always present.

anakinra

Prompt treatment with high-dose corticosteroids, IL-1 or IL-6 inhibitors, and/or cyclosporine can prevent life-threatening complications in MAS.

Oligoarticular JIA

Oligoarticular JIA is disease affecting ≤ 4 joints during the first 6 months of disease. oJIA occurs in approximately 30% of those with JIA and usually presents between 1 and 5 years of age, with an average age of onset of 1–3 years. Females outnumber males 3:1 overall, but in those with uveitis, females outnumber males 6.5:1. These patients often present with few symptoms and slow onset. About 25% do not have any pain but have incidental joint swelling. The joints most commonly involved (in most frequently seen order) are the knee, ankle, fingers/toes, elbows, and wrists, but rarely the hips. Asymptomatic temporomandibular joint (TMJ) involvement is typical in patients with oJIA and is best diagnosed by MRI. Fever, rash, and night pain are not seen in oligoarticular disease.

The 2 subtypes of oJIA are defined by the course of the arthritis after 6 months of disease. **Persistent** oligoarthritis is when the child has only ≤ 4 joints involved throughout the course of disease, and **extended** oligoarthritis (a worse prognosis) is when the child develops disease in ≥ 5 joints after the first 6 months.

Asymptomatic anterior uveitis can occur in about 30% of patients with oJIA, and ANA positivity predicts higher risk of developing uveitis. Screening frequency is based on various risk factors. Uveitis most commonly presents within the first 5–7 years of initial JIA presentation; thus, eye screening is performed more frequently in the early years following diagnosis but should continue annually in later years due to continued increased risk. In general, children with oJIA need ophthalmologic screening with slit-lamp exam:

- Every 3 months, if:
  ○ young (≤ 6 years of age at time of diagnosis),
  ○ ANA positive, and
  ○ recent onset (within 4 years).
- Every 6 months, if:
  ○ young (≤ 6 years of age at time of diagnosis),
  ○ ANA negative, and
  ○ child is 4–7 years beyond the time of diagnosis.
- Every 12 months, if:
  ○ older (> 6 years of age at time of diagnosis),
  ○ ANA negative, and
  ○ child is > 7 years beyond diagnosis.

If uveitis is found, treat aggressively to prevent synechiae (Image 20-1), cataracts, glaucoma, and blindness. Uveitis and arthritis do not necessarily happen at the same time. Even a child with no active arthritis is at risk.

Laboratory studies are nonspecific in oJIA. About 70% of children with oJIA have a positive ANA in low titer (≤ 1:320). It is very important to know that a positive ANA is not a diagnostic tool for JIA. It is used as a prognostic indicator for risk of uveitis in children with JIA. Other laboratory tests—including RF and hemoglobin—are usually normal in patients with oJIA; inflammatory markers, including ESR and CRP, can be normal in many of these patients. An elevated platelet count, which

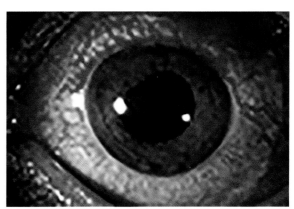

Image 20-1: Peripheral anterior synechiae

is a nonspecific marker of inflammation, can be encountered in any patient with JIA and inflammation.

Polyarticular JIA

Polyarticular JIA involves ≥ 5 joints during the first 6 months and is found in about 30–40% of those diagnosed with JIA. There is a higher prevalence in girls compared to boys, approximately 3:1. There are 2 distinct groups with polyarticular disease: those who are RF negative and those who are RF positive.

RF-negative poJIA has 2 age peaks: the first from 1–3 years of age and the second from 9–14 years old. poJIA affects large and small joints (metacarpophalangeals [MCPs] and proximal interphalangeals [PIPs]) and typically involves the cervical spine, hips, shoulders, and TMJs. Symmetrical joint involvement can occur, as in adult RA. Cervical spine fusion and micrognathia are typical late findings of polyarticular disease (for both polyarticular onset and systemic onset). Fatigue is a common presenting symptom; weight loss and rheumatoid nodules (usually RF+) can also occur.

RF-positive poJIA represents only about 4–5% of all children with JIA. RF+ disease more frequently occurs in older adolescents; the disease course corresponds to adult RA with a more aggressive course. RF positivity is a poor prognostic finding and mandates aggressive management of the patient. Anticyclic citrullinated peptide (anti-CCP) antibodies, often seen in adult RA, are also detectable in a significant proportion of RF+ JIA patients. Anti-CCP antibody is also associated with erosive arthritis in this group of patients. Most, but not all, RF+ poJIA patients are CCP+ and vice versa.

Approximately 50–80% of children with RF-negative poJIA have a positive ANA. Uveitis is less common with polyarticular onset, compared to oligoarticular onset, affecting only 10–15% with a +ANA. Uveitis is typically asymptomatic; younger children, < 7 years of age, with a +ANA and poJIA, have intermediate risk of uveitis and should be monitored more closely (as outlined previously under Oligoarticular JIA on page 20-3).

Juvenile Psoriatic Arthritis

Juvenile psoriatic arthritis (psJIA) is defined by:

- Arthritis and psoriasis
  or
- Arthritis and at least 2 of the following:
  ◦ Dactylitis
  ◦ Nail findings (pitting [Image 20-2], oil spots, or onycholysis)
  ◦ Family history of psoriasis in at least one 1st degree relative

Arthritis can precede the psoriasis by many years. Arthritis develops in about 7% of patients with cutaneous psoriasis, but it is much more likely to develop (> 30%) in those with psoriatic nail involvement. Initially, the arthritis is an asymmetric oligoarthritis of small and large joints. Distal interphalangeal (DIP) joint arthritis is also typical, and this makes psoriatic arthritis unique compared to the other JIA subtypes. Note: DIPs are the distal joints; PIPs are the middle joints; MCPs are the joints at the base of the fingers; and MTPs (metatarsal phalangeals) are the joints at the base of the toes. In some, the arthritis can involve more joints, and they can have a polyarticular pattern. Some patients have a chronic oligoarthritis or DIP arthritis and never progress to polyarthritis. Acute or chronic anterior uveitis is common, as is ANA positivity (30–50% of patients).

Dactylitis can be present and looks like a sausage digit where there is inflammation at the joints and in the soft tissue between the joints of a finger or toe.

Younger patients with psJIA are more commonly girls, whereas children presenting during adolescence are more often boys.

Enthesitis-Related Arthropathies

The enthesis is where a tendon or ligament inserts into bone. Enthesitis is inflammation and tenderness of this area. Enthesitis-related arthropathy (ERA) is enthesitis and arthritis, or either enthesitis or arthritis with ≥ 2 of the following:

1) History or presence of sacroiliac joint tenderness and/or inflammatory lumbosacral pain
2) Presence of HLA-B27 antigen
3) Onset of arthritis in a male > 6 years of age
4) Acute symptomatic uveitis
5) A 1st degree relative with ankylosing spondylitis, ERA, sacroiliitis with inflammatory bowel disease, or reactive arthritis

You may be familiar with older terminology for 1 or more of the ERAs. The ILAR recommends that the following entities (some historical) be referred to as ERAs: juvenile spondyloarthropathy; SEA syndrome (syndrome of seronegativity, enthesopathy, and arthropathy); HLA-B27-associated arthropathy and

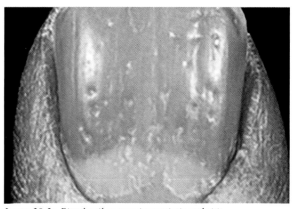

Image 20-2: Pitted nail as seen in psoriatic arthritis

enthesopathy syndrome; oligoarticular-onset JIA "Type II"; and juvenile ankylosing spondylitis.

ERA has different characteristics, compared to the other childhood inflammatory arthritides:

• Older children are affected more often.
• Males are more commonly affected.
• It is familial 10–20% of the time.
• Arthritis is typically peripheral, with lower limb involvement in an asymmetric manner.
• Enthesitis is a common finding.

Constitutional symptoms are less common, with fever and weight loss occurring in < 10% of children with ERA. Conduct a complete review of systems to be sure there is no growth delay, abdominal pain, or blood in the stools, as can be seen with inflammatory bowel disease.

Clinically, these children (usually boys) present with morning pain and stiffness that is relieved by playing or other activity. The pain is predominantly in the joints of the lower extremities and is frequently in the lower back/ buttocks and at the entheses of the heels, feet, and knees. The enthesitis at the patellar tendon can be misdiagnosed as Osgood-Schlatter disease, which is an overuse injury of the patellar ligament over the tibial tuberosity. The oligoarthritis of ERA is commonly asymmetrical. The entheses that are affected can be exquisitely tender to palpation. You can elicit sacroiliac pain by direct palpation or pelvic manipulation. Lumbar flexion is often limited and remains flat (no lumbar curvature) on exam.

Acute symptomatic iritis (i.e., an acutely painful, red eye) occurs in about 5–10% of children with ERA and requires ophthalmology referral.

ESR is normal in 50% of patients and HLA-B27 is positive in 50–90%.

Those with a chronic course are more likely to develop sacroiliitis with spondylitis and progress into adulthood with ankylosing disease of the back and sacroiliac joints.

DIFFERENTIAL DIAGNOSIS OF JIA

Joint inflammation, which manifests as heat, pain, and swelling, is required to make the JIA diagnosis. If pain occurs without evidence of inflammation, think of an orthopedic problem such as avascular necrosis, slipped femoral epiphysis, or Osgood-Schlatter disease. Also consider other conditions such as benign nocturnal limb pains of childhood ("growing pains"), benign hypermobility, and psychogenic/amplified pain syndrome. The differential diagnosis of sJIA includes various illnesses with fever, joint symptoms, rash, lymphadenopathy, and lab abnormalities such as:

• Malignancies (e.g., leukemia, lymphoma, neuroblastoma)
• Bone or joint infections
• Systemic lupus erythematosa (SLE)
• Acute rheumatic fever

• Serum sickness
• Kawasaki disease
• Sarcoidosis
• Sjögren syndrome

TREATMENT OF JIA

Nonsteroidal antiinflammatory medications (**NSAIDs**) are often used initially, typically with disease-modifying antirheumatic drugs (**DMARDs**). Many pediatric rheumatologists start a DMARD immediately after ruling out other possible diagnoses.

Intraarticular injection of triamcinolone (an injectable steroid) is an excellent local way of treating JIA, especially if only a "few" joints are affected. Remember: patients with oligoarticular joint disease can have leg length discrepancies if the knees are involved (affected leg is longer initially, particularly in younger patients). Joint injections decrease this occurrence.

The DMARD most commonly used for JIA is methotrexate. Methotrexate is administered 1×/week either as pills or injected subcutaneously. It is important that patients who take methotrexate be on folic acid supplementation to decrease risk for methotrexate side effects (liver abnormalities, oral ulcers, and cytopenias). Sulfasalazine is useful in the treatment of ERA. Cyclosporine is also used occasionally in sJIA, especially in the presence of MAS.

Biologic therapies that target a specific cytokine are commonly used for children with aggressive disease or disease refractory to DMARDs, although not all are approved by the FDA for treatment in children.

Biologic treatments for JIA:

• Tumor necrosis factor inhibitors (e.g., etanercept, adalimumab, infliximab)
• T-cell modulators (abatacept)
• IL-6 receptor blockers (tocilizumab)
• IL-1 blockers (e.g., anakinra, canakinumab, rilonacept)

TNF inhibitors (TNFi) appear to work very well for poJIA but less so for sJIA patients (who respond well to IL-6 and IL-1 inhibition). **Abatacept**, a soluble fusion protein that inhibits the costimulation of T cells, is also useful for refractory cases of poJIA.

Test for latent TB infection, hepatitis B virus (HBV), and hepatitis C virus prior to initiating biologic therapy. Once a patient is on a biologic therapy, avoid live attenuated vaccines.

Generally, do not use corticosteroids except for very severe disease, flares of disease, or systemic manifestations. Try to use the lowest doses possible (< 0.25 mg/kg/day or < 10 mg/day) to minimize side effects, which include diabetes, stunted growth, osteoporosis, infection, cataracts, glaucoma, hypertension, hyperlipidemia, mood changes, and adrenal insufficiency.

Follow patients closely every 1–3 months; remission is the goal of therapy, and patients can then be seen every 4–5 months. Physical and occupational therapy, orthotics, and splinting can be helpful for children to maintain function and prevent deformities.

OUTCOMES OF JIA

Long-term follow-up studies show that patients with JIA treated in the era before biologics had a higher rate of disability than previously thought, with 25–50% of them having functional limitations. Data shows steady improvement in functional capacity over the past 40 years due to better treatments, including medication and joint replacement. Up to 30–40% still have active synovitis as adults and require ongoing rheumatologic care. Mortality from JIA is rare, < 0.5% in the U.S. Deaths in children with sJIA related to amyloidosis, infections, and MAS have declined as a result of better disease recognition and control.

ARTHRITIS WITH INFLAMMATORY BOWEL DISEASE

PREVIEW | REVIEW

- What percentage of patients with IBD have arthritis?
- In arthritis with IBD, how do the peripheral vs. axial arthritis forms differ?
- What are the systemic symptoms of arthritis with IBD?

Arthritis occurs in about 25% of patients with inflammatory bowel disease (IBD; Crohn's or ulcerative colitis). Characteristics of this associated arthritis depend on whether it is peripheral or axial:

- If **peripheral** arthritis (more commonly affected):
  ◦ Incidence in girls = incidence in boys
  ◦ Not associated with HLA-B27
  ◦ Arthritis flares with gut flares
- If **axial** arthritis (e.g., spine, hips, sacroiliac joints):
  ◦ Incidence in boys >> incidence in girls
  ◦ Associated with HLA-B27
  ◦ Not dependent on gut flares

Look for the following systemic symptoms and signs to help diagnose arthritis with IBD: fatigue, iron deficiency anemia, a low albumin, persistently elevated inflammatory markers, weight loss, growth delay, fever, oral ulcers, abdominal pain/tenderness, diarrhea, erythema nodosum, pyoderma gangrenosum, and clubbing.

Arthritis coinciding with a gut flare (typically peripheral arthritis) usually responds to appropriate therapy for the gut disease, such as corticosteroids or oral DMARDs (sulfasalazine, methotrexate, infliximab, and adalimumab). Spinal disease sometimes needs treatment even when gut disease is inactive; typical agents used are NSAIDs and the monoclonal antibody TNF inhibitors (infliximab and adalimumab). Oral DMARDs do not help with spinal disease, only peripheral disease. The FDA added label warnings of increased risk of hepatosplenic T-cell lymphoma (HSTCL) in children who receive TNF inhibitors, especially when used in combination with azathioprine or 6-mercaptopurine (6-MP); however, HSTCL has been described in patients receiving azathioprine and 6-MP alone. NSAIDs are used sparingly because of risk for IBD flares and GI side effects.

INFECTION-RELATED ARTHRITIS

PREVIEW | REVIEW

- In infectious arthritis, what are the differing characteristics between bacterial and viral etiologies?
- Infections of which 2 systems typically occurs prior to reactive arthritis?
- What is the typical triad of reactive arthritis?
- Can urethritis occur in reactive arthritis even if the organism is of GI origin?

INFECTIOUS ARTHRITIS

Infectious arthritis is most frequently caused by the direct spread of bacteria into the joint space but can also be caused by viruses and fungi. Presenting symptoms include fever, substantial pain, and decreased range of motion of the affected, often erythematous joint. The arthritis can affect one joint or multiple joints, depending on the causative agent.

Bacteria tend to affect single, large joints, although certain pathogens (especially *Staphylococcus aureus* and *Neisseria gonorrhoeae*) can affect multiple joints. **Viral** etiologies cause a rash and commonly can have symmetric involvement of smaller joints. **Fungal** causes are rare and typically occur in the neonate or immunocompromised patient. Fungal causes have a more indolent course and occur with disseminated disease.

A good history and physical are important, with special attention given to location and number of joints affected. Diagnosis is made by isolation of the pathogen by culture or polymerase chain reaction (PCR) from synovial fluid or blood. The mainstay of treatment is drainage and lavage of the joint space and antimicrobial therapy (unless viral) targeted toward the inciting organism.

Some of the microbes that cause arthritis include:

- *S. aureus* (most common)
- *N. gonorrhoeae*
- Viruses
  ◦ Parvovirus B19
  ◦ HBV

REACTIVE ARTHRITIS

Reactive arthritis (previously postinfectious arthritis) usually occurs 1–4 weeks after:

- GI infection with
  ◦ *Yersinia*
  ◦ *Shigella*
  ◦ *Salmonella*
  ◦ *Campylobacter*
  ◦ *Clostridium difficile*
  ◦ *Giardia*
- Genitourinary infection caused by *Chlamydia (*usually lasts 3–6 weeks but occasionally remains chronic)
- Lyme disease
- Streptococcal infection

Reactive arthritis typically manifests as a triad of urethritis, conjunctivitis, and arthritis (thus the catch phrase, "can't pee, can't see, can't climb a tree"). Not all symptoms necessarily occur, or they can occur at separate times. Urethritis can occur even if the infectious trigger was GI in origin; urinalysis may show a sterile pyuria. Mucocutaneous features, including oral ulcers, genital ulcers, and papular skin lesions (such as keratoderma blenorrhagicum on the palms and soles), are common as well. Look for enthesitis, dactylitis, and arthritis that affects the large weight-bearing joints. Due to fever and the severity of the systemic symptoms, reactive arthritis can present like septic arthritis, requiring you to aspirate joint fluid.

A convincing history of infection occurring 2–4 weeks prior to onset of urethritis, conjunctivitis, and arthritis is usually enough to make the diagnosis; however, obtaining stool, urethral, conjunctival cultures, and/or blood serologies—looking for presence of current or recent infection—is recommended. The arthritis usually lasts for 3–6 weeks but occasionally can remain chronic.

Treat with NSAIDs. Resistant cases may benefit from sulfasalazine, methotrexate, and/or anti-TNF agents. Antibiotics are not required unless there is evidence of active infection.

VASCULITIDES

PREVIEW | REVIEW

- What is the most common vasculitis in childhood?
- What antibody mediates HSP?
- What is a predisposing factor in 50% of HSP cases?
- What do you do if a child with HSP has persistent, severe abdominal pain? What do you suspect as an etiology?
- What system are you concerned about for up to 6 months after diagnosis of HSP?

- Are most cases of HSP self-limited?
- How common are recurrences in HSP during the first 2 years?
- What is the nasal deformity seen in granulomatosis with polyangiitis?
- What laboratory test is useful in diagnosing granulomatosis with polyangiitis?
- What is the main cause of death in Kawasaki disease? When does this usually occur?
- What are the diagnostic criteria for Kawasaki disease?
- What gallbladder abnormality is seen in Kawasaki disease?
- What are the cardiac manifestations of Kawasaki disease?
- What is the treatment for Kawasaki disease?
- What are potential therapies available for Kawasaki disease refractory to IVIG?
- What is polyarteritis nodosa (PAN)?
- Which organ system is typically spared in PAN?
- What is Takayasu arteritis?
- What is the classic triad of Behçet disease?
- Which skin lesions are commonly seen in Behçet disease?

OVERVIEW

The vasculitic disorders are relatively uncommon in children. Severity and manifestations are dependent on the size of the vessels.

Small-vessel vasculitis, caused by immune complexes, presents with purpura. Examples of small-vessel vasculitis include drug reactions, serum sickness, Henoch-Schönlein purpura (HSP), and granulomatosis with polyangiitis (GPA; formerly known as Wegener's).

Medium-vessel vasculitis causes organ system damage and includes polyarteritis nodosa (PAN) and Kawasaki disease.

Large-vessel vasculitis can cause claudication symptoms. Takayasu arteritis is the classic form of a large-vessel disorder.

SMALL VESSEL VASCULITIDES

Henoch-Schönlein Purpura

HSP is a **small-vessel vasculitis.** It is the most common vasculitis of childhood, affecting ~ 1 in 5,000 children. The mean age at diagnosis is 4 years, and > 75% of those affected are < 7 years of age. The age range is typically 3–15 years, but HSP is seen in older adolescents and adults as well. HSP affects boys more frequently with a ratio of nearly 2:1. Seasonality is important, with more cases in the winter and spring. HSP is an immune-mediated leukocytoclastic vasculitis with neutrophil infiltration and primarily IgA (immunoglobulin A) deposition in vessel walls, along with small amounts of IgG and C3 (complement component 3).

The specific cause of HSP is unknown, but in about 50% of cases, an upper respiratory infection precedes the disease. The literature has listed a number of possible "triggers": bacteria (e.g., *Streptococcus pyogenes*, *Legionella*, *Mycoplasma*, *Yersinia*), viruses (e.g., EBV, varicella, CMV, parvovirus, HBV), drugs (e.g., penicillin, cephalosporins, thiazide diuretics), vaccines (e.g., measles, yellow fever), food additives, and insect bites.

Skin lesions (Image 20-3 and Image 20-4) are present in all HSP patients, and it is the presenting finding in about 50%. The rash begins as small wheals or red maculopapules that progress to petechial and palpable purpuric lesions. They are generally found on the dependent, pressure-bearing areas: lower extremities and buttocks. They can occur in other areas as well, particularly the face and ears in younger children. The skin lesions last anywhere from 4 days to 4 weeks. Angioedema sometimes precedes the rash.

The second most common manifestation is **joint involvement**, occurring in 50–80%. In about 25% of patients, arthritis is the initial manifestation and makes the diagnosis difficult until the rash appears. The arthritis/arthralgia is transient and mainly of the large joints, particularly the knees and ankles. Joint effusions do not usually occur. Periarthritis, with edema around the joints and inflammation involving the tendon sheaths, is the most common musculoskeletal manifestation. Chronic arthritis is not present.

The next most prevalent are the **gastrointestinal manifestations**. The most typical GI manifestation is abdominal pain that is colicky in pattern and sometimes involves vomiting as well. The pain can precede the rash (in 15–35% of cases)—again, making the diagnosis more difficult until the rash appears. Occult bleeding is common in those with abdominal pain, and melena can occur. Hematemesis can occur but is less typical. Fortunately, only about 5% have a major GI bleeding

episode. Ultrasound (U/S) may show increased echogenicity and/or thickening of the wall of the 2nd portion of the duodenum and hydrops of the gallbladder. These changes occur only if the patient has GI symptoms, which occur in about 65% of patients.

If abdominal pain is severe or persistent, perform U/S to evaluate for intussusception, which can occur in 2–14% of patients.

Renal manifestations affect between 10% and 50% of those with HSP and are usually mild and transient. Look for isolated microscopic hematuria or for hematuria and proteinuria. A renal biopsy (which is not normally performed in this disease) shows IgA deposition just as with Berger disease (a.k.a. IgA nephropathy). Generally, < 1–2% have residual renal disease, and even fewer progress to end-stage renal disease. Those at greater risk for permanent renal damage are generally children with purpura that lasts > 1 month; children with severe, persistent GI symptoms; and children who have decreased Factor 13. For more information on HSP, see Nephrology and Urology, Book 3.

Other manifestations include orchitis and pulmonary hemorrhage. Acute appendicitis is often mistakenly suspected when severe GI symptoms precede the other classic manifestations.

HSP is a clinical diagnosis without specific confirmatory laboratory tests. Nonspecific findings include high WBC counts, elevated ESR (increased in about 50% of patients), elevated IgA levels, and normal platelet and coagulation studies. Ultrasonography, as mentioned above, can be helpful.

Order serial urinalysis for at least 3–6 months after diagnosis to monitor for renal involvement.

There is no specific therapy for HSP. Supportive outpatient care is generally sufficient. Skin lesions do not need specific therapy unless they are severe and ulcerated; administer corticosteroids in these cases. Use nonsteroidals for pain control but avoid if renal disease and significant GI disease are present. Corticosteroids have

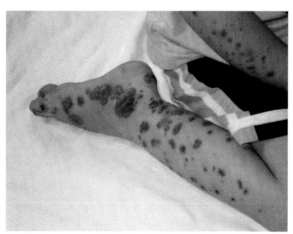

Image 20-3: HSP skin lesions on the lower extremities

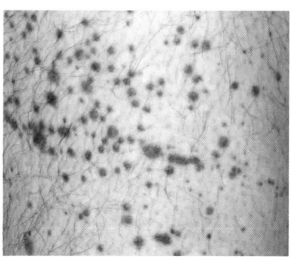

Image 20-4: HSP skin lesions; maculopapules and petechiae

been used successfully in those with severe abdominal pain or severe scrotal swelling/edema. No controlled trials to date show benefit of therapy for HSP nephritis. Most improve without specific therapy, although uncontrolled trials have used IV pulses of methylprednisolone, cyclophosphamide, and azathioprine.

Prognosis is excellent, with most of the problems stemming from acute GI bleeds early in the illness or long-term renal involvement. Otherwise, the disease tends to be self-limited and lasts 4 weeks in about 65% of children. HSP recurs in up to 40% of patients from 6 weeks to 2 years after initial presentation.

Granulomatosis with Polyangiitis

GPA (formerly known as Wegener's) is very rare in children and is characterized by necrotizing granulomatous vasculitis of small-sized vessels involving the upper and lower respiratory tracts and the kidney—pulmonary-renal syndrome. Other potentially confounding pulmonary-renal syndromes include microscopic polyangiitis (MPA), sarcoidosis, SLE, and Goodpasture syndrome. GPA can present in adolescence and affects males and females equally. Common symptoms are fever, weight loss, arthralgias or migratory large joint arthritis, cough, nasal stuffiness, epistaxis, resistant ear infections, and persistent sinusitis. Nasal deformity (saddle nose, Image 20-5) and subglottic stenosis can also occur in children with GPA and, less commonly, in relapsing polychondritis.

Lung findings (nodules, infiltrates, hemoptysis, or pleuritis) are reported in 70% of children with GPA. Ocular findings (conjunctivitis, dacryocystitis, scleritis, and proptosis) occur in about 15–20% of these children. Renal involvement is uncommon in these children at presentation but eventually occurs in 60–70%. Finding cytoplasmic ANCA (c-ANCA specific for PR3 [proteinase 3]) aids in the diagnosis. c-ANCA positivity is found in > 90% of patients with diffuse disease and only ~ 50%

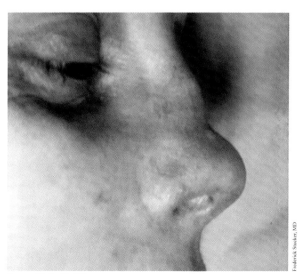

Image 20-5: Saddle nose

Frederick Stucker, MD

of those with limited (i.e., no renal involvement) disease. You must perform a biopsy to confirm the diagnosis.

Consider using steroids, methotrexate (especially for limited disease), rituximab, and cyclophosphamide. Chronic therapy with trimethoprim/sulfamethoxazole prevents relapses and decreases the risk for *Pneumocystis jiroveci* pneumonia (PCP). Relapses occur in 30–50% of patients. Long-term use of cyclophosphamide increases risk for infertility, lymphoma, hemorrhagic cystitis, and secondary cancers.

MEDIUM VESSEL VASCULITIDES

Kawasaki Disease

Kawasaki disease, a **medium-vessel vasculitis**, is the 2nd most common vasculitis of childhood. It is the leading cause of acquired heart disease in children in the U.S. It generally occurs in children < 5 years of age, affects boys more than girls (1.5:1), and occurs year-round with clusters in the winter and spring. Incidence is highest in children of Asian descent. In Japan, the incidence is 90/100,000 in children < 5 years of age, but the reported incidence in the U.S. is about 9–19/100,000. Nearly 1–3% of those affected have a recurrence. Recurrence is most likely in boys > 6 years or < 6 months of age. The etiology of this disorder is unknown. Kawasaki disease simulates an infectious disease, but no consistent organism can be identified. One theory points to staphylococcal and streptococcal superantigen stimulation of the immune system.

Myocardial infarction is the main cause of death and most commonly occurs during the 1st year from the onset of illness. Fatality rates are 0.16% in those < 1 year of age and 0.05% in those > 1 year of age.

A clinical diagnosis requires fever for at least 5 days and a minimum of 4 of the following 5 findings (Table 20-2 on page 20-10):

1) Bilateral conjunctival injection without exudate in 80–90%

2) Rash in > 90% (Image 20-6 on page 20-10)—typically macular and polymorphous in character with no vesicles, scaling, or crusting; found on the trunk and frequently more prominent in the perineal area later in the course; desquamation of the area follows

3) Changes in lips and oral cavity occur in 80–90%—red pharynx, dry fissured lips, and/or an injected, strawberry tongue (Image 20-7 on page 20-10)

4) Changes in the peripheral extremities in approximately 80%—redness and swelling of the hands/feet (Image 20-8 on page 20-10) and, later, desquamation of the fingers/toes (Image 20-9 on page 20-11)

5) Cervical lymphadenopathy in approximately 50%—typically nonfluctuant with 1 node required to be at least 1.5 cm in diameter

Diagnosis with < 4 of the 5 criteria is possible if coronary aneurysm is demonstrated on echocardiogram or angiography. Fever is an absolute requirement.

Table 20-2: Classical Clinical Criteria of Kawasaki Disease	
Frequency (%)	**Criteria**
100	Fever persisting at least 5 days
80–90	Changes in lips and oral cavity: erythema, lips cracking, strawberry tongue, diffuse injection of oral and pharyngeal mucosae
80–90	Bilateral bulbar conjunctival injection without exudate
> 90	Polymorphous exanthem
50	Cervical lymphadenopathy (> 1.5-cm diameter), usually unilateral
80	Changes in extremities Acute: Erythema of palms, soles; edema of hands, feet Subacute: Periungual peeling of fingers, toes in weeks 2 and 3

Adapted from Newburger JW, et al. AHA Scientific Statement 2004. *Textbook of Pediatric Rheumatology*, 7th ed. Ross E. Petty, et al. (eds.) Elsevier, 2015.

Think of Kawasaki disease in 3 stages:

The **1st stage**, the acute phase, is the initial febrile period, usually lasting 1–2 weeks with temperatures of ≥ 104.0° F (40.0° C) and with at least 4 of the 5 findings outlined above. Irritability is a hallmark in this stage. Look for other findings, including aseptic meningitis, acute uveitis, diarrhea, mild obstructive jaundice with elevated transaminases, hydrops of the gallbladder, and sterile pyuria. Nearly 33% have polyarthritis or polyarthralgia, typically of the knees, ankles, and hands. Edema of the hands and feet is more common than localized inflammatory arthritis. Fluid aspirated from the joint shows polymorphonuclear leukocytes (PMNs), simulating septic arthritis but with a negative culture.

Be particularly aware of cardiac manifestations. Nearly 33% have pericardial effusions, and myocarditis is also common. Coronary artery abnormalities (aneurysms are the main worry) can occur as early as day 3 of illness but are more typically seen from 10 days to 4 weeks after onset. Even with treatment, they are found in 5–9% of patients. Increased risks of coronary aneurysm include age < 1 year, male gender, fever > 16 days, cardiomegaly, arrhythmias, and fever recurrence after 48 hours of being afebrile. See more about Kawasaki disease in Cardiology, Book 3.

The **2nd stage**, the subacute phase, starts around 10–25 days after the initial fever presentation and persists until all clinical signs of inflammatory activity subside. The fever, rash, and lymph nodes usually resolve early in this phase, but irritability and conjunctival injection can persist. Skin changes occur during this stage, most commonly desquamation. Thrombocytosis generally occurs after day 7 of the illness. Coronary artery aneurysms occur in 25% of those untreated and 5–9% of those treated. Oligoarticular disease can occur in 25% during the 2nd and 3rd weeks but is self-limited.

The **3rd stage**, the convalescent phase, occurs about the 3rd or 4th week, when clinical signs disappear, and usually lasts 3–4 weeks.

Kawasaki disease is mostly a clinical diagnosis. Use laboratory tests to exclude strep or staph infection and serum sickness. Laboratory findings include leukocytosis with a left shift, platelet counts commonly > 1 million during the subacute phase of the illness, and the ESR and/or CRP typically very high. Elevation of the gamma-glutamyl transferase (GGT) can help differentiate Kawasaki disease from other fever and rash syndromes that do not have gallbladder involvement. Beware of possible multiorgan dysfunction.

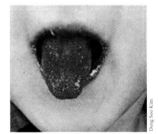
Image 20-7: Strawberry tongue

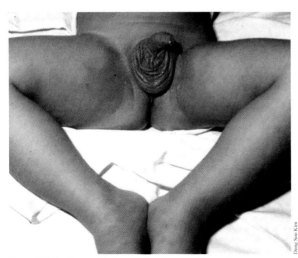
Image 20-6: Kawasaki disease showing macular rash

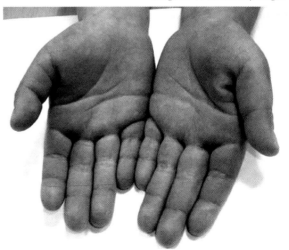
Image 20-8: Kawasaki disease with redness and swelling of hands

Approximately 1% of these patients can develop overt MAS (macrophage activation syndrome).

There is a syndrome known as atypical or incomplete Kawasaki disease, which you see in those patients who have fewer than the required 4 of 5 clinical findings needed for diagnosis. Usually missing is cervical lymphadenopathy and rash. It more often occurs in younger patients, especially infants < 1 year of age.

Treatment is well established. Traditional recommendations are to give aspirin at a dose of 80–100 mg/kg/day initially and IV immunoglobulin (IVIG) at a dose of 2 g/kg as a single infusion over 12–14 hours. The IVIG typically causes a rapid improvement in fever and clinical symptoms. If the patient has a relapse or does not respond well, repeat the dose of IVIG. Retreatment is needed in < 5–10% of cases. IVIG side effects are uncommon, but look for anaphylaxis and aseptic meningitis, which can occur 1–2 days after treatment. Corticosteroid therapy is controversial, with some studies showing some benefit even though early (flawed) studies showed an increased risk of coronary aneurysm. Consider high-dose steroid use only as "rescue" therapy in patients who are IVIG failures. Infliximab and cyclosporine have been used safely and successfully in patients who are IVIG failures. Continue high-dose aspirin for a few days until IVIG response is achieved and fever resolves. Reduce the aspirin dose to 3–5 mg/kg/day for platelet inhibition, and discontinue when you are assured there is no cardiac involvement. Because IVIG, corticosteroids, and infliximab all help treat the inflammation, some consider the high risk-to-benefit ratio of high-dose aspirin a valid reason to remove it from future standard therapy.

Every child with Kawasaki's should have an initial echocardiogram at the time of diagnosis and a 2ⁿᵈ echocardiogram performed 6–8 weeks after the initial one. Myocardial infarction, if it occurs, usually does so during the 1ˢᵗ year after the onset of illness. Fatality rates are 0.16% in those < 1 year and 0.05% in those > 1 year of age.

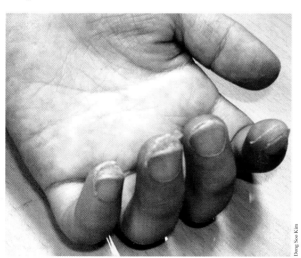

Image 20-9: Kawasaki disease with desquamation of fingers

Polyarteritis Nodosa

PAN causes inflammation of **medium-sized arteries** and results in a focal segmental necrotizing vasculitis. It is rare in children and occurs at a mean age of about 9 years, with males more frequently affected (about 2:1). The exact etiology is unknown, although documented cases have occurred after hepatitis B or strep infection, or the use of certain drugs, all of which seem to implicate immune complexes.

PAN in childhood typically presents with constitutional symptoms (e.g., fever, fatigue, anorexia), musculoskeletal findings, and renal disease. The following may be observed: red rashes, HSP-like lesions (i.e., maculopapular, purpuric), painful skin nodules (erythema nodosum), livedo reticularis (a persistent, purplish, network-patterned discoloration of the skin caused by dilation of capillaries), cutaneous ulcers, and, very rarely, infarction of digits. Musculoskeletal findings can include arthralgia, arthritis, and myositis. Renal arterial involvement occurs in about 50–60% of patients and can present as hematuria, proteinuria, or hypertension. There is an absence of lung involvement.

GI bleeding and ulcers as well as neurologic disease (mononeuritis multiplex, hemiparesis, or stroke) are seen much less often. One other thing to look for—orchitis! It occurs most commonly in those with concomitant hepatitis B infection.

Cutaneous PAN (a subset of PAN) has just the skin manifestations without the systemic findings; it responds well to oral prednisone, but expect relapses. Occasionally, peripheral neuropathy develops in these patients. Diagnosis of PAN is difficult because there is no specific PAN test. Diagnosis is usually based on criteria from the American College of Rheumatology, which includes:

- Skin lesions (e.g., purpura, livedo)
- Testicular pain/orchitis
- Mononeuritis multiplex (presenting as a foot drop)
- Renal involvement
- Hypertension
- Evidence of hepatitis B
- Weight loss
- Biopsy or angiographic findings

You can confirm diagnosis with biopsy of affected tissue (e.g., skin, kidney, muscle, sural nerve) or angiograph showing stenosis and aneurysm formation.

Treat with steroids and immunosuppressive agents. Daily steroids are most effective, and IV pulse cyclophosphamide is effective in some. Prognosis is poor without aggressive treatment.

PAN is a separate condition from MPA (microscopic polyangiitis). PAN is a medium-vessel vasculitis that causes aneurysms and stenosis, resulting in hematuria and renovascular hypertension. It does not cause glomerulonephritis; MPA does.

MPA – PANCA – MPO

MPA is a p-ANCA-associated (perinuclear antibodies to MPO [myeloperoxidase]), small-vessel vasculitis without granuloma formation. Glomerular involvement is extensive, causing rapidly progressive glomerulonephritis and a pulmonary-renal syndrome (resulting in pulmonary hemorrhage) similar to GPA.

LARGE-VESSEL VASCULITIDES

Takayasu Arteritis (Pulseless Disease)

Takayasu arteritis (TA) is very rare in children in the U.S. In Japan, TA is the 3rd most common childhood vasculitis, after HSP and Kawasaki disease.

TA is a granulomatous vasculitis of large vessels. It leads to arteritis of the aorta and its major branches, resulting in weak or absent pulses in the upper extremities. Look for coarctation of the aorta and/or hypertension with systemic findings of fever, arthritis, and myalgia. A simple, yet very useful test to help identify this as a possible diagnosis is to perform 4-extremity blood pressures. There are proposed criteria for the diagnosis of TA in children (Table 20-3); ischemic findings in children are infrequent (unlike in adults).

Think of TA as occurring in phases: the inflammatory prepulseless stage and the noninflammatory occlusive stage. During the inflammatory stage, patients can have fever, fatigue, weight loss, arthritis, and elevated markers of inflammation. During the noninflammatory stage, patients can have symptoms that are secondary to vessel involvement, such as claudication, dizziness, headaches, and vision problems. During this stage, markers of inflammation can be normal. These stages can overlap or be separated by ≥ 10 years.

Glucocorticoids and cyclophosphamide are the mainstays of therapy. Consider surgery for stenotic lesions that do not respond to immunotherapy. Also consider antiplatelet agents or anticoagulation for patients with nonsurgical but stenotic lesions. Recently, retrospective analyses suggest patients with refractory TA benefit from TNF or IL-6 blockade with biological agents.

Table 20-3: Proposed Criteria for the Diagnosis of Takayasu Arteritis in Children
Angiographic abnormalities (as demonstrated by CT or MRA) of the aorta or main branches, plus at least 1 of the following:
1) Decreased peripheral pulses and/or claudication of the extremities
2) Blood pressure difference of > 10 mmHg between arms
3) Audible bruits over aorta and/or major branches
4) Hypertension
Adapted from Tann OR, et al. Takayasu's disease: A review. *Cardiology in the Young.* June 2008;18(3):250–259.

VASCULITIDES OF > 1 VESSEL SIZE

Behçet Disease *any size vessel : CNS, renal, heart*

Behçet disease is unlike any other vasculitis in that it can involve blood vessels of any size and type (including arteries or veins). Look for the classic triad of:

1) oral ulcers (painful, recurrent),

2) genital ulcers (painful, recurrent), and

3) inflammatory eye disease.

Behçet's occurs sporadically in children in the U.S. but is much more common in children from the Mediterranean and the Far East. The key finding is recurrent buccal aphthous ulcers, which are found in nearly 100% of patients. Behçet disease can present as a periodic fever syndrome in younger children before the typical manifestations occur. Skin lesions (including erythema nodosum and necrotic folliculitis) are common. You occasionally see a positive pathergy test—prick the skin with a needle, and after 48 hours you see a pustule or papule surrounded by redness. Pathergy is found most often in individuals of Middle Eastern origin. Genital ulcers occur in about 75% of patients, and most have recurrent oral aphthous ulcers. Eye lesions also occur and can include both anterior and posterior uveitis, retinal vasculitis, and papilledema. Arthralgias or arthritis can also be seen. Rarely, GI involvement mimics Crohn disease or ulcerative colitis. When this happens, it typically presents with diarrhea and GI bleeding from ulcerations within the GI tract. It can be very difficult to distinguish between Behçet and Crohn disease, which may represent a spectrum of disease with different modes of inheritance.

The diagnosis is clinical and requires observation of recurrent oral ulceration at least 3× over a 1-year period plus at least 2 of the following: recurrent genital ulceration, eye lesions, skin lesions, or positive pathergy test. Pathology shows a neutrophilic infiltrate in affected blood vessels.

Initially, treat with corticosteroids (oral or topical). Some patients with ulcerative manifestations benefit from colchicine and pentoxifylline. Use azathioprine for severe vasculitis with CNS or eye involvement. Infliximab helps treat the colitis.

Childhood Primary Angiitis of the CNS

Central nervous system (CNS) vasculitis is an inflammatory disease affecting the blood vessels of the brain. It can be primary or secondary (e.g., another autoimmune disease, infection, drugs).

Childhood primary angiitis of the CNS (cPACNS) is a primary form of this vasculitis. This disease can present with arterial stroke in children. The etiology of this disorder is unknown, and the histopathology is nonspecific.

cPACNS is defined by the size of the artery/arteries involved and whether or not it is progressive over time. **Small-vessel** cPACNS has a normal angiography, and

medium- and large-vessel cPACNS have abnormal angiography. Medium- and large-vessel disease are further identified by exhibiting evidence of ongoing inflammatory disease (i.e., new stenosis on angiography) after 3 months from onset.

Clinical presentations vary depending on the arteries involved. In medium- and large-vessel cPACNS, patients present with headaches, focal deficits, movement disorders, arterial ischemic strokes, and cranial neuropathies. Small-vessel cPACNS patients usually have seizures, psychiatric manifestations, and/or diffuse neurological deficits.

Laboratory abnormalities vary with the type of vasculitis. Small-vessel cPACNS often has abnormal blood tests, including high ESR, CRP, thrombocytosis, anemia, elevated C3, and an elevated von Willebrand factor. Normal inflammatory markers (ESR and CRP) do not rule out medium- or large-vessel cPACNS. Elevated opening pressures on lumbar puncture, abnormally high WBC counts, and high protein on CSF analysis are not uncommon in small-vessel cPACNS. Angiography is considered the gold standard for diagnosis but is rather invasive. MRA (magnetic resonance angiography) can miss smaller lesions, and findings can mimic benign conditions, such as reversible vasoconstriction syndromes. When available, high-resolution MRA with special attention to the cross section of the wall of the affected vessel can provide information about vessel wall inflammation without an angiogram. A leptomeningeal and brain biopsy is sometimes necessary to establish the diagnosis of small-vessel cPACNS. Histology of the tissue in this group is usually one of nongranulomatous inflammation with a lymphocytic infiltration.

Treatment for small-vessel and medium-to-large vessel progressive cPACNS typically consists of high-dose steroids and cyclophosphamide. Treatment for nonprogressive disease is controversial. Children with stroke are usually given heparin, and those with small-vessel disease are treated with antiplatelet agents. Supportive treatment with typical agents used for seizures, movement disorders, and psychosis are appropriate as adjunctive therapy.

SYSTEMIC LUPUS ERYTHEMATOSUS

PREVIEW | REVIEW

- Which ethnic groups have higher rates of SLE?
- What antibodies increase the risk for neonatal lupus?
- Which cardiac complication is seen in neonatal lupus?
- Is a positive ANA common in pediatric SLE?
- With what are antiphospholipid antibodies associated?

- What is the most common cause of chorea in the U.S.?
- Which 2 autoimmune diseases are signified by the finding of a malar rash?
- Which hair finding is common in SLE?
- Where are the painless ulcerations typically located in patients with lupus?
- Which joint abnormality, common in SLE, is due to the disease itself, antiphospholipid antibody, and/or high-dose steroid usage?
- Which type of endocarditis is associated with SLE and antiphospholipid antibodies?
- Which drug class reduces lupus mortality and improves prognosis?
- What are the clinical side effects of long-term corticosteroid use in children with SLE?

OVERVIEW

Systemic lupus erythematosus (SLE) is diagnosed in children < 18 years of age with an incidence of about 10–20 new cases per 100,000/year. Incidence is higher in females (especially those of childbearing age) and in Americans of African, Asian, and Hispanic descent.

Note: Pediatric SLE is different from **neonatal lupus erythematosus**. Neonatal lupus develops as a result of transplacental passage of maternal autoantibodies. 50% of these mothers do not know they have these autoantibodies, typically anti-SSA (anti-Ro) and anti-SSB (anti-La) antibodies. The risk of developing neonatal lupus is < 5–10% but substantially increases in those whose mother has had a previous pregnancy complicated by neonatal lupus. Common features of neonatal lupus erythematosus include rash, cytopenias, hepatitis, and, most importantly, bradycardia from congenital complete heart block (occurs in 1–3%), requiring a pacemaker. In women with known positive serologies, initiate screening with fetal echocardiogram starting at week 16 of pregnancy, then every 2 weeks thereafter. If there is evidence for cardiac conduction abnormalities, dexamethasone is often given to decrease the risk for complete heart block and pacemaker dependency. Most noncardiac features resolve within 6 months as maternal antibodies disappear. Prolonged QT$_c$ syndrome can develop in children up to 12 months of age; because of this, an ECG should be repeated at least once by 12 months of age. *radiologic finding: chondrodysplasia punctata stippling of the epiphyses*

DIAGNOSIS

Overview

Patients with SLE often present with malaise, fever, and/or weight loss. Common manifestations in pediatric SLE are arthritis (80–90%), rash (70–80%), and nephritis (50–60%). Other clinical manifestations include hematologic, pulmonary, and neuropsychiatric abnormalities.

Laboratory Findings

Common laboratory findings in patients with SLE include presence of autoantibodies.

 +ANA

A positive **ANA** occurs in almost all pediatric patients with SLE (98–99%).

Anti-dsDNA antibodies are the 2nd most common (60–70% at some point during the disease course); these antibodies fluctuate with disease activity and are typical with renal disease. **Anti-Smith** antibodies are found in about 33% of SLE patients. The presence of dsDNA and anti-Smith antibodies correlates with renal involvement in SLE.

Antiphospholipid antibodies (lupus anticoagulant, anti-cardiolipin, and beta-2-glycoprotein-1 antibodies) are found in up to 50% of lupus patients. These antibodies affect pathways of coagulation and increase the risk of miscarriages, thrombocytopenia, livedo reticularis, and/or blood clots in about 25% of patients.

Anti-U1 RNP antibodies are the least produced of the antibodies listed here. They are, however, also seen in high titers in the related condition, mixed connective tissue disease.

Hypocomplementemia is another finding seen in SLE. Complement proteins are consumed during immune complex formation in active SLE, particularly with nephritis. C3 and C4 often decline with active disease and may normalize with successful treatment. Inherited C4, C2, or other complement deficiencies correlate with more severe SLE.

Table 20-4 lists the American College of Rheumatology's 11 criteria for SLE. A patient must meet 4 of the 11 criteria, but clinically this may or may not happen; and, if

Table 20-4: Criteria for Diagnosis of Systemic Lupus Erythematosus (must have at least 4 of 11)

Clinical Criteria

1) Neurologic disorder (seizures or psychosis)

2) Malar rash

3) Discoid rash

4) Photosensitive rash

5) Oral ulcers and/or nasal ulcers

6) Serositis (pleuritis, pericarditis, or peritonitis)

7) Renal disorder (proteinuria or cellular casts)

8) Arthritis

Laboratory Criteria

9) Hematologic disorder (hemolytic anemia, leukopenia, lymphopenia, or thrombocytopenia)

10) Immunologic disorder (positive antiphospholipid ab, anti-dsDNA, anti-Smith, or false-positive syphilis test—RPR or VDRL)

11) Antinuclear antibody

it does happen in adolescence, it can occur over time. Most manifestations, if they are going to occur, do so in the first 4–5 years of diagnosis. The one exception to this is CNS disease, which may not show up for many years.

Renal Manifestations

Renal involvement in SLE is very common and directly affects both morbidity and mortality. SLE with no renal involvement or with nephritis requiring a short course of steroids has a better outcome, and SLE with nephritis requiring immunosuppressive therapy has a poorer outcome.

Lupus nephritis can be classified into 6 classes—see Table 20-5.

Infectious complications from immunosuppression are a major cause of morbidity and mortality in lupus nephritis. For more information on lupus nephritis, see Nephrology and Urology, Book 3.

CNS Manifestations

CNS disease occurs in 10–30% of children with SLE. Psychiatric and mood disorders occur in about 10–20%. You must rule out psychosis or organic brain syndrome—usually by lumbar puncture—because infection or hemorrhage is possible. Seizures are also a common presentation for CNS disease. Note: SLE is the most common cause of chorea in the U.S.! Chorea in SLE is often associated with antiphospholipid antibodies. Cranial nerve involvement is more common than peripheral nerve disease. Autonomic dysfunction is common but typically mild—changes in heart rate can be the only change you observe. Cognitive difficulties are common in patients with SLE. Neurocognitive testing is helpful in evaluating whether this is secondary to SLE or not. Order serum antiribosomal P antibodies and antineuronal antibodies (from CSF) to help diagnose lupus psychosis or lupus cerebritis.

Skin Manifestations

Characteristic skin manifestations of SLE include butterfly rash (a.k.a. malar rash; Image 20-10 on page 20-16), discoid rash (uncommon in childhood SLE; Image 20-11 on page 20-16), and/or photosensitivity. A malar rash is usually due to either SLE or dermatomyositis; the rash involves the malar eminence and spares the nasolabial fold (unlike rosacea and psoriasis, which can involve the nasolabial folds). Fifth disease (parvovirus) can also present with a facial rash and is part of the differential diagnosis. Alopecia is fairly common. This can be diffuse, and generally mild, because of disease activity, scarring discoid lesions, and/or steroid use. Oral and nasal erosions can occur, as well as ulcerative lesions of the arms, legs, or ears. Oral lesions/ulcerations are usually painless and located on the hard palate or in the nares. A less common vesicular or bullous rash can develop and is associated with anti-SSA and anti-SSB

Table 20-5: Guidelines[1,2] for Management of Lupus Nephritis
Class 1: Minimal Mesangial Lupus Nephritis
Good prognosis; no immunosuppressive therapy required; short duration of steroids if needed
Class 2: Mesangial Proliferative Lupus Nephritis
Fair prognosis
No immunosuppressive therapy required; short duration of steroids if needed
Class 3: Focal Lupus Nephritis (< 50% of glomeruli)
3(A): Active lesions 3(A/C): Active and chronic lesions 3(C): Chronic lesions
Treat with steroids, CYP or MMF induction therapy; maintenance therapy with MMF or AZP.
Class 4: Diffuse Segmental or Global Lupus Nephritis (> 50% of glomeruli)
Diffuse segmental (4-S) or global (4-G) 4(A): Active lesions 4(A/C): Active and chronic lesions 4(C): Chronic lesions
Treat with steroids, CYP or MMF induction therapy; maintenance therapy with MMF or AZP.
Class 5: Membranous Lupus Nephritis
Associated with nephrotic range proteinuria
Treat with steroids, MMF—if ineffective switch to CYP; maintenance therapy with MMF or AZP.
Class 6: Advanced Sclerosing Lupus Nephritis
> 90% globally sclerosed glomeruli without residual activity Prepare for renal replacement therapy (hemodialysis/kidney transplant).

Classes 3 and 4 nephritis are associated with HTN, and risk for renal failure is high if not treated.
Class 5 can occur in combination with Class 3 or 4.
Monitor blood pressure, lipids.
Use ACE inhibitors or ARBs to decrease proteinuria and preserve renal function.
Key: AZP = azathioprine, CYP = cyclophosphamide, MMF = mycophenolate mofetil,
   ACE = angiotensin-converting enzyme, ARB = angiotensin receptor blocker, HTN = hypertension

References:
[1] Weening JJ, et al. International Society of Nephrology Working Group on the Classification of Lupus Nephritis; Renal Pathology Society Working Group on the Classification of Lupus Nephritis. The classification of glomerulonephritis in systemic lupus erythematosus revisited. *Kidney Int*. 2004;65:521–530.
[2] Hahn BH, et al. American College of Rheumatology Guidelines for Screening, Case Definition, Treatment and Management of Lupus Nephritis. *Arthritis Care Res* (Hoboken). Jun 2012;64(6):797–808.

antibodies. This condition is termed **subacute cutaneous lupus erythematosus (SCLE)** and has the same rash and antibodies as seen in neonatal lupus.

Musculoskeletal Manifestations

Look for polyarticular arthritis, especially of small and large joints, with morning stiffness. The arthritis is nondeforming. You might find it difficult to distinguish poJIA from SLE arthritis early on. Over time, poJIA can show osteopenia and joint damage on x-ray; but in SLE, the x-rays are nonerosive even after years of arthritis. Avascular necrosis (AVN) is fairly common and is due to the disease itself, antiphospholipid antibodies, and/ or high-dose steroid use. AVN presents with nighttime pain, joint or bone tenderness, and a noninflammatory effusion. AVN has a tendency to be asymptomatic: A nuclear bone scan reveals the sites of asymptomatic AVN; MRI confirms the diagnosis. Hips, knees, and shoulders are common sites of involvement. AVN is a common cause of morbidity in SLE.

Cardiopulmonary Manifestations

The most common cardiac abnormality in children with SLE is **pericarditis.** It occurs in 25–35% of patients and is associated with pleuritic disease as well. Tamponade is very rare in these patients. Myocarditis and endocarditis occur in < 10%. Valvular disease is common but is usually clinically insignificant. Libman-Sacks endocarditis (nonbacterial endocarditis with verrucous vegetations) is associated with SLE and antiphospholipid antibodies.

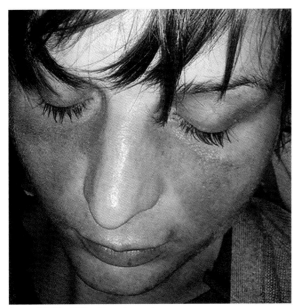

Image 20-10: SLE with malar rash

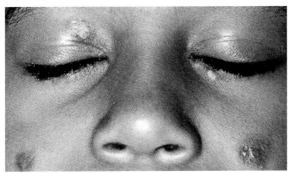

Image 20-11: SLE with discoid rash

Pulmonary manifestations can vary from something as severe as pulmonary hemorrhage or infection to a more benign, indolent, decreased diffusion capacity. Pleural disease is very common and can present as pleuritis or pleural effusion. The pain is usually sharp, stabbing, and worsens with deep inspiration.

Gastrointestinal Manifestations

Gastrointestinal manifestations occur in about 33% of patients. Abdominal pain is the most common presenting symptom. It can be due to serositis, autoimmune hepatitis, vasculitis, pancreatitis, or enteritis. Hepatomegaly is common; jaundice is rare.

Hematologic Manifestations

Cytopenias are common. Up to 75% of patients are found to have 1 or more cytopenias, including leukopenia (WBC < 4,000 cells/µL), lymphopenia (total lymphocyte count < 1,500 cells/µL), hemolytic anemia, or thrombocytopenia (platelet count < 150,000 cells/µL).

Normochromic normocytic **anemia** and hypochromic microcytic anemia are more common than Coombs-positive hemolytic anemia.

Lupus anticoagulant causes an *in vitro* prolongation of partial thromboplastin time (PTT) but not prothrombin time (PT). These patients do not bleed excessively; instead, they have an increased risk of arterial thrombosis, deep vein thrombosis, and thromboembolism.

Endocrine Manifestations

Antithyroid **antibodies** occur in nearly 50% of patients, and clinical hypothyroidism occurs in 10–20%. Graves disease can occur but is much less common than hypothyroidism.

Note

In 2012, new criteria for the diagnosis of pediatric SLE were proposed by the Systemic Lupus International Collaborating Clinics (SLICC), which provide more inclusive diagnostic criteria. Changes include:

• recognizing other cutaneous features,
• including a greater number of neurologic manifestations, and
• including low complement measurements.

These have not yet been formally accepted by the American College of Rheumatology but are likely to be important in upcoming clinical trials and longitudinal studies in SLE.

TREATMENT

Only 4 drugs are approved by the FDA to be used in SLE: low-dose aspirin, prednisone, hydroxychloroquine, and belimumab. However, rheumatologists use multiple DMARDs and immunomodulators that are not FDA approved to manage their patients (i.e., mycophenolate mofetil, methotrexate, azathioprine, cyclophosphamide, cyclosporine, leflunomide, rituximab). The reasons for lack of FDA approval of these agents to treat lupus are multiple and include heterogeneity of the disease, inadequate outcome tools to assess disease activity and treatment response, and variable background medications that patients are taking during the trials—so gauging treatment response is difficult.

The treatment mainstay for lupus is antimalarial drugs. **Hydroxychloroquine** is helpful with skin and joint manifestations and can improve fatigue in many patients. Data shows that continued use of antimalarial therapy prevents disease flares (a 3× reduction in the rate of flares when compared to those who discontinued hydroxychloroquine), decreases mortality in adult SLE patients, lowers serum cholesterol levels, and decreases the risk for neonatal lupus in mothers who take the drug. The risk of ophthalmic complications (retinal toxicity) is very low as long as average dosages of ≤ 6.5 mg/kg/day are maintained. Screen for these rare complications 1–2×/year with eye examinations performed by an ophthalmologist.

Corticosteroids are used for many aspects of disease therapy. Use a low dosage (< 0.1–0.25 mg/kg/day or < 10–15 mg/day) for joint complaints and fatigue. Serositis responds to 20–30 mg/day, but nephritis and CNS disease often require high-dose steroids (2 mg/kg/day or pulse therapy 30 mg/kg/day of methylprednisolone).

Know the common side effects from long-term use of steroids:

• AVN
• Osteoporosis with fracture or vertebral collapse
• Growth failure
• Glaucoma and cataracts
• Diabetes mellitus
• HTN
• Accelerated atherosclerosis
• Infection

Cyclophosphamide (CYP) can carry a lot of toxicity and is used mainly for initial control of aggressive disease. CYP increases the risk of infertility (10–20% risk in 25-year-old women and up to 50% infertility risk in those > 32 years of age). The risk of malignancy, especially lymphoma, is an accumulated dose-related side effect. Minimize this risk by reducing the total dose of cyclophosphamide, using monthly IV pulse therapy, and switching to a potentially less toxic agent after the first 6–12 months. The risk of bladder carcinoma is directly related to the development of hemorrhagic cystitis that is a result of bladder wall toxicity from this agent.

CYP → bladder wall toxicity → hemorrhagic cystitis → risk of bladder carcinoma.

To prevent this cystitis, administer mesna with IV cyclophosphamide.

If psychosis or organic brain syndrome is severe or life-threatening, give high-dose steroids with cyclophosphamide, and consider plasmapheresis. Remember that steroids can be the cause of hallucinations (especially auditory) and are dose dependent (increased risk if ≥ 40 mg/day). Steroid-induced neuropsychiatric symptoms typically resolve with discontinuation of steroids.

Mycophenolate mofetil (MMF) and **azathioprine (AZP)** are effective for managing SLE. MMF is noninferior to CYP in the treatment of lupus nephritis; it has less toxicity than CYP, but compliance can sometimes be an issue. Choosing MMF to induce remission in active glomerulonephritis is a decision based on the individual patient. Both MMF and AZP are useful for long-term maintenance of aggressive disease.

Note that with Classes 3 and 4 disease, prognosis is improved by aggressive management with high-dose steroids and cyclophosphamide, either daily oral or IV pulse (pulse preferred due to lower toxicity), or mycophenolate. Manage hypertension aggressively because poorly controlled blood pressure increases the risk of renal failure.

Belimumab, a fully human monoclonal antibody that inhibits the activity of B-lymphocyte stimulator (BLyS), is approved in SLE patients ≥ 18 years of age. The drug helps with moderate manifestations of SLE but has not been studied in aggressive disease (Class 3/4 nephritis or CNS disease). There is also evidence that B-cell-depleting antibody, rituximab, is of benefit in treating pediatric lupus nephritis and allowing for corticosteroid tapering.

PROGNOSIS

Morbidity in SLE is due to disease manifestations (renal and CNS manifestations) and to medication toxicity (steroid side effects and infections from immunosuppression). Late morbidity and early mortality are due to premature atherosclerotic disease > 10–20 years after onset. SLE is an independent risk factor for coronary artery disease. Risk for atherosclerosis is multifactorial and includes endothelial damage secondary to chronic inflammation and immune dysregulation.

MIXED CONNECTIVE TISSUE DISEASE

PREVIEW | REVIEW

• What is the autoantibody affiliated with mixed connective tissue disease?

• What is the main cause of mortality in mixed connective tissue disease?

Mixed connective tissue disease (MCTD) used to be *anti-U1 RNP* referred to as an overlap syndrome with features of dermatomyositis, JIA, lupus, and/or scleroderma, but it is now characterized as its own entity due to the presence of a distinctive autoantibody, anti-U1 RNP. Girls account for 80% of cases, and they characteristically present with Raynaud phenomenon, fever, arthritis, dorsal hand edema, rash, and myositis. Joint abnormalities are seen in 60–90% of children. Over time, MCTD progresses like scleroderma, and many patients develop restrictive lung disease. GI disease frequently presents; esophageal disease, especially dysphagia and abnormal esophageal function, is most typical of the GI manifestations. Cardiac findings can occur, most commonly acute pericarditis with pericardial effusion and mitral valve prolapse. Renal disease occurs in about 25% of pediatric patients, and the nephritis can be membranous, membranoproliferative, or mesangioproliferative. Erosive arthritis is rarely seen except in those who are RF+. CNS disease and eye disease are also rare with this syndrome.

Mortality most often occurs due to chronic interstitial lung disease or pulmonary HTN. Mortality also results from severe thrombocytopenia and infectious complications of immunosuppression. The prognosis is generally better than in SLE or scleroderma.

Labs show a high-titer speckled ANA, anti-U1 RNP antibodies, RF, and hypergammaglobulinemia. Diagnosis requires high-titer antibodies against U1 RNP autoantigen.

As in SLE, use antimalarials. Also, corticosteroids can be used with MCTD patients with severe disease. Many require more intensive immunosuppression, such as methotrexate for arthropathy or CYP for severe organ system involvement.

SJÖGREN SYNDROME

PREVIEW | REVIEW

- Name the diagnostic criteria for Sjögren syndrome.

- Which antibodies are frequently present in pediatric SS?

- How do most pediatric cases of Sjögren syndrome present?

- Which malignancies are patients with Sjögren syndrome at risk for?

Sjögren syndrome (SS) is a rare autoimmune exocrinopathy that causes a combination of symptoms/signs; dry eyes and dry mouth are the most notable. In pediatric cases, consider the following for diagnosis:

- Inflamed and dry eyes (keratoconjunctivitis sicca)
- Dryness of the mouth (xerostomia)
- Lymphocytic infiltrate on minor salivary gland biopsy
- Laboratory evidence of the following: RF+, ANA+, or Ro+ (SSA; 70%) or La+ (SSB; 50%) antibodies

Suspect SS in a child with recurrent parotitis in whom infection has been excluded. Girls outnumber boys 3:1. Most cases present with the recurrent parotitis and keratoconjunctivitis sicca. CNS (e.g., transverse myelitis) and renal (including renal tubular acidosis) manifestations are uncommon but do occur in children. Remember that particularly young children may not yet be symptomatic with dry eyes and dry mouth. However, excessive dental caries can represent poor saliva production. One extraglandular manifestation to look for is hypergammaglobulinemic purpura—2- to 3-mm, palpable or nonpalpable purpura that can ulcerate on the lower extremities. Annular erythema, usually seen with anti-SSA (anti-Ro) or anti-SSB (anti-La), is also sometimes observed.

Primary SS is defined as an isolated disorder, while **secondary SS** is defined as associated with another autoimmune disease. Some children with a diagnosis of primary SS go on to develop another autoimmune disorder, most commonly SLE.

Treat symptomatic patients with agents that increase moisture: artificial tears for the eyes, artificial saliva, and pilocarpine to stimulate exocrine secretions.

Antimalarial agents can be used for skin rashes and joint symptoms. Suggest dental visits at least 2–3×/year due to marked increase in caries. Chewing sugarless gum can help stimulate salivary flow. Cyclosporine ophthalmic suspension and cevimeline are approved for adults, but not children, with Sjögren syndrome.

Children generally do well, but patients with Sjögren's are at increased risk for lymphoma, especially mucosa-associated lymphoid tissue (MALT) lymphoma and non-Hodgkin B-cell lymphomas.

Note: Children born to mothers with SS who have Ro (SSA) and/or La (SSB) antibodies are also at risk for developing neonatal lupus. (See more about neonatal lupus under the SLE Overview on page 20-13.)

AUTOIMMUNE MYOPATHIES

PREVIEW | REVIEW

- Describe the classic rashes of juvenile dermatomyositis.

- The muscle weakness of juvenile dermatomyositis mainly affects which muscle groups: proximal or distal?

- What is the primary therapy for juvenile dermatomyositis?

OVERVIEW

Juvenile dermatomyositis (JDM) is a systemic connective tissue disorder with chronic skeletal muscle and skin inflammation. Its etiology is unknown, but its pathogenesis is one of autoimmune angiopathy. Polymyositis is a much less common inflammatory myositis in children (< 10% of cases) that has no skin involvement. These diseases are very rare and occur at a rate of about 1.5–5 cases/million. They affect girls more often than boys and have a bimodal pattern of incidence, peaking first at 3–7 years and again in the early teenage years.

JUVENILE DERMATOMYOSITIS

There is a seasonal clustering of the onset of JDM, suggesting a viral or bacterial trigger for this illness.

Patients present with a rash and with muscle weakness. The symptoms gradually develop over weeks to months. Rashes can be quite varied; some children have only subtle skin lesions, whereas others have severe, vasculitic, ulcerative rashes. The typical rashes include the classic heliotrope (faint purple-to-red discoloration of the eyelids, with or without periorbital edema; Image 20-12) and Gottron papules (red plaques over the extensor surfaces—most often occurring on the small joints of the hands; Image 20-13). Periungual changes, such as cuticular overgrowth and dilated tortuous capillaries by capillaroscopy, can occur. You might also observe SLE-like malar and facial redness and red rashes on sun-exposed areas. Photosensitivity is common and can precipitate flares.

The muscle weakness is always proximal and symmetric in nature. This presents with difficulty in grooming hair, getting up off the floor, and climbing stairs. Some distal weakness occurs in severe cases. When distal weakness is present early on, consider a different form of muscle disease, such as muscular dystrophy, congenital myopathies, and CNS denervation. Children with JDM can also develop muscle involvement of the GI tract, resulting in difficulty swallowing or hoarseness/dysphonia. Dysfunctional swallowing can be asymptomatic and may only be detectable with barium swallow testing. Dysphonia and dysphagia are very serious manifestations, requiring aggressive, prompt treatment.

Nearly 70% of patients have arthralgias. When true arthritis occurs, oligoarthritis (affecting ~ 65%) is more common than polyarthritis (30–35%). Contractures of large joints can occur after prolonged muscle weakness. You see fever and Raynaud phenomenon in about 25% at the onset of disease.

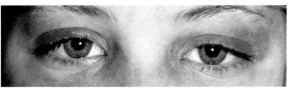
Image 20-12: Heliotrope rash

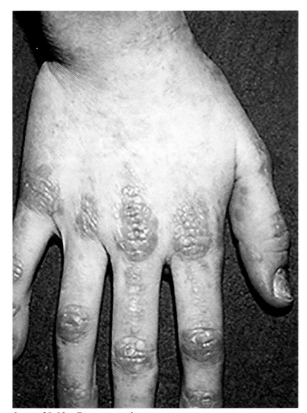
Image 20-13: Gottron papules

Be aware of the potential complications of JDM. Ulcerations are rare but can be severe if they occur. Ulcerative skin disease is a poor prognostic sign and can portend GI vasculitis—one of the most serious, life-threatening complications of JDM. Dystrophic calcification (calcinosis cutis) of the skin, subcutaneous tissue, and fascia occurs in about 33% of affected patients. Calcinosis is much less common today because of better recognition of the complication and prompt treatment. Risk factors for complications are inadequate steroid therapy and delay of therapy for > 4 months from onset of myositis. Another late complication of JDM is lipodystrophy. This is characterized by insulin resistance, hyperlipidemia, and asthenic body habitus. Muscle strength can be completely normal, or the patient can still have active myositis.

Diagnostic criteria are defined in Table 20-6. MRI (T2 or STIR images) of the thigh muscles, demonstrating inflammation as symmetrical muscle edema, has become the preferred modality over electromyography (EMG) since EMG is invasive and uncomfortable. Beware, though, as edema on MRI is not specific to inflammatory myopathies. A diagnosis of juvenile polymyositis is based on similar criteria, except that the rashes are absent.

Begin primary therapy with prednisone 2–3 mg/kg/day. In more severe cases of myositis, many rheumatologists give IV pulse methylprednisolone at 30 mg/kg/dose for ≥ 3 doses. Sunscreens, sun avoidance, and hydroxychloroquine are important adjunctive therapies for rashes. Also prescribe physical and occupational therapy. The 2nd line therapies—and therapies for severe exacerbations—include IV methylprednisolone, IVIG, methotrexate, cyclosporine, and AZP. Utilizing these adjunctive therapies frequently allows for successful

Table 20-6: Diagnosis of Juvenile Dermatomyositis
Presence of heliotrope rash or Gottron papules is required
Plus at least 3 of the following 4 findings = Definite Dx
Plus at least 2 of the following 4 findings = Probable Dx
1) Symmetric proximal muscle weakness
2) Elevated CPK, aldolase, LDH, or transaminases

3) EMG abnormalities
  a. Small amplitude, short duration, polyphasic motor-unit potentials
  b. Fibrillations, positive sharp waves, increased insertional irritability
  c. Spontaneous, bizarre, high-frequency discharges

4) Muscle biopsy abnormalities of
  a. Degeneration
  b. Regeneration
  c. Necrosis
  d. Phagocytosis
  e. Interstitial mononuclear cell infiltrate

tapering of steroids and avoidance of steroid-induced morbidities. If patients do not respond, try 3rd line therapy; combine 2nd line therapies plus:

- other immunomodulators (anti-TNFi and rituximab) or
- IV cyclophosphamide.

Prednisone and other immune modulators have reduced mortality from 40% to < 3%. About 60–80% of patients recover after their initial episode (uniphasic disease course) or after ≥ 1 recurrences. Fewer than 20% have difficult-to-control disease with persistent myositis over a long period of time. Unlike adult dermatomyositis, in which the dermatomyositis is often a paraneoplastic syndrome, childhood dermatomyositis rarely predisposes to malignancy. Therefore, screening for malignancy is not routinely indicated in children with this disease.

JUVENILE POLYMYOSITIS

Juvenile polymyositis is extremely rare and generally has a chronic course. It has the same clinical features as JDM except there is no rash. Patients can present with proximal girdle weakness. Labs indicate elevated CPK and aldolase, EMG indicates muscle irritability, and MRI shows muscle edema. Differential diagnoses include muscular dystrophy. Frequently, biopsy is indicated to clarify the diagnosis.

SCLERODERMA

PREVIEW | REVIEW

- What are the 2 main subtypes of systemic scleroderma?

- Which part of the GI tract is most commonly affected in systemic scleroderma?

- Which class of antihypertensive do you use to reduce the incidence of scleroderma renal crisis?

- Which laboratory findings are helpful in the diagnosis of systemic scleroderma?

- Anticentromere antibodies are seen in which rheumatic disorders?

- Why are corticosteroids not used in systemic scleroderma?

- What is the most common form of localized scleroderma seen in children? Explain how it can affect soft tissue and bone.

- In what disorder is *en coupe de sabre* seen?

- What are the common antiinflammatory treatments used for linear scleroderma?

OVERVIEW

Scleroderma means "hard skin." There are 2 major categories of this disease:

1) Systemic scleroderma (sclerosis) and limited cutaneous sclerosis (i.e., CREST syndrome)
2) Localized scleroderma (linear scleroderma and morphea)

Recognize that the terms sclerosis and scleroderma are used interchangeably throughout the literature. Both systemic and limited sclerodermas are rare, although other forms of localized scleroderma (linear scleroderma and morphea) are found much more often in children than in adults.

The etiology of scleroderma is unknown. Both types involve an abnormality in the regulation of fibroblasts and collagen production. Endothelin, an endothelial cell-dependent vasoconstrictor, is increased in systemic scleroderma.

SYSTEMIC SCLERODERMA

Systemic scleroderma (sclerosis) can be divided into 2 separate subtypes:

1) **Diffuse cutaneous scleroderma**: proximal and distal skin involvement with internal organ dysfunction of the GI tract, lung, heart, and kidney
2) **Limited cutaneous scleroderma**: formerly known as CREST syndrome—calcinosis, Raynaud phenomenon (Image 20-14), esophageal dysmotility, sclerodactyly, and telangiectasias (Image 20-15)

Although both of these subtypes are rare disorders in childhood, anti-SCL-70 + diffuse scleroderma is seen more than anticentromere + limited scleroderma.

Children with systemic scleroderma usually present with **Raynaud phenomenon** (spasm of the digital arteries with blanching and numbness or pain of the fingers, often precipitated by cold). Classic Raynaud's is triphasic: white, blue, and red on rewarming. Fingertip ulcerations occur frequently in children. Gradual thickening of the skin of the distal extremities occurs and slowly progresses, eventually involving the face and trunk.

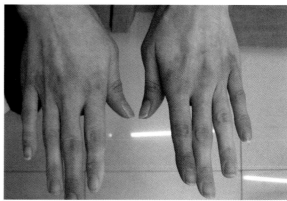
Image 20-14: Secondary Raynaud's in Sjögren syndrome

The GI tract is commonly affected, particularly the distal esophagus where systemic scleroderma affects distal smooth muscle, resulting in dysphagia. GE reflux is common.

Lung involvement is initially asymptomatic but gradually manifests in a dry cough. Alveolitis develops first; then pulmonary interstitial fibrosis worsens, most often in patients with diffuse cutaneous scleroderma. Pulmonary HTN occurs, which leads to right heart failure. This is found more frequently in those with limited cutaneous scleroderma.

Renal crisis occurs in only about 10%, and for the most part only in diffuse cutaneous scleroderma patients. Managing HTN with ACE inhibitors decreases the incidence of renal crisis.

Clinical diagnosis is dependent on findings of sclerodactyly (stiffness and tightness of the skin of the fingers), nail bed capillary findings showing periungual tortuous dilated loops (referred to as nailfold capillaroscopy), and internal organ involvement.

Laboratory testing shows that 80% of patients have a nucleolar or speckled ANA, and 50% have antibodies to SCL-70 (topoisomerase 1). Anticentromere antibodies, if they occur, are seen with limited cutaneous scleroderma and primary biliary cirrhosis. Which test is used to determine esophageal abnormalities? Esophageal manometry is the most sensitive test. Use barium swallow to show severe motor dysfunction and/or reflux.

High-resolution CT scan is a sensitive test for lung abnormalities such as fibrosis or alveolitis. Monitor patients for carbon monoxide diffusion capacity (DLCO) using pulmonary function tests (PFTs), which are highly sensitive in detecting pulmonary hypertension. It is essential to monitor patients at risk for pulmonary HTN with echocardiography to assess right-sided heart pressures and pulmonary pressures. Consider right heart catheterization in such patients.

Treatment is mainly supportive. Order aggressive physical and occupational therapy to prevent progression to flexion contractures. Raynaud phenomenon responds to calcium channel blockers (nifedipine)

and alpha-blockers (doxazosin). Corticosteroids are relatively contraindicated due to the increased risk of renal crisis. ACE inhibitors to prevent (and treat) renal crisis and anti-GE reflux agents are important adjunctive therapies. If it is necessary to use corticosteroids, as in myositis, try to use dosages ≤ 10 mg/day. You can use methotrexate, although avoid it in patients with significant interstitial lung disease. CYP reverses alveolitis and stabilizes, if not reverses, severe scleroderma lung disease; MMF may have a role as well. Systemic vasodilators, such as sildenafil and iloprost, are used for pulmonary HTN, as well as endothelin receptor antagonists. Prognosis is poor for those with internal organ involvement; those with limited cutaneous scleroderma generally do better.

LOCALIZED SCLERODERMA

This is the most common form of scleroderma and occurs with an incidence in children of about 50/100,000. It is also known as morphea, plaque morphea, generalized morphea, linear scleroderma (Image 20-16), and deep morphea (Image 20-17 on page 20-22).

Plaque morphea occurs gradually and is characterized by an oval or circular area of cutaneous induration with a central ivory color surrounded by a purplish halo. If the plaques become more extensive and involve 3 separate anatomic sites, it is called **generalized morphea**. If generalized full-thickness skin involvement occurs, it is

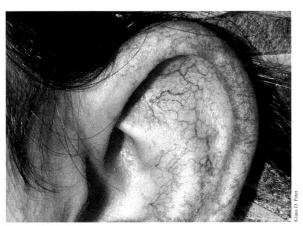

Image 20-15: Telangiectasias

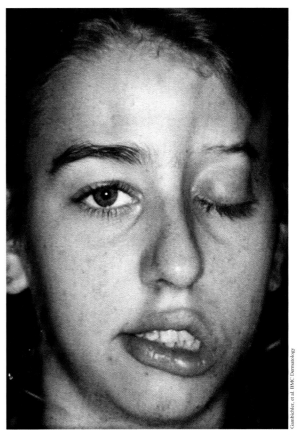

Image 20-16: Frontal linear (localized) scleroderma

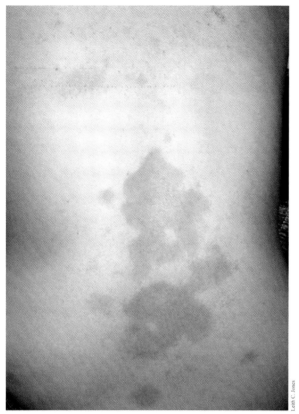

Leith C. Jones

Image 20-17: Deep morphea (localized scleroderma)

called **deep morphea**. Typically, this involves the scalp, face, trunk, and extremities.

Linear scleroderma (formerly known as linear morphea) is the most common localized scleroderma seen in children. It is characterized by linear streaks of the upper or lower extremity that usually are dermatomal. If the streaks cross a joint, flexion contractures can develop. The streaks become more indurated and gradually extend deeper into underlying muscle and bone (melorheostosis). Streaks involving the face are known as *en coupe de sabre*—like a depression due to a dueling stroke from a sword. These patients can have associated ipsilateral CNS findings, seizures, uveitis, dental defects, and facial abnormalities, including Parry-Romberg syndrome.

Base diagnosis of these forms of localized scleroderma on clinical findings of the skin lesions; some cases require biopsy. Depth of disease determines the subtypes: plaque morphea is confined to the dermis, while linear scleroderma can go to muscle and bone. Laboratory testing is not helpful; antibodies to centromere, SCL-70, nuclear RNP, Smith, and SSA are not present. Occasionally, antibodies to single-stranded DNA are present in linear scleroderma.

Before you begin treatment, remember that localized scleroderma is generally a benign condition that resolves in 3–5 years. Although localized scleroderma is relatively benign and self-limited, it can lead to significant limb growth abnormalities when there is extensive subdermal involvement; this sometimes requires systemic therapy including steroids and/or methotrexate. If a joint is involved, prescribe physical therapy to prevent contractures.

SARCOIDOSIS

PREVIEW | REVIEW

- List the most common systems affected in sarcoidosis.
- What is the triad of clinical manifestations typically seen in Blau syndrome?
- Describe the skin findings in sarcoidosis.

Sarcoidosis is an uncommon multisystem granulomatous disease (with increased relative prevalence in the southeastern U.S.) that mainly affects the lungs, lymph nodes, eyes, and skin. The etiology is unknown but results from an immunologic response that causes accumulation of inflammatory cells (granulomas). Symptoms vary depending on the system affected. Most, however, present with fatigue, fever, and weight loss. A familial form of sarcoidosis, Blau syndrome, typically presents with uveitis, rash, and "boggy" arthritis.

Lung involvement is common and presents with a persistent dry cough. Chest x-ray reveals hilar infiltrates and sometimes parenchymal infiltrates. PFTs demonstrate restrictive changes. See more on sarcoidosis in Pulmonary Medicine, Book 2.

Granulomatous infiltration of the liver, spleen, and lymph nodes is typical and presents as hepatomegaly, splenomegaly, and lymphadenopathy (peripheral but especially hilar/mediastinal) respectively. Most are asymptomatic, but monitoring liver functions is warranted.

The most common skin findings are nodules on the face, neck, back, and extremities (e.g., erythema nodosum). The lesions are red-brown, maculopapular, and < 1 cm in diameter.

Eye involvement includes uveitis and conjunctival granulomas. All patients with sarcoidosis require complete ophthalmological examination.

Diagnosis is made by biopsy of the affected tissue demonstrating noncaseating granulomatous lesions. A patient with sarcoidosis must be monitored with serial testing, including chest x-ray, PFTs, LFTs, renal function tests, and ophthalmologic slit-lamp examination. Serum angiotensin-converting enzyme and lysozyme levels are often elevated during active disease.

Corticosteroids are the mainstay of treatment. Duration is 8–12 weeks, followed by a 6–12 month wean. Immunosuppressive drugs, such as methotrexate, are also used. Monoclonal antibodies to TNF are also effective.

PAIN SYNDROMES

PREVIEW | REVIEW

- Is morning pain a common finding with growing pains?
- Are unilateral findings common in growing pains?
- Describe some of the tasks that can be attempted to determine if a child has hypermobility syndrome.
- If you find hypermobility syndrome, which traits do you look for to determine if a hereditary syndrome might be present?
- What is a recommended exercise activity for hypermobility syndrome?
- What are the clinical findings in patients with AMPs?
- What is common regarding school attendance in patients with AMP syndromes?

GROWING PAINS

Growing pains are the most common cause of recurrent limb pain in children. Rheumatologists refer to this as "benign nocturnal limb pains of childhood." Actually, the pain is not due to growing. The name was probably coined because the pain occurs in children (who are growing).

We do not know what causes growing pains. Musculoskeletal symptoms may be prevalent in the families of these children, but a true familial tendency has not been proven. These symptoms may also be associated with emotional disturbances.

So then, what are they? Classically, growing pains are characterized as a deep aching located in nonarticular areas, generally within muscle groups, especially thighs and calves but rarely back or forearms. Pain is bilateral and typically occurs late in the day or evening, and commonly awakens a child from sleep. Limping and mobility problems do not occur. Usually, there are no objective findings. Unilateral symptoms require further evaluation.

Beware: The other diagnosis that causes nighttime bone pain (since it is difficult for most patients to differentiate between bone and muscle pain) is malignancy. Perform a thorough review of systems, including whether the child is experiencing weight loss, night sweats, or daytime pain as well. Bone pain from metastases can also include other areas (spine, ribs, and skull), which are not typical for growing pains.

Laboratory testing is not indicated in situations where the clinical picture is compatible with growing pains, except to rule out other etiologies. ESR, WBC, CPK, and all serologic tests are normal.

Treat symptomatic patients with heat, massage, and acetaminophen or ibuprofen for pain. Sometimes, a dose of these medications before bed for children with frequent episodes can decrease the severity of the spells. Normally, it just takes time. If the pain is persistent, explore psychological stressors as well as family dynamics. Growing pains occur most commonly in preschool and elementary age children. Growing pains generally disappear by 12–13 years of age.

HYPERMOBILITY SYNDROMES

Benign hypermobility joint syndrome is fairly common and is seen in 4–13% of children, with girls more commonly affected. Most of these children are asymptomatic. You can demonstrate hypermobility by having the child attempt 5 tasks:

1) Extend the wrist and metacarpophalangeal joints so that the fingers are parallel to the dorsum of the forearm (bilateral).
2) Passively oppose the thumb to the flexor aspect of the forearm (bilateral).
3) Hyperextend the elbows 10° or more (bilateral).
4) Hyperextend the knees 10° or more (bilateral).
5) Flex the trunk with the knees fully extended so the palms rest on the floor.

The ability to perform the above tasks in ≥ 5 locations (a point for each side of the body plus flexing the trunk) indicates hypermobility on the Beighton scale. If found, look for other signs of inherited diseases of connective tissue, such as high-arched palate, ocular/cardiac lesions, skin hyperelasticity, arachnodactyly, and velvety skin texture. Variants of Ehlers-Danlos syndrome or Marfan syndrome are most common.

Joint and muscular pain, as well as transient joint effusions, can occur in those with benign hypermobility syndrome. The knees and the hands are most commonly affected.

Treat pain with NSAIDs or acetaminophen. Swimming and other low- to no-impact sports are good recommendations. Psychological factors seem to exacerbate or prolong the course. Premature osteoarthritic changes can occur in some of these children, but generally, the prognosis is good. If Marfan syndrome (i.e., tall stature, high-arched palate, lens dislocation) or Ehlers-Danlos syndrome (i.e., velvety, loose skin with thin, widened scars) is suspected, perform cardiac screening with echocardiography, and consider the involvement of a genetics specialist.

AMPLIFIED MUSCULOSKELETAL PAIN SYNDROMES

Amplified musculoskeletal pain (AMP) syndromes cause noninflammatory musculoskeletal pain in children. These syndromes include juvenile fibromyalgia, complex regional pain syndrome, localized pain without autonomic changes, and intermittent pain.

In general, AMP episodes are the result of an amplified pain signal. The 3 primary causes include injury, illness, and psychological stressors. The most common psychological stressors include those from family or school issues, but it can be complicated from the stress of having chronic pain and not having an accurate diagnosis and/or appropriate plan for improvement.

AMP syndromes can present with one affected limb (e.g. a distal lower extremity) but can be anywhere on the body and can also be diffuse. Most children describe the pain as being constant, but it can be intermittent in some. The pain patients experience is real.

Juvenile fibromyalgia is a subset of AMP syndromes. Children often fail to fulfill the diagnostic criteria for fibromyalgia outlined for adults. However, children do have tender points. Figure 20-1 shows the 18 total trigger points that can be found by digital palpation (as used for the adult criterion). Juvenile fibromyalgia has a high familial association.

It is important to remember that patients with fibromyalgia do not have evidence of articular swelling, loss of motion, or muscle weakness. If these are present, look for another diagnosis. However, keep in mind that secondary fibromyalgia can develop in individuals with JIA or SLE.

Complex regional pain syndrome (CRPS; formerly reflex sympathetic dystrophy) is another subtype of AMP syndromes. The characteristic features of CRPS include allodynia (pain aggravated by light touch) and/ or hyperalgesia. Patients have localized autonomic dysfunction with edema, coolness or excess warmth, mottling, and/or sweatiness. CRPS may be preceded by a soft tissue injury, such as a sprain, but often there is no identifiable preceding trauma.

Appropriate therapy includes aggressive physical and occupational therapy, preferably by a therapist with experience in treating this diagnosis. In many cases, physical therapy includes desensitization to textures, pressure, and temperatures (particularly in those with allodynia). Treatment results are often better when professional psychological support is provided. Improvement and resolution of symptoms is better in children than in adults and is particularly good in those children who partake in an aggressive treatment program.

School absenteeism can be a big problem in patients with AMP syndromes. Be sure to ask about attendance as you are trying to understand if a patient has AMP; many children with an inflammatory or autoimmune disease do not miss school as frequently as children with AMPs do.

Because fatigue and pain can be seen in some patients with an autoimmune disorder, such as SLE, Sjögren's, and JIA, be sure to check appropriate laboratory tests (e.g., CBC, ESR, RF, ANA, anti-SSA and anti-SSB antibodies, CPK, thyroid function tests) to rule out these conditions.

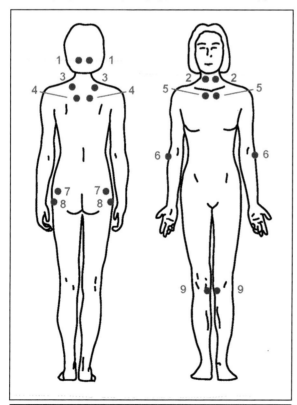

Figure 20-1: Tender Points

AMYLOIDOSIS

PREVIEW | REVIEW

- What are some diseases that cause amyloid deposition?
- What is the most serious manifestation of amyloid deposition?

Amyloidosis is the extracellular accumulation of protein fibrils, which then interfere with specific organ functions. You can see amyloid by staining with Congo red under polarized light and then looking for green-yellow birefringence.

Amyloid accumulation occurs with many diseases, including infectious diseases (tuberculosis, leprosy, and chronic osteomyelitis), familial Mediterranean fever, inflammatory bowel disease, Behçet disease, and SLE. In the past, amyloidosis was found in children with long-standing JIA (typically systemic disease), particularly in Europe. This complication has virtually disappeared with the advent of better, aggressive therapies.

Renal disease is the most prevalent and serious manifestation of amyloid deposition. Patients present with proteinuria, with rapid progression to nephrotic-range proteinuria, and then eventually renal failure. Renal vein thrombosis due to proteinuria is also common. Hepatosplenomegaly can occur but usually does not cause abnormalities.

There is no specific "amyloidosis blood test," but look for markedly increased ESR, C-reactive protein, and serum amyloid A levels if active inflammation, proteinuria, and hypoalbuminemia are present. The key is to find amyloid deposition in tissue. Rectal biopsy, gingival biopsy, or aspiration of subcutaneous abdominal fat are potential sites for tissue acquisition.

Prevention is much more effective than treatment. As such, aggressive therapy for diseases that predispose to amyloidosis is important. For example, the use of colchicine is effective in treating familial Mediterranean fever and preventing amyloidosis. Renal transplant is successful in some patients, but there is recurrence in some of those who have had transplants.

RECURRENT FEVER SYNDROMES

PREVIEW | REVIEW

- What is PFAPA syndrome?
- Which recurrent fever syndrome does not have a known genetic abnormality?
- Where is the gene responsible for familial Mediterranean fever? What is the product of the gene?
- How do you treat FMF?
- What is TRAPS?
- Define the genetic defect in hyper-IgD syndrome.
- What is CAPS?
- Name the 3 periodic fever syndromes due to cryopyrin abnormalities.
- What is the neutrophilic pattern in cyclic neutropenia?

OVERVIEW

Fever is a common cause of presentation to the pediatrician. Recurrent fevers are most often due to repeated infections, frequently viral. Fever of unknown origin (documented fever for > 2 weeks with no etiology identified on routine evaluation) is often due to infections but can also be due to malignancies and rheumatic diseases such as systemic JIA or SLE.

Recurrent fever syndromes are defined as ≥ 3 episodes of unexplained fever in a 6-month period. This group of disorders can follow a definitive periodic pattern or can have variable intervals between attacks. Initially, you may think these children have recurrent infections. The periodicity is ultimately recognized before these diagnoses are considered. Specific genetic abnormalities have been identified for many of these disorders.

PFAPA

PFAPA (**p**eriodic **f**ever, **a**phthous stomatitis, **p**haryngitis, and cervical **a**denitis) is a benign syndrome that occurs in children between the ages of 6 months and 7 years (mean age ~ 3 years). It is a relatively common disorder with no known genetic cause.

PFAPA has no recognizable Mendelian inheritance pattern. It is not prominent in any ethnic group and is not associated with amyloid deposition. Children with PFAPA have normal growth parameters and are in good health between episodes.

There are no laboratory tests to diagnose PFAPA. The diagnosis is based on the fever pattern and physical exam. In contrast to familial Mediterranean fever (FMF; see below), the fever generally lasts longer in PFAPA—from 5 to 7 days. Some children can manifest joint pain, abdominal pain, rash, headache, vomiting, or diarrhea. The flares respond quickly to prednisone (1 mg/kg/dose [tx: prednisone] × 3 doses given 12 hours apart), which also helps to point to PFAPA as the disease. The periodicity is usually ~ 4 weeks and is unaccompanied by any sign of infection.

Although episodes are typically very responsive to steroids, the interval to the next episode can decrease with steroid use. The decision to treat often depends on whether the symptomatology is interfering with the family's work or school routines. In some children who do not respond to the short course of steroids, consider cimetidine and/or tonsillectomy. The fever cycles generally stop recurring by the teenage years.

FAMILIAL MEDITERRANEAN FEVER

FMF is an autosomal recessive disorder mainly seen in Armenians, Turks, Levantine Arabs, and Sephardic Jews. The responsible gene (*MEFV*) is localized to chromosome 16. The product of this gene is an amino-acid protein called pyrin (a.k.a. marenostrin), which is responsible for the regulation of PMN inflammatory response and biochemically interacts with TNF, IL-1, and other cytokines. Patients have benefited from therapy with newer anticytokine biologic agents (specifically IL-1 inhibition). Curiously, some patients with documented FMF have only 1 *MEFV* gene or even none, prompting researchers to investigate for other possible loci or mediators for this disease.

Children usually present with symptoms before 10 years of age. Most children have attacks of fever that can last from several hours to 5 days. The fever typically recurs in predictable cycles: for 3–5 days every month for one patient, for example, or several times a year for another patient. Severe abdominal pain occurs with the fever. Pleuritis, pericarditis, and scrotal swelling also can occur. An erysipelas-like rash can appear around the ankles. Arthritis, arthralgia, and myalgia are common.

Make your diagnosis based on the clinical pattern, family history, and response to colchicine. Laboratory results are nonspecific, but ESR, CRP, fibrinogen, and WBC counts are usually quite high during the episodes and can normalize between flares. Genetic testing is diagnostic in > 50%, but not all gene defects have been identified.

Treat FMF with daily colchicine, which treats acute attacks, prevents future attacks, and prevents development of amyloidosis. The most common side effects are diarrhea and bone marrow suppression (particularly if renal disease is present). Colchicine prevents amyloidosis in all patients and prevents attacks in about 65% of patients. Increasing the dose to 2 mg a day in 2 divided doses prevents attacks in 95% of patients with FMF. Amyloidosis is of high concern in those not treated. Drugs that target IL-1 are being used to treat patients with disease refractory to colchicine.

TRAPS

TRAPS, or TNF receptor-1–associated periodic syndrome (formerly known as familial Hibernian [Irish] fever or familial periodic fever), is an autosomal dominant disorder with incomplete penetrance. It is due to a genetic defect in the gene that encodes the 55-kDa receptor for TNF. Diagnosis is based on history and physical exam, as in other fever syndromes, but genetic testing is helpful in this case. Episodes last longer than those of PFAPA—a minimum of 5 days and commonly longer than 2 weeks. Conjunctivitis and periorbital edema are common. Abdominal pain can occur and can be confused with FMF, but the fever episodes are much more prolonged in TRAPS. Additional findings include focal migratory myalgias and single or multiple erythematous patches on extremities.

TRAPS does not respond to colchicine but is treated with NSAIDs, prednisone, etanercept, and anakinra. Amyloidosis is a potential consequence, so it is important to diagnose and treat appropriately.

HYPER-IgD SYNDROME

Hyperimmunoglobulin D syndrome is an autosomal recessive disorder that affects mainly those of Dutch or French descent. It is due to a mutation in the *MVK* gene that encodes mevalonate kinase, which likely results in excess production of IL-1. A majority of patients present by 1 year of age, and the fevers generally last 3–7 days. Fever episodes usually occur every 1–2 months. Clinically, these patients can have abdominal pain, nausea/vomiting, and nondestructive large-joint arthritis. They can also have a diffuse nonmigratory erythematous macular rash. Lymphadenopathy, headaches, oral/vaginal ulcers, and splenomegaly also can occur during febrile episodes. Characteristically, as expected, IgD is often elevated (> 100 IU/mL) but not always, and IgA is also elevated in most cases. This helps differentiate this disease from other periodic fever syndromes. Amyloidosis is rare in this disorder.

Treatment can include colchicine, prednisone, IVIG, NSAIDs, etanercept, and anakinra.

CRYOPYRIN-ASSOCIATED PERIODIC FEVER SYNDROMES

Cryopyrin-associated periodic syndromes (CAPS) are a group of autoinflammatory diseases with an autosomal dominant inheritance with variable expression.

There are 3 periodic fever syndromes resulting from inheritable abnormalities in cryopyrin (*CIAS1* gene). These include **f**amilial **c**old **a**utoinflammatory **s**yndrome (**FCAS**), Muckle-Wells syndrome, and **n**eonatal-**o**nset **m**ultisystem **i**nflammatory **d**isease (**NOMID**). These disorders have overlapping clinical presentations, including fever, acute-phase inflammation, a neutrophilic urticarial skin rash, and joint involvement.

The diagnosis is made by genetic testing. Other tests include skin biopsy of the rash, an eye examination, hearing tests, lumbar puncture, and imaging of the brain and inner ears by MRI.

Cryopyrin is involved with the activation of IL-1beta. Targeted inhibition of the IL-1 pathway has resulted in new treatments for these diseases. Approved drugs include rilonacept, anakinra, and canakinumab.

OTHER CAUSES OF PERIODIC FEVERS

Consider cyclic neutropenia (really an immunodeficiency syndrome) in your evaluation of recurrent fevers. This can be autosomal dominant or sporadic in inheritance. It usually presents in early childhood. Absolute neutrophil counts of < 500 cells/µL occur every 21 days (with a range of 14–36 days) like clockwork, with each episode lasting 3–10 days. Clinical symptoms include fever, malaise, lymphadenopathy, and mouth sores. Blood counts 3×/week every 6–8 weeks is sometimes necessary to make the diagnosis.

THE MEDSTUDY HUB: YOUR GUIDELINES AND REVIEW ARTICLES RESOURCE

For both the review articles and current Pediatrics practice guidelines, visit the MedStudy Hub at

medstudy.com/hub

The Hub contains the only online consolidated list of all Pediatrics guidelines! Guidelines on the Hub are continually updated and linked to the published source. MedStudy maintains the Hub as a free online resource, available to all physicians.

MedStudy®

OPHTHALMOLOGY & ENT

SECTION EDITOR

Julieana Nichols, MD, MPH
Assistant Professor of Pediatrics
Associate Director of Academic General
 Pediatric Fellowship
Baylor College of Medicine
Texas Children's Hospital Clinical Care Center
Houston, TX

MEDICAL EDITOR

Jenny Way, MD, MS
Bellevue, WA

REVIEWER

Erik Langenau, DO, MS
Chief Academic Technology Officer
Philadelphia College of Osteopathic Medicine
Philadelphia, PA

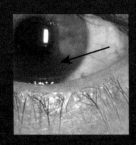

Table of Contents

OPHTHALMOLOGY & ENT

OPHTHALMOLOGY / ENT

NORMAL VISUAL DEVELOPMENT

PREVIEW | REVIEW

- At what age does visual fixation achieve accuracy?
- Are most infants nearsighted or farsighted at birth?

Some important basics:

- Visual fixation can be demonstrated soon after birth and achieves accuracy by 6–8 weeks.
- By 2 months of age, infants should track across midline. Object tracking to 180° and conjugate gaze should be present by 4 months of age.
- Optokinetic nystagmus (defined as nystagmus induced by looking at objects moving across the visual field) and vestibular ocular reflex are normal involuntary eye movements that provide stability of visual images.
- Stereopsis, known as binocular depth perception is when 2 separate images from both eyes are combined into 1 image in the brain. Stereopsis and binocular visual function develop between 3 and 7 months of age.
- Accommodation is the ability to focus the intraocular lens for near-viewing and is present at birth; however, it is not accurate until 2–3 months of age.
- Due to its size and shape, the normal eye at birth is often hyperopic (farsighted). As the visual system matures, the eye elongates and becomes less hyperopic. Although most newborn full-term infants are normally mildly farsighted, premature and low-birth-weight infants tend to be either less hyperopic or even myopic (nearsighted) and often also have some degree of astigmatism (misshapen cornea resulting in improperly refracted light and blurred vision). Approximately 45% of premature infants are myopic compared to 20% of full-term infants.
- Color discrimination occurs by 2 weeks of age and improves over the next 3 months.

EYE DISORDERS

PREVIEW | REVIEW

- What are some abnormalities that can cause an abnormal red reflex?
- What is strabismus?
- What are the causes of amblyopia?
- What is the incidence of color vision abnormalities in boys compared to girls?
- Which brain lesion is suggested by upbeating jerk nystagmus? Downbeating?

- What are the symptoms of a corneal abrasion? How do you diagnose it?
- What are the most common risk factors for ROP?
- What is the most prevalent malignant ocular tumor in childhood?
- How does retinoblastoma usually present?
- What is hyphema?

OVERVIEW

Common visual disorders include amblyopia, strabismus, significant refractive error, color vision defects, and ocular disease. In the U.S., the leading causes of blindness in children are cortical visual impairment, retinopathy of prematurity, and optic nerve hypoplasia. The leading cause of "acquired" blindness is ocular trauma, most often following a sports-related injury or an accidental or intentional injury by another child.

An abnormal red reflex can indicate a number of abnormalities (e.g., strabismus, cataracts, glaucoma, retinoblastoma, high refractory error); refer immediately.

STRABISMUS

Strabismus is the continuous or intermittent malalignment of one or both eyes, in which one or both eyes are turned in (esotropia), out (exotropia), up (hypertropia), or down (hypotropia). In childhood, the most common forms are infantile and accommodative esotropia. Physical exam reveals an asymmetric corneal light reflex and abnormal cover/uncover test (i.e., movement of the uncovered eye that is fixated on a target when the other eye is covered). While ocular instability of infancy is frequently present in normal newborns during the first few months of life, refer for possible pathologic strabismus if it persists past 4 months of age.

Pseudoesotropia (pseudostrabismus) is the result of a wide nasal bridge and/or epicanthal folds, which obscure the nasal sclera, particularly when the child looks to the right or left. On formal testing, a symmetric light reflex is demonstrated on both examination of the corneal light reflex and the cover/uncover test, thereby confirming that the child has pseudostrabismus. (See more about vision screening in Preventive Pediatrics, Book 1.)

AMBLYOPIA

Amblyopia, a functional reduction in visual acuity ✓acuity caused by disuse or misuse of visual pathways, occurs in 1–4% of 3-year-olds. It also affects depth perception and binocularity and is often due to strabismus (strabismic amblyopia). Amblyopia is the most common cause of visual loss in individuals < 45 years of age. It can result from early childhood refractive disorders, strabismus, cataracts, corneal opacities, or anisometropia (an unequal refractive error between the eyes).

Have the child use the amblyopic eye by patching the better-seeing eye with a patch or cycloplegic eye drops.

COLOR VISION DEFECTS

The ability to match colors is present by 2 years of age. Abnormal color vision occurs in ~ 8–10% of boys and < 0.5% of girls; it is due to X-linked protan and deutan deficits (red-green color blindness). While most color vision defects are congenital, acquired color vision abnormalities can occur, though rare, and are caused by retinal and optic nerve abnormalities.

CORTICAL VISUAL IMPAIRMENT

Damage to the geniculostriate pathway (composed of the visual cortex and optic radiations) causes cortical visual impairment. There is reduced vision and absence of optokinetic nystagmus, but pupillary light reflexes are intact. Hypoxia is the most common cause, but other etiologies include meningitis, encephalitis, metabolic disease, head trauma, and hydrocephalus. Generally, children with cortical visual impairment have other associated abnormalities, including cerebral palsy, seizures, or paralysis.

NYSTAGMUS

Nystagmus is an involuntary oscillation of the eyes. The movements can be pendular (like a pendulum) or jerk.

Pendular nystagmus has a sinusoidal oscillation. It is typically acquired, and it is due to visual loss or can be a late unremitting sign of multiple sclerosis. The sinusoidal oscillation can occur in any direction, but it is usually horizontal.

Jerk nystagmus has 2 components: slow and fast. The eyes "drift" (= slow component) and try to quickly recover (= fast component). The fast direction defines the direction of the nystagmus. The nystagmus is sometimes (but not always) associated with vertigo. Jerk nystagmus is most common in vestibular disorders but does not indicate whether the lesion is within the central nervous system or if it involves the cranial nerve itself. **Upbeating jerk nystagmus** usually indicates a lesion in the pons but can be seen in lesions of the medulla or cerebellum (i.e., infratentorial). **Downbeating jerk nystagmus** indicates a lesion at the cervicomedullary junction.

Most congenital nystagmus is horizontal and conjugate, and it is often associated with visual loss. This type usually has a blending of jerk and pendular waveforms.

Gazing in particular directions precipitates the abnormal eye movements in certain types of nystagmus. For instance, drugs (e.g., antiepileptic medications) can cause **horizontal** and **vertical gaze–evoked nystagmus** (occurring when the person looks right, left, or up)—in other words, it is present "in all directions."

[handwritten left margin: upbeating ↑ higher up lesion in pons; downbeating ↓ lower down lesion in cervico-medullary jxn.]

[handwritten bottom margin: Spasmus nutans: an acquired nystagmus of unknown etiology. Presenting w/in the 1st 0-2mo of life. Spontaneous resolution w/in months-years. characterized by horizontal, rapid pendicular nystagmus + associated w/ torticollis + slow head nodding]

Isolated vertical gaze–evoked nystagmus typically indicates disease in the posterior fossa.

PAINFUL ERYTHEMATOUS EYE

Overview

The painful red eye is a typical primary-care complaint. Although conjunctivitis is the usual cause, consider also corneal abrasion, foreign body, subconjunctival hemorrhage, glaucoma, iritis, keratitis, and scleritis. Evaluate with history, visual acuity testing, and penlight examination:

- If there is mild or no pain and normal or mildly blurred vision, consider:
  ○ Viral conjunctivitis (most common, watery discharge, very contagious)
  ○ Bacterial conjunctivitis (usually thick discharge, very contagious)
  ○ Subjunctival hemorrage (bright red patches)
- If there is moderate-to-severe pain with vision abnormalities, distorted pupil, or corneal involvement, refer urgently to ophthalmology for further evaluation, as there is likely to be a serious underlying cause.

Conjunctivitis

Conjunctivitis is an inflammation of the conjunctiva; it can be either infectious (bacterial or viral) or noninfectious (typically allergic). Allergic conjunctivitis is covered in Allergy & Immunology, Book 4, so we will concentrate on infectious etiologies here. The most common infectious etiology is adenovirus. Bacterial causes include *Streptococcus pneumoniae*, *Haemophilus influenzae*, and *Moraxella catarrhalis*. Both viral and bacterial conjunctivitis are very contagious and spread by direct contact. *[handwritten: URI bugs]*

The patient with conjunctivitis presents with red conjunctiva and a gritty sensation in the eye that often accompanies an upper respiratory infection. Viral conjunctivitis usually produces a waterier discharge and tends to start in one eye, spreading to the other within 24–48 hours. Bacterial conjunctivitis produces a purulent discharge and tends to be unilateral, although it can be in both eyes.

Although there is no specific treatment for viral conjunctivitis, many patients get some relief with lubricant drops.

Treatment for bacterial conjunctivitis often includes erythromycin ophthalmic ointment or trimethoprim-polymyxin ophthalmic drops 4×/day for 5–7 days. Use fluoroquinolone drops in contact lens wearers due to the increased incidence of *Pseudomonas* in these patients.

[handwritten: pseudo → Cipro]

Corneal Abrasion

Corneal abrasions are very common; most superficial abrasions heal quickly without sequelae. Symptoms include pain, tearing, photophobia, and blurry vision. Infants can present with inconsolable crying. Corneal ulcers are uncommon but potentially much more serious; contact lens wearers are at risk. Be sure to look for a foreign body.

Diagnosis is best made with fluorescein dye and either a Wood's lamp or the blue light of a slit lamp (Image 21-1). An abrasion is transparent on gross examination without fluorescein, whereas an ulcer is opaque; both light up under fluorescein.

Treat corneal abrasions with a topical antibiotic ointment and oral analgesia. Topical anesthetics are helpful in the emergency department or office to provide temporary pain relief and allow examination, but do not send the patient home with anesthetic drops—they can be toxic to the cornea with repeated use, and the child may retraumatize the eye. Semipressure patches have not been found to reduce pain or help healing in most patients.

Multiple vertical abrasions suggest a foreign body retained in the upper eyelid; the lid must be everted to see and remove the object. Remove superficial foreign bodies with a cotton swab (after topical anesthesia, of course). Refer to an ophthalmologist for removal of deeper foreign bodies.

Recheck corneal abrasions for resolution in 24–48 hours. Corneal ulcers should also be treated by ophthalmology.

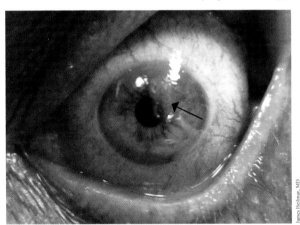

Image 21-1: Corneal abrasion with fluorescein staining

ORBITAL AND PRESEPTAL CELLULITIS

Preseptal cellulitis is an infection of the eye involving tissues anterior to the orbital septum (i.e., anterior to the orbital contents), while **orbital cellulitis** is an infection involving structures behind the orbital septum. It is imperative to distinguish between preseptal cellulitis, which is typically mild, and the far more serious orbital cellulitis. Although both present with eye pain and a red swollen eyelid, only orbital cellulitis causes pain with eye movement, ophthalmoplegia, chemosis, and/or proptosis.

Diagnose preseptal cellulitis by history and physical exam, but a CT scan is required if there is any question of possible orbital cellulitis. Preseptal cellulitis is typically caused by contiguous spread of infection from surrounding soft tissue due to trauma or from sinusitis. *Staph+ strep* The usual pathogens are *Staphylococcus aureus* and *Streptococcus pyogenes* when the infection originates from local trauma and *S. pneumoniae* when it originates from sinusitis. Treatment is usually outpatient and consists of 7–10 days of:

- clindamycin or
- combination therapy of trimethoprim/sulfamethoxazole (TMP/SMX) plus 1 of the following:
  - amoxicillin,
  - amoxicillin/clavulanic acid,
  - cefpodoxime, or
  - cefdinir.

Hospitalize patients who are < 1 year of age.

If suspected clinically, use CT scan to diagnose orbital cellulitis. It typically originates from sinusitis, particularly ethmoidal sinuses. Orbital cellulitis is usually caused by multiple organisms, but the most commonly identified pathogens are *S. aureus* and streptococci. Admit the patient for parenteral antibiotic therapy with vancomycin plus ampicillin-sulbactam or for parenteral antibiotic therapy with ceftriaxone. Once the patient improves, typically within 3–5 days, switch treatment to the same oral drug regimen used for preseptal cellulitis. Treat with a total duration of combined antibiotic therapy (both IV and oral) of at least 2–3 weeks. Surgery is sometimes required if the patient does not respond to antibiotic therapy. Possible complications include orbital abscess, subperiosteal abscess, and intracranial extension.

CHALAZION / STYE
infected

A chalazion is a localized bump at the edge of the eyelid caused by a blockage of the meibomian glands, which produce oil. If it becomes infected, it is referred to as a stye or hordeolum. Styes are red and painful for 3–5 days before they rupture, and then they heal in about a week; hasten rupture with warm compresses. A chalazion does not grow as rapidly as a stye and often is not painful. Chalazions typically resolve without treatment within a few months; if still persistent, refer to an ophthalmologist for incision and curettage.

NASOLACRIMAL DUCT OBSTRUCTION (DACRYOSTENOSIS)

Dacryostenosis is caused by obstruction of the nasolacrimal duct and is very common in newborns. The main symptom is persistent tearing in the affected eye. Treatment consists of lacrimal sac massage; 90% of cases resolve by 6 months of age. Refer to an ophthalmologist for possible duct probing if the condition persists after 6–7 months of age.

CATARACTS

A cataract refers to an opacification of the lens.

Congenital cataracts are caused by abnormal lens development *in utero* and are present at birth, although they sometimes go undetected for a period of time. A unilateral cataract is usually sporadic and not associated with a systemic disease. Bilateral cataracts, however, can be caused by autosomal dominant (AD) inheritance, trisomy syndromes (i.e., 21, 13, 18), metabolic disorders (e.g., galactosemia), and intrauterine infections (i.e., **TORCH** [**t**oxoplasmosis, **o**ther, **r**ubella, **c**ytomegalovirus, and **h**erpes]). Cataracts in older children can occur following ocular trauma, glucocorticoid treatment, and ionizing radiation.

The simultaneous red reflex test is the most useful assessment to detect lens opacity. If abnormal, a complete eye examination must be done by an ophthalmologist. Not all cataracts are visually significant, but those that are centrally located and > 3 mm require immediate removal to prevent vision loss. Smaller ones can be observed for a period of time but must be removed at the 1st indication of visual interference.

PAPILLEDEMA

Papilledema refers to optic nerve swelling due to increased intracranial pressure. It is imperative to urgently recognize and evaluate papilloma. Underlying causes include a mass lesion, cerebral edema, obstructive hydrocephalus, and pseudotumor cerebri. Symptoms can include headache, nausea and vomiting, and pulsatile tinnitus. Often visual symptoms are absent, but if they occur, they include diplopia and brief visual obscurations that are often unilateral.

Diagnosis is made by funduscopic examination, and findings can range from loss of spontaneous venous pulsations to obscured disc margins, venous congestion, and papillary hemorrhages. Once the diagnosis of papilledema is made, neuroimaging, preferably MRI, is required to determine the cause. If the MRI is normal, evaluate opening pressure and spinal fluid with a lumbar puncture. Treatment varies and depends upon the underlying etiology.

RETINOPATHY OF PREMATURITY

Retinopathy of prematurity (ROP) is a developmental proliferative vascular disorder that occurs in the retina of preterm infants with incomplete retinal vascularization. Prematurity is the most important risk factor for ROP, followed by low birth weight. Other risk factors include elevated arterial oxygen tension, assisted ventilation for > 7 days, surfactant therapy, hyperglycemia, insulin therapy, and cumulative illness severity.

Severe ROP occurs mainly in infants born at ≤ 28 weeks of gestation and with a birth weight of < 1,250 grams.

Screen all infants weighing ≤ 1,500 grams at birth or with a gestational age of < 30 weeks. Also, screen those with a birth weight between 1,500 and 2,000 grams or a gestational age ≥ 30 weeks whose clinical course places them at increased risk for ROP. The ROP screening should be performed with a dilated eye exam by a pediatric ophthalmologist.

OPTIC NERVE HYPOPLASIA

Optic nerve hypoplasia is a nonspecific finding due to damage of the visual system prior to full development. It is characterized by pallor of the disc, loss of substance of the nerve head, and enlargement of the disc cup.

Intracranial tumors and hydrocephalus are the most common causes of optic atrophy in children. Other causes are hypopituitarism, hypothyroidism, growth hormone deficiency, and/or neonatal hypoglycemia.

Maternal risk factors are diabetes, alcohol abuse, and exposure to toxins.

Optic nerve hypoplasia is an example of a midline facial defect; other defects include a single central incisor, cleft lip/palate, and a male with a microphallus or undescended testicle.

RETINOBLASTOMA

Retinoblastoma is the leading malignant ocular tumor of childhood, with an incidence of 3.7 cases per million. It can be genetic or sporadic. About 60% of cases are unilateral and nonhereditary; 15% are unilateral and hereditary; all remaining cases are both bilateral and hereditary. Bilateral involvement is most common in those < 1 year of age. Germinal retinoblastoma is the result of inactivation of the *RB1* gene on chromosome 13q14 and is inherited in an AD pattern.

There is a significant risk of secondary malignancies, especially osteosarcoma, soft tissue sarcomas, and malignant melanoma. The tumor arises from the primitive retinal cells—most present at < 4 years of age.

Retinoblastoma typically presents with a white pupillary reflex—leukocoria; however, strabismus can also be the initial presenting complaint.

Treatment depends on the size and location of the tumor. Options include enucleation, chemotherapy, radiation therapy, laser therapy, and cryotherapy.

HYPHEMA

Hyphema is the presence of blood in the anterior chamber of the eye. Usually, it occurs after blunt or penetrating injury. It appears as a bright or dark red fluid level between the cornea and iris (Image 21-2); early

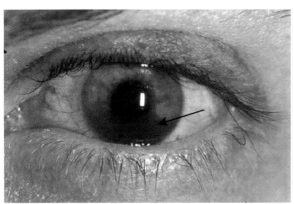

Image 21-2: Hyphema

injuries sometimes show diffuse murkiness before the blood settles. Complete opacification of the anterior chamber ("eight ball hyphema") can occur in more severe injuries. Ophthalmologic consult is required. Consider ruptured globe and intraocular foreign body if the history or physical are concerning—e.g., struck by a sharp object (such as knife or scissors) or shot with a BB. A clue to a ruptured globe is a teardrop-shaped or eccentric pupil. Protect any serious eye injury from further trauma with a rigid shield, and consult ophthalmology.

Treatment includes topical steroid and cycloplegic drops. There is little evidence for the previous standard treatment of bed rest with elevation of the head 30° to 45°. Use ondansetron and analgesics to alleviate vomiting and/or pain, which can otherwise further elevate intraocular pressure. Although most children with minor hyphemas do well, they are at risk of rebleeding (usually in the 1st week after initial injury); this increases the risk for long-term complications such as glaucoma. Prevent secondary bleeding with antifibrinolytic therapy (e.g., aminocaproic acid). Closely monitor intraocular pressures.

ORBITAL BLOWOUT FRACTURE

Blunt trauma to the eye (such as being punched or struck by a baseball) can cause fracture of the orbital walls or floor. Herniation of orbital contents into a paranasal sinus can entrap extraocular muscles and other structures. Orbital floor fractures are the most common. Symptoms can include vertical diplopia, cheek numbness, and limited upward gaze. Other findings can include circumferential ecchymosis, subconjunctival hemorrhage, hyphema, and enophthalmos (eye appears sunken in).

Consult ophthalmology and get a CT scan of the orbits (Image 21-3). Advise these patients to avoid blowing their nose, and prescribe antibiotics to prevent infection. Refer early to a maxillofacial surgeon, as operative treatment will likely be needed; exact timing depends on the severity of entrapment and other findings.

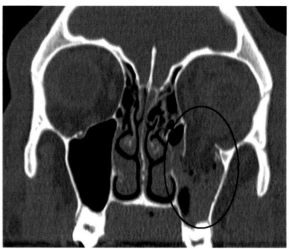

Image 21-3: Orbital blowout fracture

EAR DISORDERS

PREVIEW | REVIEW

- A child with a preauricular pit is at increased risk for what kind of impairment?
- What are the most common bacterial pathogens of acute otitis media?
- What is the pattern of inheritance for the majority of inherited deafness cases?
- What are the most common causes of conductive hearing loss in children?
- What is the most likely etiology for severe and profound hearing loss?
- What is the most common infectious cause on congenital deafness?
- Interpret common tympanogram results.

PREAURICULAR SINUSES AND PITS

A preauricular sinus/pit is a common congenital abnormality. There is an increased risk of hearing impairment, so all affected patients need an audiologic examination. There is no increased risk of renal abnormalities with isolated preauricular sinus/pit. However, if there are other dysmorphic features or malformations or hearing loss, order a renal ultrasound to rule out associated syndromes. See Genetics, Book 5, for more on associated syndromes with preauricular sinus/pit.

EXTERNAL EAR

Otitis Externa

Otitis externa (a.k.a. swimmer's ear) is inflammation of the outer ear canal. It is common in swimmers, as water remaining in the ear canal provides a favorable environment for bacterial overgrowth. Although bacterial infection is the most common cause of otitis externa, allergic reactions and fungal infections can also cause otitis externa.

Symptoms include pruritus, pain, drainage, redness, and muffled hearing. On physical exam, the ear canal is red, swollen, and often scaly. A key finding is worsening pain with manipulation of the pinna, which doesn't occur with otitis media. The most common etiologies are *Pseudomonas aeruginosa* and *S. aureus*, although cultures are typically not done.

Treatment is aimed at the most likely causes and consists of a combination of a topical antibiotic and glucocorticoid. The fluoroquinolones (ofloxacin and ciprofloxacin) are preferable because they provide excellent coverage against both common pathogens. Aminoglycosides and polymyxin B are alternatives. Treat for a minimum of 7 days, and up to 2 weeks. Fluoroquinolone drops are given 2×/day, whereas the other antibiotic classes are given 3–4×/day.

Foreign Body

Most foreign bodies of the external ear canal occur in children ≤ 6 years of age and can include beads, food, toys, rocks, and insects. Although a foreign body can cause pain and/or decreased hearing, many are asymptomatic, and found incidentally on exam, or are brought to medical attention by a caretaker who saw the patient place an object into the ear. Diagnosis is made by otoscopy. Removal techniques include irrigation and instrumentation under direct visualization. Mineral oil or lidocaine can be placed in the ear canal to kill live insects prior to removal. Referral to ENT is necessary if proper instruments are not available or if removal is difficult.

Hematoma

Auricular hematoma is caused by blunt trauma to the auricle; accumulation of blood between the cartilage and the perichondrium interrupts the blood supply to the cartilage. Drain as soon as possible to prevent necrosis and a cauliflower ear. Refer to ENT if drainage is delayed > 7 days.

MIDDLE EAR

Acute Otitis Media

Acute otitis media (AOM) is an acute inflammation of the middle ear caused by infection. Most episodes of AOM are triggered by an upper respiratory infection causing blockage of the eustachian tube. The typical pathogens are viruses, *S. pneumoniae*, nontypeable *H. influenzae*, and *M. catarrhalis*. Risk factors include age (6–18 months), family history, day care attendance, lack of breastfeeding, and tobacco smoke exposure. The most common symptom is ear pain, but in younger children, the symptoms are nonspecific and can include fever, anorexia, irritability, and tugging at

the ears. Complications of AOM include mastoiditis. Diagnosis of AOM is made by pneumatic otoscopy when the following criteria are met according to the 2013 AAP guidelines: bulging tympanic membrane (TM), middle ear effusion, and opaque TM.

High-dose (80–90 mg/kg/day) amoxicillin is the drug of choice for AOM. If patients fail to respond within 48 hours, broaden coverage to include penicillin-resistant *S. pneumoniae*, beta-lactamase-producing *H. influenzae*, and *M. catarrhalis*, by switching to amoxicillin/clavulanate or a 2nd or 3rd generation cephalosporin. In 2013, the AAP published updated guidelines for the diagnosis and management of uncomplicated AOM in children 6 months to 12 years of age. These guidelines base initial antibiotic treatment on:

- age (6 months to 2 years vs. > 2 years),
- severity of symptoms,
- unilateral vs. bilateral disease, and
- presence of otorrhea.

For children 6 months to 2 years of age with unilateral AOM without otorrhea, and for children ≥ 2 years of age with unilateral or bilateral otitis without otorrhea, start with observation only and monitor for symptom resolution. However, follow up closely, and start antibiotics if the child worsens or fails to improve within 48–72 hours from onset.

Recurrent Acute Otitis Media

Recurrent AOM is defined as ≥ 3 episodes in a 6-month period or ≥ 4 episodes within a 12-month period. Treat with prophylactic antibiotics or tympanostomy tubes. Typical antibiotic regimens are amoxicillin 40 mg/kg/day or sulfisoxazole 50 mg/kg/day.

Otitis Media with Effusion

Otitis media with effusion (OME) is a middle ear effusion without clinical signs of infection. It is typically seen during the resolution of AOM or with eustachian tube dysfunction. OME is often asymptomatic but can present with some hearing loss. Spontaneous resolution usually occurs within 6 weeks. Tympanostomy tube placement is recommended for patients with persistent OME. ⟩ 3 mo

Chronic Suppurative Otitis Media

Chronic suppurative otitis media (CSOM) refers to a perforated tympanic membrane with chronic drainage lasting > 6 weeks. Typical causes include recurrent AOM, injury, or tympanostomy tube placement. The patient presents with painless drainage and possibly decreased hearing. The most common pathogens are *Pseudomonas* and *Proteus*. Treatment consists of ototopical therapy with a quinolone (5 drops 3×/day for 2 weeks). This can be combined with ear wicking, suctioning of the otorrhea, or using gauze to absorb the drainage.

Complications of Otitis Media

Cholesteatoma is an abnormal growth of squamous epithelium in the middle ear; progressive enlargement can destroy the nearby ossicles, thus causing hearing loss. It can also cause cranial nerve palsies and vertigo. Cholesteatoma occurs most commonly in children with recurrent or chronic otitis media, cleft palate, Down syndrome, and Turner syndrome. Diagnosis is made on otoscopy exam when a white mass is seen behind an intact ear drum. Surgical removal is required, but there is > 50% recurrence rate within 5 years of surgery.

Mastoiditis occurs when the mastoid air cells of the temporal bone, which are contiguous with the middle ear cavity, become infected. The most common pathogens include *S. pneumoniae*, *S. pyogenes*, and *S. aureus*. Physical features include fever; postauricular erythema, tenderness, and swelling; and protrusion of the auricle.

Immediate diagnosis and treatment can prevent serious complications (e.g., meningitis, osteomyelitis). Treat uncomplicated cases with IV vancomycin +/– ceftazidime or cefepime, until culture results from tympanocentesis are back. Switch to oral antibiotics once improvement is seen and sensitivities are known. If needed, additional drainage of the middle ear can be achieved with myringotomy. Treat complicated cases the same as above, but also arrange for a mastoidectomy to remove the infected mastoid cortical bone.

HEARING PROBLEMS

Deafness is defined as hearing loss at > 90 dB, which results in the inability to distinguish between elements of spoken language. "Mild" hearing loss is defined as a 25-dB loss, but even a 15-dB loss can result in problems with speech perception, especially during early childhood.

Deafness is inherited in ~ 50% of cases. Of these, 80% are inherited as autosomal recessive (AR), 18% as AD, and 2% as X-linked recessive. Deafness can be due to either an isolated event or associated with a syndrome (e.g., Treacher-Collins, Alport, Crouzon, Waardenburg, Usher, or trisomy 21). One form of the prolonged QT syndrome (Jervell and Lange-Nielsen syndrome) is associated with sensorineural hearing loss—syncope and a history of hearing loss are important clues to this diagnosis!

According to the CDC, 1–3/1,000 children have hearing loss. Hearing loss is generally classified into 1 of 3 categories: conductive, sensorineural, or cortical.

Conductive hearing loss (more common) is due to disruption of mechanical components required for the transduction of sound wave energy. Cerumen impaction, ossicular chain fixation, and fluid in the middle ear—due either to acute suppurative otitis media or otitis media with effusion—are the most common causes of conductive hearing loss. With a middle ear effusion, sounds

are distorted by the fluid, leading to problems in early language discrimination.

About 65% of children have, at various points in time, some degree of intermittent conductive hearing loss, usually limited to sounds at 50 dB or lower; sounds louder than this can be conducted directly by bone to the cochlea.

Sensorineural hearing loss (less common) is caused by dysfunction of the sensory epithelium, cochlea, or neural pathways leading to the auditory cortex via cranial nerve 8 and other connections. Severe and profound hearing loss is always sensorineural and most often affects higher frequencies.

The most common infectious cause of congenital deafness is cytomegalovirus (CMV), which causes sensorineural hearing loss in 60% of symptomatic and 7% of asymptomatic infants. Other congenital infections that can cause sensorineural hearing loss include toxoplasmosis, rubella, and syphilis. Routine immunization with *H. influenzae* Type b and pneumococcal vaccines has decreased the rate of bacterial meningitis and the resulting hearing loss. Other causes of acquired sensorineural hearing loss include prolonged exposure to loud noise (a typical cause of high-pitched hearing loss in adolescents), ototoxic drugs (e.g., aminoglycosides, salicylates, loop diuretics), and trauma.

Cortical dysfunction can also result in hearing loss due to an impaired ability to perceive or process sounds.

Table 21-1 lists risk factors for neonatal hearing loss as identified by the Joint Committee on Infant Hearing. Around 50% of infants with sensorineural hearing loss have ≥ 1 risk factor. However, do hearing screening for all infants, not just those at potential risk. (See Preventive Pediatrics, Book 1.) Screening is performed with either otoacoustic emissions (OAE) or an automated auditory brainstem response (ABR) test.

In children with persistent middle ear effusions, closely monitor language development for any delay because prolonged hearing loss during the critical period of speech acquisition can lead to significant impediments.

Table 21-1: Risk Factors for Hearing Loss in Neonates

Family history of sensorineural hearing loss (AR)

Congenital infection—especially CMV

Presence of craniofacial anomalies

Birth weight < 1,500 g

Neonatal jaundice resulting in exchange transfusion

Ototoxic medications (e.g., furosemide, aminoglycosides) gent

Bacterial meningitis

Apgar scores of ≤ 3 at 5 minutes

Physical findings consistent with a syndrome associated with hearing loss

The key to success in treating hearing loss is early diagnosis and intervention (e.g., hearing aids, implants).

TYMPANOGRAMS

Tympanometry is an objective tool in testing middle ear function. It measures the changes in the acoustic impedance of the middle ear in response to changes in air pressure.

Common tympanograms:

Type A, normal tympanogram (Figure 21-1):

- Peak +50 to –150 decaPascals (daPa)
- Peak compliance (*y* axis) between 0.2 and 1.8 cc
- Absence of middle ear pathology
- Intact and mobile tympanic membrane (TM)
- Normal eustachian tube function
- If hearing loss, likely sensorineural

Type A(s), shallow (Figure 21-2): *S: Scarring Sclerosis*

- Peak pressure curve normal in position
- Peak compliance very low (below 0.2 cc)
- Occurs with ossicular fixation or TM scarring
- Can be caused by otosclerosis
- Not due to middle ear effusion
- Can result in hearing loss

Type A(d), disarticulation (Figure 21-3):

- Peak pressure between +50 and –150 cc (normal)
- Peak compliance very high
- Occurs with ossicular disarticulation
- Can result in hearing loss

Type B, retracted, poorly mobile (Figure 21-4):

- Peak is absent or poorly defined.
- Negative middle ear pressure (peak pressure is shifted left)
- Maximum compliance below normal
- Suggestive of fluid behind the middle ear or perforation of eardrums
- Conductive hearing loss likely

Type C, negative pressure (Figure 21-5):

- Clear peak
- Negative middle ear pressure (left shift: peak pressure negative)
- Peak compliance may be normal
- Diagnosis: eustachian tube dysfunction
- Conductive hearing loss likely

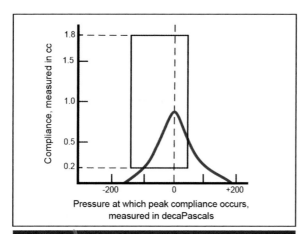

Figure 21-1: Type A, Normal Tympanogram

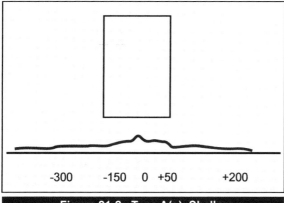

Figure 21-2: Type A(s), Shallow

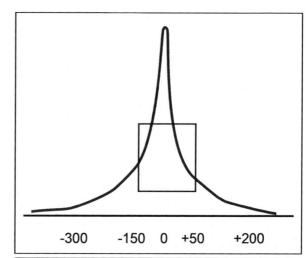

Figure 21-3: Type A(d), Disarticulation

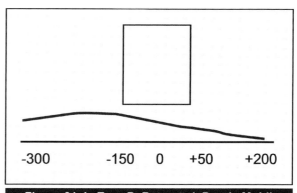

Figure 21-4: Type B, Retracted, Poorly Mobile

Coloboma: a keyhole like or notch like defect of the iris, ciliary body, retina, choroid, + or optic nerve, often associated w/ nystagmus + microphthalmia

CONGENITAL DISORDERS OF THE NOSE

PREVIEW | REVIEW

- What is the most common congenital anomaly of the nose?

- What is CHARGE syndrome?

CHOANAL ATRESIA

Choanal atresia is the most common congenital anomaly of the nose and occurs in ~ 1/7,000 newborns. It is characterized by a bony (90%) or membranous (10%) septum between the nose and the pharynx, unilaterally or bilaterally. Nearly half of these infants have other associated congenital anomalies. Look for **CHARGE** syndrome (**c**oloboma, **h**eart disease, **a**tresia of the choanae, **r**etarded growth and development, **g**enital anomalies, and **e**ar anomalies/deafness).

Symptoms vary, depending upon the infant's ability to breathe through the mouth and the severity of the atresia. These infants can appear initially normal with mouth breathing or crying, but, because infants are primarily nose breathers, they typically show symptoms early on. Infants with bilateral atresia frequently suck in their lips when they inspire, and they have respiratory distress and cyanosis. Even infants who are able to adequately breathe through their mouths still have difficulty with breathing when fed. Symptoms improve with crying. Infants with unilateral choanal atresia can be asymptomatic until the nonaffected nares become blocked, for example, with secretions.

Diagnosis is suggested by the inability to pass a firm catheter through each nostril past a depth of about 3–4 cm. Confirm with CT scan. Due to the high association of other anomalies, cardiology and ophthalmology consultations are warranted.

Treat initially by providing an adequate oral airway, which also allows the infant to feed. Usually, an orogastric tube is sufficient for infants who can breathe by mouth. Consider performing corrective neonatal surgery

if the infant does not have other associated defects. Infants with severe bilateral involvement who cannot breathe effectively by mouth require a tracheotomy until reconstructive surgery can be safely performed. Unilateral correction can usually be delayed for several years. Restenosis after surgery is common.

OTHER LESS COMMON DISORDERS

Congenital perforation and/or deviation of the nasal septum is rare. If they occur, most are due to birth trauma.

Pyriform aperture stenosis is an abnormality of the anterior nasal aperture that is rare and has symptoms that mimic choanal atresia.

Congenital midline nasal masses can include dermoids, gliomas, and encephaloceles. Nasal dermoids can have a dimple or pit on the nasal dorsum and sometimes contain hair.

Intracranial extension of any defect increases the risk of recurrent intracranial infections. Use high resolution CT or MRI scan to evaluate for intracranial involvement. Resection is indicated if intracranial extension is found with any of these lesions.

ACQUIRED DISORDERS OF THE NOSE

PREVIEW | REVIEW

- What do you suspect in a child who presents with a unilateral, foul-smelling nasal discharge?

- What is the most common etiology for epistaxis?

- Ask an adolescent with epistaxis about which type of illicit drug usage?

- Which studies do you do for a child with recurrent or severe epistaxis?

- If you find nasal polyps in a child < 12 years of age, what diagnosis do you consider first?

- What is an effective treatment of nasal polyps?

FOREIGN BODY

The nose is the toddler's playground. Various items can end up there without anyone's knowledge as to how they got there. These include crayons, various foods, toys, erasers, paper, beads, beans, stones, and pencils. Suspect a foreign body when a child presents with a unilateral purulent nasal discharge. Over time, the drainage (and the child) becomes foul smelling.

You can frequently see the foreign material with good lighting and an otoscope or nasal speculum. Do not push the foreign body further into the nose.

Outpatient treatment includes topical anesthetics and forceps or nasal suction. In some cases, general anesthesia is required.

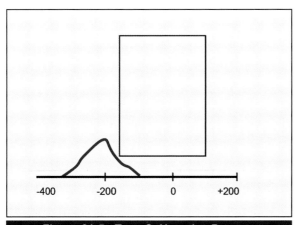

Figure 21-5: Type C, Negative Pressure

-400   -200   0   +200

EPISTAXIS

Epistaxis (nose bleed) is common in children. The most frequent cause is "nose picking." Nose bleeds usually occur during the dry, winter months. Besides nose picking, other causes include trauma (during sports, particularly), foreign bodies, and neoplasms (nasopharyngeal carcinomata, rhabdomyosarcomas, and lymphomata) of the nose. Question any adolescent with epistaxis regarding drug use. Mucosal irritation is often seen in those who inhale cocaine, resulting in nosebleeds. Coagulopathies can obviously predispose to prolonged epistaxis. Hereditary hemorrhagic telangiectasia (HHT) can also present with recurrent epistaxis.

Most bleeding originates from the Kiesselbach plexus (anterior portion of the nasal septum); treat by pinching the nose for 5–10 minutes to compress the nasal alae, putting pressure on this area. If bleeding does not stop, try other therapies, including vasoconstrictor nose sprays or cautery of the bleeding site with silver nitrate. If bleeding still persists, refer the patient to an ENT specialist for nasal packing and further monitoring.

Search for other underlying conditions if epistaxis continues to recur or is difficult to correct. In these cases, order coagulation and hematologic studies. Also, fully evaluate the nasal passages, and look for nasal masses or other causes of epistaxis.

NASAL POLYPS

Nasal polyps are benign tumors that form in the nasal passages and are usually due to chronically inflamed nasal mucosa. One of the most common causes in children is cystic fibrosis (CF). With any child < 12 years of age who has nasal polyps, evaluate for CF—even in the absence of other findings for CF. Other predisposing conditions include chronic sinusitis and allergic rhinitis. Note: There is also a condition called aspirin-exacerbated respiratory disease (AERD), which is diagnosed in patients who have (1) asthma and chronic sinusitis with nasal polyposis and (2) acute respiratory tract reactions to ingestion of aspirin and other cyclooxygenase-1 (COX-1) inhibitors.

Children with nasal polyps present with mouth breathing and a nasal-sounding voice. Polyps are sometimes visible using an otoscope or nasal speculum (Image 21-4). However, diagnosis of smaller polyps requires nasal endoscopy or CT scan. The polyps look like gray, grape-like masses found between the nasal turbinates and septum.

Nasal decongestants are not effective in decreasing polyp size. Nasal steroids, however, are quite effective for many polyps, especially in children with CF. Surgically remove polyps if they do not respond to steroids

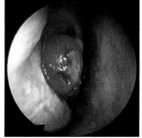

Image 21-4: Nasal polyps

and cause symptomatic obstruction, recurrent sinus infection, or nasal deformity. Nasal polyps can recur after surgery.

NASAL FRACTURES

Nasal fractures are rare in children < 5 years of age. Incidence of fractures increase after this and peak in the later teen years. Nasal fractures usually result from sports and play.

Most of these injuries are minor, but check all patients for associated injury of the cervical spine, orbit, maxilla, and teeth. Order x-rays as needed.

If the patient has diplopia, decreased visual acuity, or any sensory or motor defects, immediately get an ophthalmology or neurology consult.

Do a thorough palpation of the nasal bones and facial bones, especially the maxilla and orbital rim. Check for broken teeth and malocclusion. Palpate the mandible.

Specialized training is needed to perform closed reduction of a nasal fracture. Usually it is done in the ED. Immediate follow-up is not necessary if closed reduction is done—schedule it for 3–5 days later.

NASAL SEPTAL HEMATOMA

Nasal septal hematoma, caused by nasal trauma, can potentially compromise the blood supply to the septum, resulting in septal perforation, saddle-nose deformity, or abscess. Diagnose by physical examination findings of a swollen, fluctuant, and tender septum. Immediately drain the septal hematoma and follow with oral clindamycin, which can be changed if needed once sensitivities are known. Typical pathogens include *S. aureus, H. influenzae,* and *S. pneumoniae.* Close follow-up with an otolaryngologist is needed.

CONGENITAL DISORDERS OF THE MOUTH AND PHARYNX

PREVIEW | REVIEW

- True or false? Cleft palate is typically associated with a genetic disorder.
- How is tongue-tie usually managed?
- What is the most common location for an ectopic thyroid?
- What are some characteristics of a thyroglossal duct cyst?
- What is the significance of thyroglossal duct cysts?

CLEFT LIP AND PALATE

A cleft lip is caused by the incomplete fusion of embryonic structures that surround the primitive oral cavity

OPHTHALMOLOGY / ENT

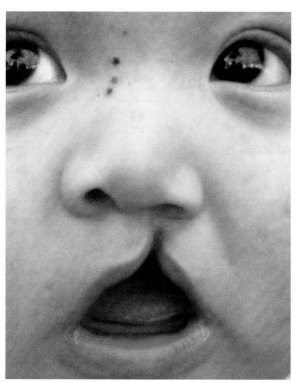

Image 21-5: Cleft lip

([Image 21-5]). It can be unilateral or bilateral. Cleft palate involves the soft palate and sometimes includes the hard palate as well ([Image 21-6]). A cleft palate can have soft tissue and/or bony involvement and often connects to a cleft lip. This disorder can run in families; however, the majority of cases are not associated with any genetic syndrome.

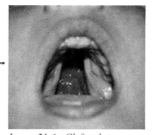

Image 21-6: Cleft palate

Submucosal cleft palate is often not obvious until several years of age. The uvula is usually bifid. Occasionally, a blue line is visible in the midline of the soft palate due to a lack of midline musculature; this is known as a zona pellucida. A notch of the posterior hard palate can sometimes be palpated.

Treatment requires a multifaceted approach and includes craniofacial teams, speech pathologists, and occupational therapists. Address feeding issues first. Lip repair usually occurs later, around 10 weeks of age, and palate repair between 9 and 12 months of age.

LINGUAL ANKYLOGLOSSIA (TONGUE-TIE)

Lingual ankyloglossia ([Image 21-7]) is a common disorder in which the lingual frenulum limits the movement of the anterior tongue tip. Infants have difficulty extending the tongue past the alveolar ridge, which can make breastfeeding difficult. Most newborns can adjust and do well without operative intervention. Speech difficulties, especially with the English language, are rare. However, one very important social activity—licking an ice cream cone—may be impossible for a child to do.

Some infants and children require frenulectomy, which is done in the outpatient office setting by a dentist or oral surgeon.

LINGUAL THYROID

A lingual thyroid is the most common location for an ectopic thyroid (90% of cases). It occurs more frequently in girls than in boys; thyroid tissue fails to descend into the neck from its site of origin in the tongue base. Usually, the lingual thyroid appears as a raised, violaceous mass visible at the base of the tongue. Of those with lingual thyroid, > 70% do not have a normally located thyroid gland, and ~ 30% present with hypothyroidism. The lingual thyroid can enlarge with upper respiratory infections during puberty or during pregnancy, causing dysphagia or airway obstruction. Use thyroid hormone to attempt reduction of the size of the thyroid remnant. Because the ectopic thyroid may be the patient's only thyroid tissue, a thorough evaluation is required prior to surgical evaluation.

THYROGLOSSAL DUCT CYSTS

Thyroglossal duct cysts, often seen with ectopic thyroid glands, are cystic masses in the midline of the neck. The cysts typically move with swallowing or movement of the tongue. Generally, these cysts are asymptomatic unless they become infected. If infection occurs, a cyst can rapidly increase in size and cause respiratory compromise. Surgically remove thyroglossal duct cysts. However, if infection is involved, treat with antibiotics first, and once infection is resolved, perform surgery.

CLEFT TONGUE

Cleft tongue is part of the X-linked **oral-facial-digital syndrome Type I**. It presents with cleft tongue, hypoplasia of the nasal alar cartilages, medial cleft of the upper lip, asymmetric cleft of the palate, digital

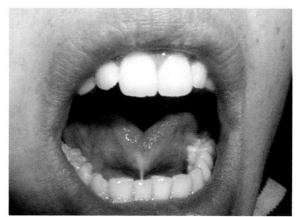

Image 21-7: Lingual ankyloglossia (tongue-tie)

malformations, and mild intellectual disability. About 1/2 of patients have a hamartoma between the lobes of the divided tongue.

Mohr syndrome is an AR disorder with lobulated nodular tongue, conductive hearing loss, cleft lip, high-arched palate, hypoplasia of the mandible, polydactyly, and syndactyly.

TEETH

See Preventive Pediatrics, Book 1, for information on teeth.

INFECTIONS OF THE MOUTH, NOSE, PHARYNX, AND UPPER RESPIRATORY TRACT

PREVIEW | REVIEW

- Does secondhand smoke increase the risk of having a URI?
- Which viruses most typically cause URIs?
- Is routine viral testing appropriate in children with URIs?
- Are antihistamines recommended for URI therapy in children?
- Does green nasal discharge in the first few days of a URI indicate that bacterial sinusitis is likely?
- If a child presents at day 9 of a URI with new fever, worsening nighttime cough, and increased sinus drainage, what do you suspect?
- A child with severe immunosuppression presents with a suspected sinus infection. What is the best way to diagnose the infection and treat appropriately?
- What is Pott's puffy tumor?
- In a diabetic adolescent with uncontrolled serum glucose and the finding of a black eschar in the nose, what infection do you suspect?
- What is the most common cause of acute pharyngitis in children?
- Is the older child who has a sore throat, conjunctivitis, runny nose, and hoarseness likely to have *S. pyogenes*?
- In a 1-year-old with sore throat accompanied by runny nose, hoarseness, cervical lymphadenitis and poor appetite, is *S. pyogenes* the likely etiology?
- Does treatment with penicillin shorten the disease course in acute pharyngitis?
- How soon can a child return to school after being treated for acute pharyngitis?

- In a retropharyngeal abscess, what does the lateral x-ray show?
- How is the voice described in peritonsillar abscess?
- What are the indications for tonsillectomy?
- Does tonsillectomy help with chronic otitis media? Does adenoidectomy help?

THE COMMON COLD

Viral upper respiratory infections (URIs), usually called common colds, are the most frequently occurring illnesses in children. Most children have between 3 and 8 "colds" a year, most often in the fall and winter months. Certain factors increase a child's risk for developing a cold: attending day care, inhaling secondhand smoke (or actively smoking), lower socioeconomic status, and overcrowding.

The majority of URIs are viral. **Rhinoviruses** cause nearly 33% of cases, followed by **coronaviruses**, **adenoviruses**, and **coxsackieviruses**. After each viral infection, the child develops lifelong immunity to that serotype. The problem is that each virus has potentially hundreds of other serotypes to which immunity is not conferred. Some viruses that cause URIs can spread to the lower respiratory tract, most notably the **parainfluenza** viruses, human **metapneumovirus**, and respiratory syncytial virus (**RSV**). Viruses that cause URIs rarely cause acute bloodstream infection or viremia.

URIs clinically present with low-grade fever, malaise, and upper respiratory symptoms of runny nose, cough, and congestion. Viral shedding peaks at 2–7 days after initial symptoms and can last as long as 2 weeks.

Viruses that cause URIs are transmitted in 1 of 3 ways:

1) Large-particle droplets, which can travel through coughing or sneezing and spread to another person
2) Small-particle aerosols, which travel longer distances and can directly enter the alveoli
3) Secretions that get on hands or other surfaces (fomites), which can transmit the virus by direct physical contact (The recipients inoculate themselves by touching their nose or other mucous membranes with their contaminated hands/fingers.)

Do not order laboratory tests in children with URIs unless the diagnosis is unclear or if the history/physical is incompatible with a diagnosis of URI.

Treat symptoms as needed; acetaminophen is used most often. No pharmacologic therapy has shown to reduce the duration of a URI. Additionally, for children < 2 years of age, certain medications (pseudoephedrine, carbinoxamine, and dextromethorphan) have resulted in death. Thus, do not use antitussives or decongestants for relief of cold symptoms in children < 2 years of age; instead use saline nose drops with a gentle bulb syringe to loosen secretions. Also, avoid antihistamines for most children because they decrease cilia movement and can delay mucus clearance. Guaifenesin, a mucolytic agent, helps to thin secretions and improve ciliary function. Topical decongestants can relieve nasal congestion in older children; however, limit the duration (maximum of 5 days) because of the risk of rebound congestion (rhinitis medicamentosa).

The most common complication of a typical cold is AOM. Other complications can include sinusitis, asthma exacerbation, and pneumonia. Thick, "green" nasal discharge by itself in the first few days of a URI does not mean the patient has bacterial sinusitis; it usually signifies an increase in the number of inflammatory cells.

ACUTE SINUSITIS

Almost all cases of sinusitis are viral in origin. The common bacterial causes of acute sinusitis are *S. pneumoniae*, *M. catarrhalis*, and non-typeable *H. influenzae*. With chronic sinusitis (symptoms > 30 days), you sometimes find *S. aureus*, α-hemolytic streptococci, or anaerobes. Risk factors include nasal polyposis, anatomic abnormalities, URIs, allergic rhinitis, asthma, and exposure to cigarette smoke.

Children with sinusitis usually present clinically with cough, nasal discharge, and halitosis. The more "adult-like" presentation is seen in adolescents and includes facial pain, tenderness, and facial edema. In children, the cough is bad in the daytime and worsens with supine position. Nasal discharge can be clear or green. Sore throat is common from postnasal drainage. Fever occurs more typically in older children.

Clinically, viral sinusitis is almost indistinguishable from bacterial sinusitis. One clue is the duration of symptoms. Most URIs improve in 7–10 days. Suspect bacterial sinusitis if sinus symptoms last > 10 days or when sinus symptoms worsen during the course of a resolving URI. Occasionally, severe sinusitis occurs in the initial 7 days of the illness, but these children typically have high fever and headache.

Sinus x-rays and CT scans are usually not reliable. Obtain valid bacterial cultures by aspirating the sinus by direct maxillary antral puncture or endoscopic middle meatal aspiration; however, reserve these only for those who have life-threatening illness, are immunocompromised, or have illness that is unresponsive to empiric therapy.

Treatment is aimed at the most common etiologies. Most centers still recommend amoxicillin; however, many use amoxicillin/clavulanic acid, extended-spectrum macrolides, or 2nd and 3rd generation cephalosporins because of the increasing rate of β-lactamase production by *H. influenzae* and *M. catarrhalis*. High-dose amoxicillin (80–90 mg/kg/day) therapy is often used, due to a dramatic rise in *S. pneumoniae* resistance to amoxicillin and TMP/SMX. Treatment duration is 10–21 days. Saline nose drops and/or saline nasal sprays are recommended.

Decongestants, antihistamines, or nasal corticosteroids are not recommended.

Complications of sinusitis are relatively rare but very important. These include:

- Preseptal (periorbital) cellulitis: mild complication characterized by swelling and erythema of the lids and periorbital area; no proptosis or limitation of eye movement
- Orbital cellulitis: pain with eye movement, conjunctival swelling (chemosis), proptosis, limitation of eye movements (ophthalmoplegia), diplopia, vision loss
- Septic cavernous sinus thrombosis: bilateral ptosis, proptosis, ophthalmoplegia, periorbital edema, headache, change in mental status
- Meningitis: fever, headache, nuchal rigidity, change in mental status
- Osteomyelitis of the frontal bone with a subperiosteal abscess (**Pott's puffy tumor**): forehead or scalp swelling and tenderness, headache, photophobia, fever, vomiting, lethargy
- Epidural abscess: papilledema, focal neurologic signs, headache, lethargy, nausea, vomiting
- Subdural abscess: fever, severe headache, meningeal irritation, progressive neurologic deficits, seizures, signs of increased intracranial pressure (e.g., papilledema, vomiting)
- Brain abscess: headache, neck stiffness, changes in mental status, vomiting, focal neurologic deficits, seizures, deficits in cranial nerves 3 and 6, papilledema

For any of these complications, order a CT scan and hospital admission for IV antibiotics. The exception to treating with IV antibiotics is preseptal cellulitis in a child > 1 year of age who shows no signs of systemic toxicity. This situation can be managed on an outpatient basis as long as close follow-up is ensured. *S. aureus* and streptococci must be covered, so treat with either:

- clindamycin or
- TMP/SMX plus
  - amoxicillin/clavulanic acid or
  - cefdinir.

Unusual organisms can cause sinusitis, depending on underlying conditions. In children with prolonged neutropenia due to chemotherapy, the risk of *Aspergillus* or *Candida* sinusitis is increased. Mucormycosis is another fungal disease that can be life-threatening. It occurs in poorly controlled diabetes and can present as a black eschar on the nasal turbinate. It is dangerous because it frequently "grows backward" into the bone and brain.

CHRONIC SINUSITIS →Staph

Chronic sinusitis is one of the most common chronic disorders in the U.S. It is defined as an inflammatory process affecting the paranasal sinuses that lasts at least 12 weeks despite medical therapy. Often it is a

© 2017 MedStudy

OPHTHALMOLOGY / ENT

continuation of acute sinusitis but can also be caused by mechanical obstruction or allergic edema.

Chronic sinusitis is frequently seen in children with chronic cough. Common symptoms include muco-purulent discharge (anterior and/or posterior nasal), congestion, and facial pain/pressure, in addition to cough. These patients often have received multiple short courses (5–7 days) of oral antibiotics that improve symptoms, but the symptoms return upon discontinuation. A clue to diagnosis is cough that worsens upon lying down and upon awakening due to postnasal drainage of secretions. Halitosis is also frequently noted.

Diagnose with history, physical exam, and objective evidence of inflammation. Diagnosis requires at least 2 of the following findings: cough, mucopurulent drainage, congestion, and facial pain/pressure. Evidence of inflammation can be obtained by CT scan or nasal endoscopy.

Treatment consists of reducing mucosal inflammation, promoting sinus drainage, and clearing infection. This requires a combination of nasal or oral steroids, sinus irrigation, and antibiotic therapy. Most cases of chronic sinusitis are polymicrobial and include anaerobes, so 1st line therapy for most patients is amoxicillin/clavulanate. For penicillin-allergic patients or cases in which methicillin resistance is a concern, clindamycin is used. Antimicrobial therapy for chronic sinusitis is given for a duration of 3–10 weeks. Patients who worsen or fail to show improvement within 1 week of therapy need referral to an otolaryngologist for culture and evaluation.

[handwritten margin note: Staph aureus is most common cause (unlike acute – h flu, moraxella, strep pneumo)]

LUDWIG ANGINA

Ludwig angina is an aggressive, rapidly spreading, bilateral polymicrobial (oral flora including anaerobes) cellulitis of the submandibular and sublingual spaces. It is most often a complication of an infection of the 2nd and/or 3rd mandibular molar teeth. Patients appear very ill, with fever, severe dysphagia, difficulty opening the mouth (trismus), and stiff neck. As the infection progresses, patients often purposely lean forward in an attempt to maximize airway space and improve, at least temporarily, their respiratory status. The cellulitis has a characteristic "brawny" or "woody" texture and is often associated with palpable crepitus within the submandibular and sublingual spaces.

CT is the imaging modality of choice in patients with deep neck–space infections such as Ludwig angina. Monitor closely for evidence of airway compromise such as cyanosis and increasing stridor.

Treat immunocompetent patients with intravenous ampicillin-sulbactam, or a combination of penicillin G plus metronidazole or clindamycin. Patients who do not improve with appropriate antimicrobial therapy, or in whom fluctuance is identified, require surgical intervention and drainage. Additionally, extract any tooth implicated as the source of infection.

ACUTE PHARYNGITIS ("SORE THROAT")

Acute pharyngitis peaks between 4 and 7 years of age; it is rare in children < 1 year of age. The most common cause of acute pharyngitis is viruses. Clinical features suggestive of viral etiology include concurrent conjunctivitis, coryza, cough, hoarseness, anterior stomatitis, discrete ulcerative lesions, viral exanthems, and/or diarrhea. You can culture other bacteria during a viral infection, but rarely, if ever, are they the etiology of the pharyngitis.

S. pyogenes (group A *Streptococcus* [GAS]) is the most frequent bacterial cause, but it makes up only 15% of cases of acute pharyngitis! Other, less common, bacterial causes include:

- *Mycoplasma*
- *Arcanobacterium haemolyticum*
- *Neisseria gonorrhea*—consider in the case of sexually active adolescents
- *Corynebacterium diphtheriae* (discussed in Infectious Disease, Book 4)

Streptococcal pharyngitis frequently begins with non-specific complaints of headache, abdominal pain, or vomiting. Fever is usually quite high. After these initial symptoms, patients develop a sore throat; they can also have exudates, pharyngeal redness, enlarged tonsils, and petechiae of the soft palate. Tender, enlarged anterior cervical lymph nodes are common. Fever can last 1–4 days.

The most helpful clues to *S. pyogenes* infection are physical examination findings of diffuse erythema of the tonsils and tonsillar pillars, petechiae of the soft palate, and absence of URI symptoms. In patients < 2 years of age, be familiar with this clinical presentation: coryza with postnasal discharge, fever (can last up to 8 weeks), pharyngitis, poor appetite, and tender cervical lymphadenitis. This is called **streptococcosis** and is a persistent illness in these younger children.

Diagnose with a rapid detection method (e.g., optical immunoassay, chemiluminescent DNA probes). The AAP recommends following up with a throat culture if the rapid test is negative.

Be most concerned with the 2 complications of *S. pyogenes* infection:

1) Rheumatic fever, which can be prevented if antibiotic treatment is given within 9 days after onset of symptoms. (Remember that rheumatic fever occurs only after pharyngitis—not skin infections!) See Cardiology, Book 3.

2) Poststreptococcal glomerulonephritis can occur regardless of therapy and regardless of source of primary infection (i.e., pharynx or skin).

Treat with penicillin. Children defervesce within 24 hours of antibiotic initiation, and penicillin shortens the disease course by an average of 1.5 days. Amoxicillin 1×/day (750 mg × 10 days) has also been shown to be effective. Use erythromycin, clindamycin, or azithromycin for those allergic to penicillin.

A common question: How soon can children go back to school? In other words, when are they no longer infectious? The answer is: A child is considered noninfectious after completing 24 hours of antibiotic therapy and can return to school or day care at that point.

Recurrence is possible and can be retreated with the same antimicrobial agent, an alternative oral drug, or an IM dose of penicillin G (especially if nonadherence to oral therapy is likely). The 2015 Red Book does not recommend any 1 of these agents as more appropriate than the other in this setting.

RETROPHARYNGEAL ABSCESS

Retropharyngeal abscess can occur as a complication in children with bacterial pharyngitis, or as an extension from a wound infection following a penetrating injury (e.g., pencil injury to the posterior pharynx). The most typical causes are GAS, oral anaerobes (most commonly *Fusobacterium* or *Prevotella*), and *S. aureus.*

Toddlers and children (most typically affected are 2–4 years of age) present with an abrupt onset of high fever and difficulty swallowing. This occurs during the acute pharyngitis phase, and they develop the following symptoms in the midst of the infection: refusal to eat, severe throat pain, neck stiffness, hyperextension of the head, and gurgling respirations. Drooling soon develops. Stridor can also occur and simulate croup. Patients might not want to open their mouths because of pain (trismus); however, if they do, an erythematous "bulge" is sometimes visible in the posterior pharyngeal wall.

In cases with no respiratory distress and where suspicion is low, a lateral x-ray of the neck is the initial study and can show a widened retropharyngeal space with anterior displacement of the airway; in addition, the retropharyngeal soft tissue is > 50% of the width of the adjacent vertebral body. However, false positives are common. In high-suspicion cases, a CT with contrast is the preferred method. If the patient is in moderate-to-severe respiratory distress, forego the CT and evaluate the patient in the operating room with a physician present who is experienced in airway management.

A retropharyngeal abscess is a medical emergency. Without prompt treatment, pus can extend into fascial planes or rupture into the pharynx, which can lead to aspiration.

In the prefluctuant phase, prevent suppuration by treating with nafcillin for *S. aureus* and clindamycin for anaerobic coverage. Single-agent therapy with ampicillin-sulbactam is an alternative. Admit to the hospital and monitor closely. Continue IV antibiotic therapy until the patient is afebrile and clinically improved, and then complete therapy with oral amoxicillin/clavulanate or clindamycin to provide a total of 14 days of therapy. If the abscess is fluctuant, drainage is necessary.

PERITONSILLAR ABSCESS

Peritonsillar abscesses (PTAs) are often polymicrobial. The predominant bacterial species are GAS, *S. aureus* (including methicillin-resistant *S. aureus* [MRSA]), and respiratory anaerobes (including *Fusobacterium, Prevotella,* and *Veillonella* species). The abscess occurs either with, or following, an acute pharyngotonsillitis. Fever (as high as 105.0° F [40.5° C]) can abate for several days and then recur or be continuous. The patient, often an adolescent, presents with severe pain and trismus and refuses to speak or swallow. Many describe the patient as having a "hot potato" voice. The uvula is often displaced to the side opposite the swelling (typically unilateral). The differential diagnosis includes retropharyngeal abscess, which occurs in younger children and lacks peritonsillar and unilateral findings.

Use CT scan with IV contrast to distinguish peritonsillar abscess from peritonsillar cellulitis and to evaluate for the spread of infection to contiguous deep neck spaces. Monitor carefully during transportation and scanning; sedation and positioning can exacerbate mild airway distress. Do not order CT scanning in children with moderate-to-severe respiratory distress, particularly when sedation is necessary; evaluate these children in the operating room, where an artificial airway can be established if needed.

Management is dependent on the child's age and cooperativeness. For most patients without a history of sore throat or recurrent pharyngitis, simple incision and drainage is best done in the operating room. If there is a history of previous recurrent pharyngitis or a prior PTA, then a tonsillectomy is recommended. Treat with the same antibiotics as used for retropharyngeal abscess. (See Retropharyngeal Abscess, above.) Surgery can be postponed for 12–24 hours pending response to antibiotics if there is no evidence of airway compromise, septicemia, severe trismus, or other complications. For patients < 7 years of age, antibiotic therapy alone may be effective if they have had fewer episodes of tonsillitis (i.e., < 3/year) and have smaller abscesses (i.e., approximately 9 cm² or less).

CHRONIC TONSILLITIS

Indications for tonsillectomy:

- Recurrent pharyngitis (7 episodes in the past year, 5 in each of the last 2 years, or 3 in each of the past 3 years)
- Marked/Severe adenotonsillar hypertrophy (exclude tumor)
- Severe sleep apnea (Adenotonsillectomy is the 1st line treatment in children with obstructive sleep apnea.)

Tonsillectomy does not help prevent or treat acute or chronic sinusitis or chronic otitis media. Tonsillectomy does not help prevent URIs! Wait 2–3 weeks after any uncomplicated infection has resolved before performing a tonsillectomy. Assess for risk factors of persistent sleep

OPHTHALMOLOGY / ENT

apnea, and consider overnight postoperative observation for cases with significant sleep-related hypoxemia.

CHRONIC ADENOIDAL HYPERTROPHY

Indications for adenoidectomy:

- Persistent mouth breathing
- Repeated or chronic OME (otitis media with effusion)
- Hyponasal speech
- Adenoid facies
- Persistent or recurrent nasopharyngitis when it seems to be temporally related to hypertrophied adenoid tissue

Do not perform a tonsillectomy for these problems.

NECK

PREVIEW | REVIEW

- What is the most common cause of acute bilateral lymphadenopathy?
- What are some causes of hoarseness in children?
- Which findings indicate possible malignancy when working up a neck mass?

CERVICAL LYMPHADENOPATHY

Cervical lymphadenopathy (LA) is very common in children. LA is defined as a cervical node > 1 cm. If the swelling is due to inflammation rather than infection, the condition is called lymphadenitis. While usually representing a self-limited viral or bacterial infection, it is sometimes a sign of a more serious disease process.

The most common lymph nodes involved are the submandibular and deep cervical nodes.

Viral lymphadenitis, which does not require treatment, typically causes acute bilateral LA. Viral causes of cervical lymphadenopathy include URI, cytomegalovirus (CMV), Epstein-Barr virus (EBV), rubeola, varicella-zoster virus, coxsackievirus, herpes simplex virus, HIV, and Kawasaki disease.

Bacterial causes of lymphadenopathy include pharyngitis with GAS (*S. pyogenes*), *S. aureus*, *M. pneumoniae*, *A. haemolyticum*, diphtheria, tuberculosis, and cat scratch fever. In very young infants, also consider *Streptococcus agalactiae* (Group B *Streptococcus* [GBS]). Remember that GBS is a common cause of postpartum infections and the most common cause of neonatal sepsis.

Acute unilateral disease most commonly results from *S. pyogenes* or *S. aureus* infection and generally responds to oral antibiotics, including amoxicillin/

clavulanate or clindamycin. Unilateral subacute/chronic LA is most typically caused by nontuberculous mycobacteria or *Bartonella henselae* (cat scratch fever), whereas bilateral subacute/chronic disease is usually the result of EBV or CMV.

More than 25% of malignant tumors in children occur in the head and neck with the cervical lymph nodes being the most common site. The most common **malignant** causes of cervical lymphadenopathy are:

- Neuroblastoma
- Leukemia
- Rhabdomyosarcoma
- Non-Hodgkin lymphoma

Other causes of lymphadenopathy:

- Juvenile rheumatoid arthritis
- Collagen vascular diseases
- Drugs
- Serum sickness
- Post-vaccination

Initial workup of cervical lymphadenitis includes CBC with differential, tuberculin skin testing, and serologic testing for *B. henselae*, CMV, EBV, and HIV. If the above tests do not identify the etiology, arrange excisional biopsy to rule out malignancy or to evaluate for nontuberculous mycobacteria.

LARYNGITIS / HOARSENESS

Hoarseness in children is typically benign and can be caused by nodules, polyps, infection, papillomas, hypothyroidism, foreign body, congenital anomalies, and vocal fold granulomas (from gastroesophageal reflux disease [GERD], intubation, and vocal cord misuse). Radiologic evaluation is usually not necessary unless a foreign body or mass is suspected. Refer to otolaryngologist if hoarseness lasts > 2 weeks.

NECK MASS

A neck mass can be congenital, inflammatory, or malignant:

- Mumps (parotid glands cross angle of jaw)
- Thyroglossal cyst (midline between hyoid bone and suprasternal notch; moves with swallowing)
- Branchial cleft cyst (fluctuant mass at lower anterior sternocleidomastoid muscle)
- Sternomastoid tumor
- Cervical ribs (extra rib arising from C7; occurrence of 1:200 births)
- Lymphatic malformation (previously cystic hygroma; multilobular cyst filled with lymph; transilluminates well)
- Hemangioma (red or bluish vascular malformation)

- Laryngocele (laryngeal saccule is abnormally large, expanding either internally with possible respiratory obstruction or externally forming an air sac on anterior of larynx
- Dermoid cyst (solid and cystic midline cyst; poor transillumination)
- Thyroid mass

A thyroglossal duct cyst is a remnant of the thyroglossal tract left during development and presents as a midline mass, commonly during childhood, when the cyst becomes infected. Diagnose with ultrasound or CT scan. Manage by treating the infection followed by surgical removal of the cyst.

A branchial cleft cyst is also an embryonic epithelial remnant. It usually presents in childhood or young adulthood when the cyst becomes infected during an upper respiratory illness. It presents as a solitary mass anterior to the sternocleidomastoid muscle. Diagnosis and treatment are the same as with thyroglossal duct cysts.

Clues on physical exam suggestive of a malignancy include hard, irregular, firm, immobile lymph nodes; nodes > 2 cm; and supraclavicular location. Investigate these findings further with lab work, ultrasound, CT scan, and fine needle biopsy. Treatment is dependent on the results.

Evaluate a thyroid mass with thyroid stimulating hormone (TSH) and ultrasound testing. If the TSH is low, order thyroid scintigraphy. If the TSH is normal or elevated, arrange needle biopsy. If biopsy confirms cancer, treatment is thyroidectomy followed by radioactive iodine to destroy any remaining thyroid or cancer cells. Thyroid hormone replacement therapy is required. Sometimes external radiation is also used.

OBSTRUCTIVE SLEEP APNEA

PREVIEW | REVIEW

- What are possible long-term complications of untreated OSA?
- What are some risk factors for OSA?
- How is OSA diagnosed?

Obstructive sleep apnea (OSA) is characterized clinically by repeated episodes of prolonged upper airway obstruction during sleep despite continued or increased respiratory effort, resulting in complete or partial cessation of airflow and disrupted sleep.

The prevalence of OSA, documented by overnight sleep studies, is 1–3%. Increased weight, anatomic abnormalities, and poor pharyngeal or laryngeal tone increases the risk of OSA. If left untreated, long-term sequelae of this condition, with frequent episodes of intermittent hypoxia and sleep arousals, include hypertension, pulmonary hypertension, arrhythmias, and heart failure.

Anatomic, physiologic, and metabolic abnormalities that can predispose to OSA:

- Nasal (e.g., choanal stenosis/atresia, deviated septum, rhinitis, polyps)
- Oropharyngeal (e.g., adenotonsillar enlargement, macroglossia, cleft palate repair, masses)
- Craniofacial (e.g., micrognathia, trisomy 21, Pierre Robin sequence, achondroplasia)
- Neuromuscular conditions (e.g., muscular dystrophies, hypotonic cerebral palsy, other hypotonics)
- Metabolic (e.g., obesity, hypothyroidism)

Nocturnal symptoms of OSA:

- Loud, frequent, and disruptive snoring
- Breathing pauses
- Choking or gasping arousals
- Restless sleep
- Nocturnal diaphoresis
- Partial arousal parasomnias (e.g., sleepwalking, night terrors)

Daytime symptoms of OSA:

- Daytime sleepiness and drowsiness (but much less common in children than adults)
- Mouth breathing/dry mouth
- Chronic nasal congestion or rhinorrhea
- Hyponasal speech
- Morning headaches
- Poor appetite
- Difficulty with morning awakening
- Poor academic performance

Mood changes of OSA:

- Irritability
- Mood instability
- Frustration
- Depression
- Anxiety

Signs and symptoms often overlap with diagnostic criteria for attention-deficit/hyperactivity disorder. (See Behavioral Medicine and Substance Abuse, Book 1.)

The gold standard for diagnosis is an overnight polysomnogram. In children, there is no standard treatment. In those with adenotonsillar hypertrophy, adenotonsillectomy is generally the 1st line therapy. Obesity, hypotonia, and craniofacial anomalies increase perioperative and postoperative risks; encourage weight loss in obese individuals. Other interventions include continuous or bilevel positive airway pressure (CPAP or BiPAP), topical nasal steroids, short-term use of topical decongestants, antihistamines, and, when indicated, repair of craniofacial anomalies.

THE MEDSTUDY HUB: YOUR GUIDELINES AND REVIEW ARTICLES RESOURCE

For both the review articles and current Pediatrics practice guidelines, visit the MedStudy Hub at

medstudy.com/hub

The Hub contains the only online consolidated list of all Pediatrics guidelines! Guidelines on the Hub are continually updated and linked to the published source. MedStudy maintains the Hub as a free online resource, available to all physicians.

MedStudy

GENETICS

SECTION EDITOR

Pamela Trapane, MD
Clinical Professor, Stead Family Department
 of Pediatrics
Program Director, Medical Genetics
 Residency Program
Medical Director, Division of Medical Genetics
University of Iowa Hospitals and Clinics
The Sahai Family Professor of Medical
 Education, Carver College of Medicine
Iowa City, IA

MEDICAL EDITOR

Jonathan S. Caudill, MD
Oxford, MS

REVIEWER

Reem Saadeh-Haddad, MD
Assistant Professor
Clinical Geneticist
Department of Pediatrics
MedStar Georgetown University Hospital
Washington, DC

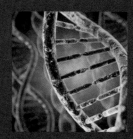

Table of Contents

GENETICS

GUIDELINES AND REVIEW ARTICLES AVAILABLE
ON THE MEDSTUDY HUB AT: medstudy.com/hub

KEY DEFINITIONS IN GENETIC DISORDERS

PREVIEW | REVIEW

- Define the following terms: congenital, hereditary, familial, genotype, phenotype, variable expressivity, mosaicism, heterozygous, homozygous, autosome, and syndrome.

At first glance, you might think that congenital, hereditary, and familial all mean the same thing. But they don't. For example: Trisomy 21, infection with rubella, and amniotic bands are all congenital conditions. **Congenital** refers to a condition or anomaly present at birth. Of the three, though, only trisomy 21 is a genetic condition. **Hereditary** refers to conditions that are genetically transmitted from parent to offspring. All hereditary conditions are genetic, but some individuals with genetic disorders are a result of a new mutation in the family and are unable to reproduce, thus not all genetic conditions are hereditary. **Familial** refers to conditions that "cluster" in families and can include genetic as well as nongenetic (e.g., attention-deficit/hyperactivity disorder [ADHD], high blood pressure) conditions. All hereditary conditions are familial, but not all genetic conditions are familial. As examples: achondroplasia is congenital, hereditary, and familial. Breast cancer is not congenital, can be familial, and a small portion is hereditary due to mutations in *BRCA1* or *BRCA2*. Trisomy 21 is congenital and, in the majority of cases, not hereditary and not familial because the individual is usually the first case in the family and does not reproduce. (Keep in mind that ~ 5% of trisomy 21 cases are due to unbalanced translocations, which can be hereditary and familial if passed down to more than one individual.) A **balanced translocation** occurs with an even exchange of material, resulting in no extra or missing genetic information (and ideally full functionality). An **unbalanced translocation** occurs when there is unequal exchange of chromosome material, resulting in extra or missing genes.

Genotype refers to the genetic constitution or different forms of a gene (alleles) at a given locus on a chromosome. Although each individual has only 2 alleles, there may be more gene variants in the population. **Phenotype** refers to observed expression (physical, biochemical, or physiological findings) of the genotype or gene mutation. Genotype may or may not be apparent in an individual's phenotype.

Penetrance is the ability of a known disease-causing genotype to exhibit the disease phenotype. Reduced or incomplete penetrance means that some people with the disease-causing genotype do not have evidence of the disease. A common example is retinoblastoma. About 10% of people who have an autosomal dominant (AD) retinoblastoma-causing mutation do not actually develop retinoblastoma. Thus, the penetrance for this condition is 90%.

Variable expressivity is when individuals have the same genetic condition (even the exact same genotype) but have varying degrees of the phenotype. For example, Treacher-Collins syndrome is an AD, craniofacial malformation syndrome. Within the same family, some individuals with the Treacher-Collins gene have cleft palate, whereas others with the exact same mutation do not.

In **genomic imprinting**, expression of the gene depends on whether the gene was inherited from the mother or father. Imprinting turns off genes. Thus, if a gene is paternally imprinted, the allele derived from the father is inactive and only the maternally derived allele is expressed. If a gene is maternally imprinted, only the paternal allele is expressed. Examples: Prader-Willi syndrome and Angelman syndrome.

Pleiotropic refers to genes that produce many effects. An example is Marfan syndrome, which can affect the eyes, cardiovascular system, and skeletal system.

Mosaicism is the presence of ≥ 2 genetically different sets of cells in the same person caused by an error in mitosis. Examples: majority of Turner syndrome cases.

Heterozygous refers to 2 different alleles at a gene locus on a pair of homologous chromosomes, whereas **homozygous** refers to identical alleles at a particular gene locus. A **mutation** is the term used to describe a change in the DNA code.

Autosome refers to all chromosomes except the X and Y chromosomes. There are 22 autosomes, chromosome numbers 1–22, and 2 sex chromosomes, X and Y. The majority of the population has a total of 46 chromosomes: 2 copies of each autosome and either XX (female) or XY (male) to determine the sex of the person.

Nondisjunction occurs when the homologous chromosomes or chromatids fail to separate, resulting in **aneuploidy**—an abnormal number of chromosomes in the daughter cells.

In clinical genetics terminology, an **anomaly** is a structural birth defect or congenital malformation. Multiple anomalies can form recognized patterns of malformation known as complex, syndrome, association, or sequence:

- **Complex**: anomalies of several different structures that are near each other during embryonic development (developmental field); example: limb-body wall complex
- **Syndrome**: a recognizable pattern of structural defects, due to a known single genetic etiology, with a predictable natural history that remains relatively consistent across unrelated patients; examples: Cornelia de Lange syndrome, Williams syndrome
- **Association**: anomalies seen together that do not have a known single genetic or developmental etiology; example: **VACTERL** association (**v**ertebral defects, **a**nal atresia, **c**ardiac defects, **t**racheoesophageal fistula, **r**enal anomalies, **l**imb abnormalities)

GENETICS

• **Sequence**: a pattern of multiple anomalies caused by a single identifiable event in development; example: Pierre Robin sequence

CHROMOSOMAL DEFECTS

PREVIEW | REVIEW

- What is the genetic abnormality in trisomy 21?

- What is considered to be the etiology of trisomy 21?

- What is the only factor shown to increase the risk of trisomy 21?

- Which screening tests indicate an increased risk of trisomy 21?

- What are some of the classic physical findings in children with trisomy 21?

- What are the common congenital heart defects found in a child with trisomy 21?

- Which GI defects are associated with trisomy 21?

- Which glandular disorder should you annually screen for in children/adults with trisomy 21?

- A 30-year-old mother has a child with trisomy 21 with three complete copies of chromosome 21. What is her risk of having another child with trisomy 21?

- Is trisomy 18 more common in boys or girls?

- What are the classic features of a child with trisomy 18?

- What are the classic features of a child with trisomy 13?

- Describe a boy with Klinefelter syndrome.

- Describe a girl with Turner syndrome.

- What are the classic features of a child with 4p deletion?

- What are the classic features of a child with 5p deletion?

- What is a classic finding in 18q deletion?

- Which deletion syndrome is associated with trigonocephaly?

- Describe a child with Angelman syndrome, and explain the genetic mechanisms that caused it.

- Describe a child with Prader-Willi syndrome, and explain the genetic mechanisms that caused it.

- Describe a child with Williams syndrome.

- What characterizes WAGR syndrome?

- Describe the classic findings in Alagille syndrome. What are the most common cardiac abnormalities?

- List the classic findings in 22q11.2 deletion syndrome.

AUTOSOMAL TRISOMY SYNDROME

Trisomy 21 (Down Syndrome)

Incidence / Screening

Trisomy 21 is the most common autosomal chromosome trisomy in humans, occurring in 1/800 live births. The incidence at conception is more than 2× the incidence at birth because > 50% of those with trisomy 21 at conception spontaneously abort during early pregnancy. Approximately 95% of those with Down syndrome have 3 copies of the whole chromosome 21 (Figure 22-1); around 3–4% have only part of the long arm due to translocations with chromosomes 13, 14, or 15; and the remaining 1–2% have mosaicism.

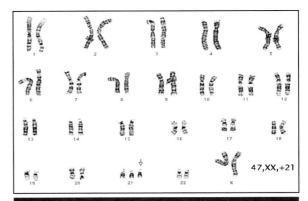

47,XX,+21

Figure 22-1: Trisomy 21 Karyotype

Trisomy 21 is caused by the "extra" copy of chromosome 21, thought to be due to nondisjunction during meiosis. The only factor shown to increase the risk of having a child with Down syndrome from nondisjunction is increasing maternal age (especially mothers ≥ 35 years of age). No environmental factors have been implicated.

Prenatal screening (e.g., quad screen [quadruple marker test]) is commonly performed in pregnant women during the second trimester to assess for Down syndrome risk. A concerning maternal serum screen shows low maternal serum α-fetoprotein, low unconjugated estriol, elevated hCG, and elevated inhibin levels.

Many providers add early ultrasound with measurement of the baby's nuchal translucency (neck thickness) and serum markers to the prenatal screening to improve sensitivity and specificity.

DNA-based maternal blood screening using free fetal DNA (the baby's DNA!) found in the mother's blood is available as well. It has much higher sensitivity and specificity than the above screening methods, but it is not perfect. Use of this technology is rapidly increasing and will likely replace serum marker screening entirely in the future.

Presentation

Down syndrome presents with a classic phenotypic pattern, but, if taken singly, many of the findings are minor anomalies or nonspecific. (For example, if you have a single transverse palmar crease, as 10% of you do, that doesn't mean you have Down syndrome.) You need the "whole picture" to make an accurate diagnosis.

Typical features:

- Hypotonia
- Poor Moro reflex
- Intellectual disability
- Brachydactyly: short, broad fingers and toes (Especially note the broad space between the 1st and 2nd toes! See Image 22-1.)
- Upslanted palpebral fissures
- Flat midface
- Full cheeks
- Protruding tongue
- Epicanthal folds
- Single transverse palmar crease (Image 22-2)

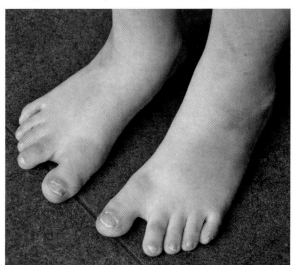

Image 22-1: Trisomy 21, brachydactyly and broad space between 1st and 2nd toes

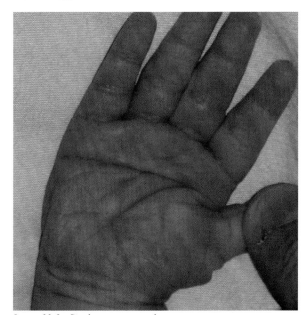

Image 22-2: Single transverse palmar crease

- Speckled irises (Brushfield spots)
- High-arched palate
- Hypoplasia of the middle phalanx of the 5th finger/clinodactyly

Heart Defects

Heart defects are common in Down syndrome, occurring in nearly 50% of patients. Atrioventricular (AV) canal defects account for 1/3 of these, and 1/3 are ventricular septal defects (VSDs). The other 1/3 have atrial septal defects (ASDs) of the secundum variety and tetralogy of Fallot. Remember that AV canal defects frequently do not have an associated murmur. Because ~ 50% of children with Down syndrome have congenital heart defects, echocardiogram is mandatory for all children with suspected Down syndrome.

GI Defects

Duodenal atresia and Hirschsprung disease occur in 5–10% of infants with Down syndrome. Look for the classic double-bubble sign (Image 22-3), indicating duodenal atresia on abdominal x-rays (see Gastroenterology, Book 2).

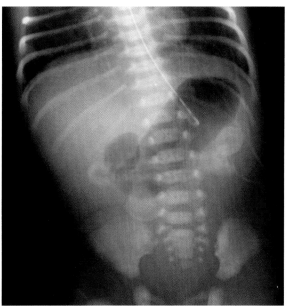

Image 22-3: Double-bubble sign in duodenal atresia

Ocular Problems

Congenital cataracts occur in about 5% of newborns with Down syndrome, but other problems, such as strabismus and refractive errors, increase with age; therefore, ensure that careful, routine ophthalmologic evaluations take place.

Developmental Disorders

Children with Down syndrome have developmental delay with mean IQ scores ranging from 50–70; however, social performance is beyond that expected for the

GENETICS

mental age. Almost all children learn to walk and communicate, and most progress at a steady but slower pace than usual. Encourage early intervention programs to accelerate milestones in the younger years.

Other Problems of Down Syndrome in Childhood

Other problems in childhood can include:

- Hypothyroidism
- Atlantoaxial instability
- Leukemia (particularly acute lymphocytic leukemia)

ALL

Check thyroid function studies at birth (included on newborn screen); at 3, 6, and 12 months; and then annually.

A unique condition that can occur in patients with Down syndrome is **transient myeloproliferative disorder** (a.k.a. transient leukemia). This type of leukemia occurs in up to 10% of all infants with trisomy 21 and occurs within the first 3 months of life. A mutation in the *GATA 1* gene is the cause. Transient myeloproliferative disorder is characterized by the presence of blast cells (most commonly megakaryoblasts) in the peripheral blood, which can number as high as 200,000/μL. In contrast to acute megakaryoblastic leukemia, the percentage of blasts in patients with transient myeloproliferative disorder is lower in bone marrow than in peripheral blood. Bone marrow cytogenetic analysis is negative for all clonal abnormalities other than trisomy 21.

Most patients are asymptomatic with the exception of vesiculopustular skin lesions, which contain cells similar to blast cells. Patients usually undergo spontaneous resolution within the first 3 months of life as the numbers of blast cells gradually decrease. A small number of patients, especially those born prematurely, can experience severe complications, including hepatic fibrosis, generalized edema, multiple effusions, and cardiopulmonary failure. In these patients, treatment with chemotherapy is warranted. Closely monitor patients with a history of transient myeloproliferative disorder as they grow older because there is a 10- to 20-fold increased risk of developing acute myeloid leukemia.

Problems of Older Patients with Down Syndrome

Patients with Down syndrome can develop problems later in life—in their 3rd, 4th, or 5th decades. However, because many pediatricians remain the primary care physician for some patients with Down syndrome even after they advance to adulthood, remember to vigilantly monitor for these long-term complications:

- Type 2 diabetes
- Thyroid disorders (both hypo- and hyperthyroidism)
- Atlantoaxial subluxation (perform screening x-rays prior to sports participation)
- Cataracts
- Leukemia
- Seizures
- Cognitive dysfunction (during the patient's 40s)
- Dementia or early-onset Alzheimer disease

Health Supervision Guidelines

The AAP publishes health supervision guidelines with anticipatory guidance for children with Down syndrome. These include:

- All routine immunizations
- Cardiac evaluation with echocardiogram in the newborn period
- Ophthalmologic evaluation before 6 months of age
- Hearing evaluation during newborn screening and again by 6 months of age
- Thyroid studies: newborn screening for hypothyroidism, then annual T_4 and TSH throughout childhood and adulthood
- Vision screening at 4 years of age

Future Risk of Sibling with Down Syndrome

If the child has 3 complete copies of chromosome 21 and the mother is < 35 years of age, her risk of having another child with trisomy 21 is 1%. If the mother is > 35 years of age, the risk is similar to the age-specific risk. (Remember: Risk for having a child with Down syndrome increases with increasing age of the mother.)

If the child with trisomy 21 has Down syndrome due to an unbalanced translocation, the future risk depends on whether one of the parents has an abnormal chromosome. For example, if a parent has a 21:21 translocation, the risk of having an offspring with Down syndrome is 100%. Besides the 21:21 translocation, if the father has a balanced translocation between 21 and another chromosome, the recurrence risk is 1–2%; if the mother has a balanced translocation, the recurrence risk is 10–15%. Although trisomy 21 is most commonly a sporadic condition (95%), it is hereditary when due to an unbalanced translocation inherited from the parent. Obtain a karyotype to determine the recurrence risk.

Trisomy 18 (Edwards Syndrome)

Trisomy 18 is the 2nd most common autosomal trisomy and occurs in about 1/6,000 live births, with a much higher incidence of stillbirths. The ratio of girls to boys born with Edwards syndrome is 4:1.

The characteristic findings of trisomy 18 are:

- Intrauterine growth restriction
- Intellectual disability
- High forehead
- Microcephaly
- Small face and mouth
- Rocker bottom feet (Image 22-4)
- Overlapping fingers (fingers 2 and 5 over 3 and 4) and clenched fist (Image 22-4)
- Short sternum
- Hypoplastic nails
- Structural heart defects (90%): most often a VSD with multiple dysplastic valves

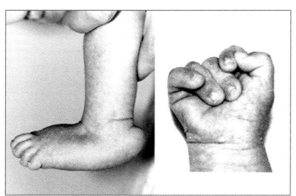

Image 22-4: Trisomy 18, rocker bottom feet and clenched fist

The risk of having an offspring with trisomy 18 increases as maternal age increases (especially mothers ≥ 35 years old). Statistics vary, but about 80% of cases are due to 3 copies of chromosome 18, with the other 20% due to mosaicism or partial trisomy of the long arm of 18. The risk of recurrence for future pregnancies is < 1% (less than for full trisomy 21 cases) for mothers < 35 years of age; it is age specific for older mothers. About 50% of affected children die in the 1st week of life, with another 40% dying by 1 year of age. Most die because of central apnea. Children with trisomy 18 do not learn to walk or develop language skills. Those who survive past 1 year of age typically function at the level of a 6- to 12-month-old, although some develop skills up to a 2-year-old level.

Trisomy 13 (Patau Syndrome)

Trisomy 13 is the 3rd most common autosomal trisomy in humans and occurs in about 1/20,000 to 1/25,000 live births. 80% of children with trisomy 13 have 3 complete copies (i.e., meiotic nondisjunction) and the remaining have 3 copies of the long arm of 13 due to an unbalanced translocation. Very few trisomy 13 children are mosaic. Recurrence risk for trisomy 13 is presumed to be very low and similar to trisomy 18: < 1% for a mother < 35 years of age and age specific for older mothers.

Common clinical findings in trisomy 13 include (think midline defects!):

• Orofacial cleft (often midline cleft lip; Image 22-5)
• Microphthalmia
• Postaxial polydactyly of the limbs (Image 22-6)
• Holoprosencephaly (cyclopia to premaxillary agenesis)
• Heart malformations (80%)
• Hypoplastic or absent ribs
• Genital anomalies
• Abdominal wall defects
• Aplasia cutis congenita
• Rocker-bottom feet
• Clenched hands

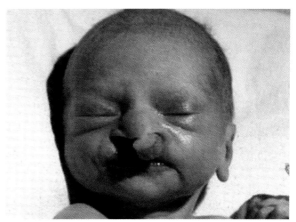

Image 22-5: Trisomy 13, cleft lip

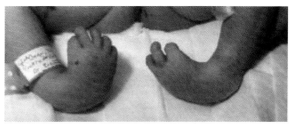

Image 22-6: Trisomy 13, postaxial polydactyly

Survival is poor, with a median survival of 2.5 days. About 70% will die in the first three months of life, and 95% will die by 3 years of age. Survivors have severe intellectual disability, seizures, and failure to thrive (FTT), and they rarely live past 10 years of age.

SEX CHROMOSOME SYNDROMES

Incidence

About 1/500 neonates has an abnormality of either the X or the Y chromosome. 80% of this group is made up of 47,XXY (Klinefelter syndrome); 47,XYY; and 47,XXX. 45,X (Turner syndrome) is much less common, occurring in only ~ 1/2,500 to 1/5,000 neonate females.

47,XXY (Klinefelter Syndrome)

47,XXY (Klinefelter syndrome) presents with a male phenotype and an extra X chromosome (Figure 22-2 on page 22-6).

Most cases are not associated with advanced maternal age. Meiotic nondisjunction is a common cause, with the extra X chromosome mostly of maternal origin. Typically, these patients are quite tall with gynecomastia, and secondary sex development is delayed. They almost always have azoospermia and small testes, and are infertile. Klinefelter syndrome is discussed in more detail in Endocrinology, Book 3.

Other Extra X Chromosome Syndromes

There are many other syndromes in which ≥ 1 extra X chromosome occurs: 47,XXX; 48,XXXX; 49,XXXXX;

GENETICS

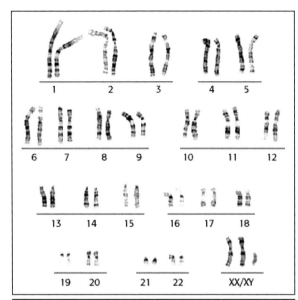

Figure 22-2: Klinefelter Syndrome (47,XXY) Karyotype

48,XXXY; and 49,XXXXY. Frequently, they are mosaic with a "normal" 46,XX and an abnormal cell line (e.g., 46,XX/47,XXX). As the number of X chromosomes increases, the degree of phenotypic abnormality increases; specifically, the neurologic problems are worse.

47,XYY Male

47,XYY occurs in about 1/1,000 live births. This is no longer considered a true syndrome. XYY males are generally taller than average, but otherwise these males are not different from the general population. Earlier studies that suggested a greater number of behavior problems in this population are now considered flawed.

45,X (Turner Syndrome)

Turner syndrome is discussed in detail in Endocrinology, Book 3. See Image 22-7 and Figure 22-3.

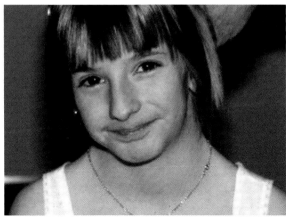

Image 22-7: Turner syndrome (45,X)

These girls are phenotypically female and have short stature and ovarian failure/gonadal dysgenesis, with subsequent lack of secondary sexual development.

Other chromosome abnormalities found in patients with Turner syndrome include:

- Xp deletion, Xq deletion, ring X (r(X))
- 46,X,i(Xq) (i(Xq) is a long arm isochromosome; i.e., it is an abnormal X chromosome resulting from the duplication of the long arm and loss of the short arm)
- Mosaics: 45,X/46,XX; 45,X/46,X,i(Xq); 45,X/46,XY

Also remember that about 50% of these girls have cardiovascular anomalies, including bicuspid aortic valves, and 15–20% have coarctation of the aorta. Other findings:

- At birth: broad, webbed neck (from fetal cystic hygroma), shieldlike chest, posteriorly rotated ears, lymphedema of the hands and feet, short 4th metacarpals, and cubitus valgus
- In childhood or adulthood: chronic autoimmune thyroiditis (a.k.a. Hashimoto disease), alopecia, carbohydrate intolerance, vitiligo, and gastrointestinal disorders

About 5–10% have some Y chromosome material in all or some cells, which puts them at risk for gonadoblastoma. These patients require removal of internal streak gonads.

Diagnosis is made by karyotype analysis. 99% of fetuses with Turner syndrome spontaneously abort.

LARGE DELETION SYNDROMES
Overview

Deletions occur when a piece of chromosome is missing. It can occur as a simple "stand-alone" deletion or as a deletion with duplication of another chromosome segment. Most deletion syndromes present as intellectual disability with associated phenotypic anomalies. If the

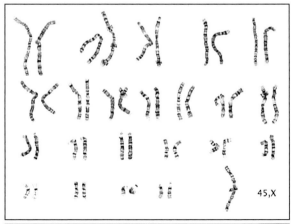

Figure 22-3: Turner Syndrome (45,X) Karyotype

Short arm = p   long arm = q

deletion comes from the short arm of the chromosome, it is denoted as a "p deletion"; from the long arm, it is denoted as a "q deletion."

4p Deletion (Wolf-Hirschhorn Syndrome)

A 4p deletion occurs in about 1/50,000 births and is more common in girls. Most (~ 87%) cases are *de novo,* while 13% are due to 1 of the parents having a balanced chromosome translocation. In a small percentage of cases, 4p deletion occurs as a result of a ring chromosome 4 where material is lost.

Features:

• Distinctive facial features: ocular hypertelorism, prominent glabella, frontal bossing, short philtrum, and relative smallness of the lower part of the face, particularly the jaw (The term "Greek helmet" is used to describe the facial features, specifically the prominent glabella. Today, this is considered inappropriate and derogatory, as are many similar "older terms." It is mentioned because it might help you remember the facial features of the syndrome.)
• Severe growth deficiency
• Microcephaly
• Kidney problems, including hypertension and renal failure
• Hypotonia
• Congenital cardiac anomalies (50%)
• Seizures (90%)
• Variable developmental delay, which can be severe

5p Deletion (Cri-Du-Chat Syndrome)

5p deletion, or cri-du-chat syndrome, is due to a deletion of the short arm of chromosome 5. This is often asked on exams, so be sure to know it! It is well known because of the association with the distinctive "cat's cry," which is due to an anatomic change in the larynx.

Characteristics of 5p deletion syndrome:

• "Moon face" with telecanthus (widely spaced eyes) in infancy and early childhood
• Down-slanting palpebral fissures
• Hypotonia
• Short stature
• Microcephaly
• High-arched palate
• Wide and flat nasal bridge
• Intellectual disability, typically severe
• Cardiac manifestations in about 33% of affected children

18q Deletion (de Grouchy Syndrome)

The long arm of chromosome 18 is deleted in 18q deletion syndrome, a.k.a. de Grouchy syndrome.

Features:

• Microcephaly
• Developmental delay
• Atretic or narrowed ear canals (classic)
• "Froglike" position with legs flexed, externally rotated, and in hyperabduction
• Depressed midface
• Protruding mandible
• Deep-set eyes
• Everted lower lip (carplike) mouth)
• Intellectual disability

OTHER DELETIONS

There are numerous other deletions, but those listed above are the ones most frequently found on exams. Others listed in major pediatrics textbooks include:

• **9p deletion**—trigonocephaly (triangle head), discrete exophthalmos, arched eyebrows, short neck with pterygium colli (a bilateral web or tight band of skin of the neck, extending from the acromion to the mastoid), long fingers and toes, and cardiac abnormalities.
• **13q deletion**—low birth weight, FTT, severe intellectual disability; ocular manifestations are common; hypoplastic hands and absent thumbs with syndactyly.
• **18p deletion**—mild intellectual disability and minor anomalies; some, however, may have severe ocular and brain abnormalities (including holoprosencephaly), more severe intellectual disability, cleft lip/palate, and IgA deficiency.
• **21q deletion**—large/low-set ears, micrognathia, hypertonia, downward-slanting palpebral fissures, skeletal abnormalities.

MICRODELETION OR CONTIGUOUS GENE SYNDROMES

Overview

Microdeletions are small chromosome deletions that are too small to detect even with the highest quality standard karyotype. They require additional technology, such as **FISH** (fluorescent *in situ* hybridization), which looks specifically at a predefined region, or **chromosomal microarray** (CMA), which is also referred to as cytogenetic microarray, cytogenomic microarray, array comparative genomic hybridization (aCGH), or single nucleotide polymorphism array (SNP array). CMA provides whole genome coverage.

Oligonucleotide microarray (usually ~ 60 base pairs long) technology and the SNP array can identify extremely small deletions or duplications anywhere in the genome. These usually provide at least 10× better resolution than a high-quality standard karyotype. However, unlike a standard karyotype, they cannot detect balanced rearrangements (where there is no actual gain or loss of material).

GENETICS

These microdeletions often involve several genes (contiguous gene deletion syndromes) and cause a fairly classic syndrome. (Several examples are shown below; e.g., Angelman and Prader-Willi syndromes.) They can also cause a more complex version of a typical "single gene" disorder, such as deletions involving the gene that causes neurofibromatosis Type 1, which have a more severe phenotype than those caused by gene mutations. Microdeletions can also "uncover" a recessive gene if the gene on the nondeleted matching chromosome is mutated.

15q11–13 Deletion (Angelman and Prader-Willi Syndromes)

Overview

Although we mentioned these syndromes earlier as examples of genomic imprinting, 15q11–13 microdeletion deserves special attention because it is such a common topic on exams. Remember: This deletion's phenotypic appearance depends solely on whether it is derived maternally (Angelman) or paternally (Prader-Willi).

Maternally Derived 15q11–13 Deletion or Lack of Expression (Angelman Syndrome)

Classic findings:

- Jerky ataxic movements (the "happy puppet"; but do not use this nomenclature except as a memory device!)
- Inappropriate bouts of laughter
- Microcephaly
- Characteristic gait
- Hypotonia
- Fair hair
- Midface hypoplasia
- Prognathism (large chin, mandible)
- Seizures
- Severe intellectual disability
- Absent or severely delayed speech

Paternally Derived 15q11–13 Deletion or Lack of Expression (Prader-Willi Syndrome)

Classic findings (see Image 22-8):

- **Infancy**
  - Severe hypotonia at birth
  - Feeding difficulties
- **Childhood**
  - Hyperphagia with development of severe obesity

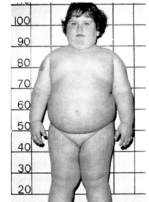

Image 22-8: Prader-Willi syndrome

- Short stature
- Small hands and feet
- Hypogonadism
- Usually mild intellectual disability
- Behavior disorders

7q11.23 Deletion (Williams Syndrome)

Williams syndrome, due to microdeletion on the long arm of chromosome 7, has the following characteristic features and facies (Image 22-9):

- Broad forehead; medial eyebrow flare; shortened, upturned nose associated with a flattened nasal bridge; elongated philtrum with prominent, down-turned lower lip (i.e., elfin facies)
- Friendly, "cocktail party" personality
- Stellate pattern of the iris
- Strabismus
- Supravalvular aortic stenosis
- Intellectual disability
- Hypercalcemia
- Connective tissue anomalies: joint laxity, soft skin
- Growth delay and short stature

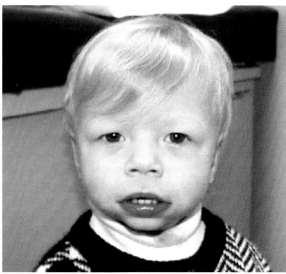

Image 22-9: Williams syndrome

In ≥ 95% of the cases studied, individuals having Williams syndrome are missing the elastin gene from 1 of their 2 copies of chromosome 7. Supravalvular aortic stenosis and connective tissue anomalies arise from this deletion.

The absent elastin gene is detected using FISH: A blood sample from the child is treated with 2 specifically colored markers that fluoresce when exposed to ultraviolet light. One of the markers attaches to each of the 2 copies of chromosome 7 in a cell. The other colored marker attaches to the elastin gene. In the normal state, each chromosome 7 shows 2 fluorescence markers: 1 identifying it as chromosome 7 and the other indicating the elastin gene is present. In the case of Williams syndrome, 1 of the chromosome 7s is completely missing the fluorescence at the elastin location.

Williams syndrome is also readily detected by CMA. (For more on CMA, see the Overview for this topic on page 22-7.)

11p13 Deletion (WAGR Syndrome)

11p13 deletion results in **WAGR** syndrome: **W**ilms tumor, **a**niridia, **g**enitourinary malformations, and intellectual disability (mental **r**etardation). It occurs due to the absence of 2 genes, *PAX6* and *Wilms tumor 1* (*WT1*).

Characteristics of WAGR syndrome:

- Wilms tumor (Wilms tumor occurs in up to 50% of cases, most often by 3 years of age.)
- Aniridia (absence of the iris, which is the colored part of the eye)
- Male genital hypoplasia (hypospadias, cryptorchidism, small penis, and/or hypoplastic scrotum)
- Intellectual disability (varies widely from IQ < 35 to normal functioning)
- Gonadoblastoma
- Long face
- Upward-slanting palpebral fissures
- Ptosis
- Beaked nose
- Poorly formed ears

20p12 Deletion (Alagille Syndrome)

20p12 deletion, a.k.a. Alagille syndrome, has AD inheritance and is caused by absence of or mutation in the *Jagged-1* (*JAG1*) gene.

Characteristics include:

- Triangular facies with pointed chin
- Long nose with broad midnose
- Bile duct paucity with cholestasis
- Pulmonary valve stenosis and peripheral pulmonic stenoses
- Ocular defects (posterior embryotoxon—a developmental abnormality marked by a prominent white ring of Schwalbe and iris strands that partially obscure the chamber angle)
- Skeletal defects: butterfly vertebrae

Hepatic involvement in patients with Alagille syndrome usually presents in the first 3 months of life as cholestasis, jaundice, and pruritus. Some patients develop liver failure. Biopsy shows a paucity of bile ducts.

Cardiac manifestations include peripheral and branch pulmonic stenoses (67% of patients) and tetralogy of Fallot (7–16% of patients).

The ocular defects (ring of Schwalbe and iris strands) and butterfly vertebrae do not generally cause symptoms.

22q11.2 Deletion (Velocardiofacial / DiGeorge Syndrome)

The 22q11.2 deletion syndrome includes phenotypes referred to as DiGeorge syndrome. (This is also covered in Allergy & Immunology, Book 4.) It is the most prevalent microdeletion syndrome, with ~ 1/6,000 live births affected.

A good mnemonic is **CATCH 22** (**c**left palate, **a**bsent **t**hymus, **c**ongenital **h**eart disease, on **22**nd chromosome)—but this is another old term and should not be used with patients.

Characteristics include:

- Cleft palate, velopharyngeal incompetence
- Thymus agenesis or hypoplasia (immunodeficiencies; see Allergy & Immunology, Book 4)
- Parathyroid gland hypoplasia/agenesis (hypocalcemia with possible tetany)
- Hypoplasia of the auricle and external auditory canal
- Cardiac abnormalities in decreasing order of frequency: tetralogy of Fallot > interrupted aortic arch > VSD > truncus arteriosus
- Short stature
- Behavioral problems

This is a developmental defect of derivatives of the 3rd and 4th pharyngeal pouches, resulting in agenesis or hypoplasia of the thymus and parathyroid gland, conotruncal heart defects, and branchial arch defects (small chin, cleft palate, abnormal ears). A majority of patients with 22q11.2 deletion have hypotonia in infancy and learning disabilities, with nonverbal learning disability in ~ 66% of patients and ~ 20–30% having intellectual disability. Presentation varies widely even within families, ranging from isolated psychiatric disorders or learning problems to severe congenital heart defects.

Given that this is a microdeletion condition, diagnostic confirmation relies on abnormal FISH or microarray analysis for 22q11.2

SINGLE GENE DEFECTS

PREVIEW | REVIEW

- Know how to differentiate a pedigree: AD, AR, and X-linked disorders.
- What is germline mosaicism?
- Which form of classic Mendelian inheritance does not have male-to-male transmission?
- Which form of classic Mendelian inheritance has a father passing the disease allele to all of his daughters and none of his sons?

GENETICS

• What is genomic imprinting? Describe an example.

• How is mitochondrial inheritance unique?

PATTERNS OF INHERITANCE

Classic Mendelian Inheritance

Overview

Mendelian inheritance refers to the strong link between genotype and phenotype in single gene traits. A botanist, Gregor Mendel, made observations of plants during cross-breeding experiments that revealed predictable, reproducible results and described the Mendelian inheritance patterns of phenotype. These patterns include autosomal dominant, autosomal recessive, X-linked dominant, and X-linked recessive.

Autosomal Dominant Disorders

Autosomal dominant (AD) disorders are caused by a mutation in only 1 copy of a gene (Figure 22-4). Although AD disorders are common as a group, each individual disorder is still rare; therefore, it would be uncommon—but not impossible—for 2 people with the same AD disorder to mate. A heterozygous parent has a 50% chance of passing the disorder to each child. Examples of AD disorders include Marfan syndrome and classic Ehlers-Danlos syndrome.

Spotting AD inheritance on pedigree:

• Both sexes are equally affected.
• Both sexes transmit to offspring.
• Present in all generations. Know: An individual may have been undiagnosed due to mild phenotype,

incomplete penetrance, or age-related penetrance (e.g., *BRCA* mutations present in adulthood at incomplete penetrance).

• Every affected child has a parent with the disorder. (Any affected individual has a 50% risk of passing on the gene mutation to offspring.)

• Fathers can transmit to sons. (This excludes X-linked and mitochondrial inheritance.)

AD disorders have a high "spontaneous" mutation rate. For example, in neurofibromatosis Type 1, 50% of cases are due to new dominant mutations. These individuals do not have an affected parent. Some factors, such as older paternal age, increase the risk of new dominant mutations. For example, the older the father, the more likely he is to have a child with achondroplasia, neurofibromatosis, or Marfan syndrome.

Germline mosaicism needs to be considered when an apparently new AD trait develops—one affected child, unaffected parents, and no other affected family members. This is most likely a "spontaneous" mutation. However, it could be germline mosaicism; i.e., the parent carries the gene mutation in gonadal tissue and germline cells, but not in the somatic cells—so they do not show signs of the disease. However, future offspring are at an increased risk (up to 50%) to inherit this condition. Suspect germline mosaicism when an apparently normal parent has more than 1 child affected with an AD condition. Note: Germline mosaicism can occur with any pattern of inheritance, but it appears to be less common in recessive disorders.

Autosomal Recessive Disorders

Autosomal recessive (AR) disorders produce a disease phenotype only when both alleles carry mutations (Figure 22-5). AR disorders are less common than AD disorders in most populations, but heterozygote carriers (having only 1 mutated allele) are much more common in the general population.

Spotting AR inheritance on a pedigree:

• No history of disease in prior generations.
• Males and females are equally affected.
• Males and females can each transmit the altered allele.

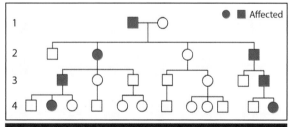

Figure 22-4: Autosomal Dominant Inheritance

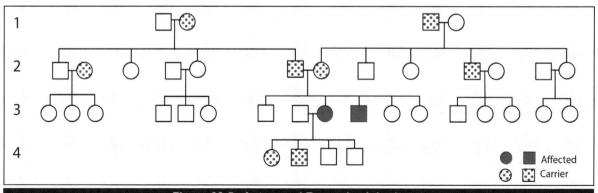

Figure 22-5: Autosomal Recessive Inheritance

- The risk for 2 heterozygotes to have an affected offspring is 1/4. (However, 2 heterozygotes also can have offspring who are all affected or all unaffected!)
- Consanguinity increases the risk of having an offspring with an AR disorder (Figure 22-6).

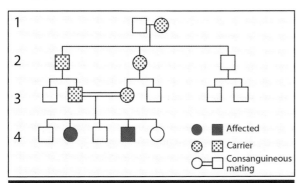

Figure 22-6: AR with Consanguinity

Affected / Carrier / Consanguineous mating

Know how to calculate probabilities or population frequencies for various diseases. Here's how to do some of these calculations.

Cystic fibrosis (CF) follows an AR inheritance pattern. CF has an incidence of ~ 1/1,600 births, with a relatively high carrier frequency (~ 1/20) in the general Caucasian population. Therefore, the general population risk for a randomly selected Caucasian couple to have a child with CF is $1/20 \times 1/20 \times 1/4 = 1/1,600$.

Another calculation using hair color:

Let's say we have an allele for black hair (B) and one for white hair (b), such that B is an AD trait. Any B in a genotype confers black hair, and the only way to have white hair is to have genotype bb.

Then let's say that, at a 2-allele locus, the frequency p of the dominant allele B is 0.80. This means that 80% of the sperm cells and 80% of the egg cells in a population have allele B. The sum of the 2 possible allele frequencies must equal 1. Therefore, the frequency q of the recessive allele b is $1 - p = q$, or $1 - 0.8 = 0.2$.

Using this equation, the chance that a sperm containing the dominant allele B unites with an egg carrying the dominant allele B is $p \times p = 0.8 \times 0.8 = 0.64$. Likewise, the probability of producing an offspring with both recessive genes or having the bb genotype is $q \times q = 0.2 \times 0.2 = 0.04$.

Two things can happen to produce a heterozygote:

1) a sperm with B can unite with an egg carrying b,

or

2) a sperm with b can unite with an egg carrying B.

So, the frequency with which heterozygosity occurs is the sum of the product of each possibility: $(p \times q) + (p \times q) = 2 (p \times q) = 2 (0.8 \times 0.2) = 0.32$.

Putting it all together, what is the frequency of white hair in the community? It is 0.04, or 4%. Note: The frequencies must add up to 1. Thus, $0.64 (BB) + 0.32 (Bb \text{ or } bB) + 0.04 (bb) = 1$.

This is different from asking: What is the probability of 2 carriers (heterozygotes) producing a child with white hair, a child who is heterozygous, and a child who is homozygous for black hair?

Here, we know that mom is Bb and dad is Bb. Thus, mom's egg is either a B egg or a b egg, and dad's sperm is either a B sperm or a b sperm.

So, the chance that junior will be white-haired (bb) is (the chance that dad's sperm is b) $\times$ (the chance that mom's egg is b), which is $1/2 \times 1/2 = 1/4$; in other words, a 25% chance.

If mom and dad already have 2 children with white hair (bb), what is the chance that the next baby will have white hair (bb)? Exactly the same: 1/4, or 25%—the mom's egg and the dad's sperm for making this new baby are not affected by what happened to the earlier kids.

Again, this risk calculation (for the 3rd child) is different from the risk calculation for all 3 as a group; i.e., asking before they have any children: "What is the chance that if they have 3 kids, all 3 will have white hair?" Answer: $1/4 \times 1/4 \times 1/4 = 1/64$.

X-Linked Disorders

X-linked traits can have either a dominant or recessive pattern of inheritance. X-linked recessive is more common and predominantly affects males. X-linked dominant traits are seen in both sexes but are typically more severe in the male population due to the absence of a normal X chromosome.

The X chromosome is twice as large as the Y chromosome and has thousands of genes compared to the Y, which has ~ 25 identified genes localized to it, including 1 especially important gene—the sex-determining region Y (*SRY*) gene. Many well-known pediatric diseases are caused by mutations in genes on the X chromosome, including:

- Hemophilia A
- Duchenne and Becker muscular dystrophy
- Red-green color blindness

Over 100 different phenotypes associated with intellectual disability have been mapped to the X chromosome (e.g., fragile X syndrome).

So, you are wondering: "Females have 2 copies of X and males have only 1 copy of X, so do females have a lot more X-linked gene products?" The answer is "no" because of **dosage compensation**, which is produced by the inactivation of 1 of the X chromosomes in each cell early in female embryonic life. It usually begins ~ 2 weeks after fertilization. This is a random process, so the inactivated X chromosome could come

GENETICS

from either the mother or the father. Somatic cells in the female embryo each have a 50% chance that the active X came from mom and 50% chance that it came from dad. **Somatic mosaicism** is the result, with females having 2 different populations of cells. If the maternally and paternally derived X chromosomes produce different products, the mosaicism might be visible in the patient! For example, women who are "carriers" for X-linked ocular albinism have patches of pigmented and nonpigmented cells, depending on whether it is the disease-bearing X chromosome (nonpigmented) or the normal X chromosome (pigmented) that is active in that cell.

In some cases, the "extra" X chromosome is not completely inactivated, and the genes in several regions continue to be transcribed. So, at a given locus, females can be homozygous for a disease, heterozygous (1 disease allele and 1 normal allele), or homozygous normal.

Males have only 1 X chromosome and are considered **hemizygous** for every allele at each locus on the X chromosome. Thus, if a male inherits an X-linked recessive allele for a disease, he will be affected—but a female inheriting such an allele would not be affected unless she also received a 2nd copy from her father. On the other hand, an X-linked dominant disease can cause disease in either males or females because the presence of only 1 copy of an altered allele is sufficient for disease to occur.

For males with X-linked recessive disorders, the frequency of the disease in males = the frequency q of the gene. This is because all males with the altered gene have the disease condition. For females, the frequency of the gene condition is $q \times q$ because they need both alleles to express the disease.

For example, let's say that being a red Smurf (as opposed to the normal blue) is an X-linked recessive trait and that the prevalence in males is about 1/500 ($q = 0.002$). Thus, you will see affected females in $q \times q = 0.002 \times 0.002 = 0.000004$—or 1/250,000 females.

Duchenne muscular dystrophy is an example of a disorder with X-linked recessive inheritance. Important features are:

- Progressive muscle weakness with delayed motor milestones
- Calf hypertrophy
- Gowers sign at ~ 2 years of age
- Wheelchair dependency generally by 12 years of age

Other findings are cardiomyopathy, progression to respiratory failure, and risk for cognitive delays.

Spotting X-linked recessive inheritance on a pedigree (Figure 22-7):

- There is never male-to-male transmission.
- If a generation has only females, the disease will appear to have "skipped" that generation.

- An affected father transmits the disease allele to all his daughters but none of his sons. (The daughters are **obligate carriers** but typically are unaffected.)
- Carrier females have a 50% chance of transmitting the disease to each son.

Why do some female "carriers" have some or all manifestations of an X-linked recessive disorder? There are 3 possibilities:

1) Remember: Because inactivation of the X chromosome occurs randomly within each cell, differing proportions of normal alleles versus disease alleles are affected. If a much greater proportion of X chromosomes with normal alleles are inactivated, females will manifest a given disease (called manifesting heterozygotes) but usually have a milder form compared to males with the condition. A common example is seen in hemophilia A, where 5% of women who carry one of the alleles for hemophilia A have Factor 8 levels low enough to exhibit mild forms of the disease.

2) Some females have only a single X chromosome (Turner syndrome).

3) Deletions or rearrangements in an X chromosome and another non-X chromosome (autosome) can result in affected females, which is rare.

Atypical Patterns of Inheritance

Overview

Some single gene disorders do not follow the AD, AR, or X-linked patterns of inheritance (classic Mendelian inheritance). In classic Mendelian inheritance for autosomal chromosomes, the expression of the disease is independent of which parent contributed the disease-causing allele. The following situations are examples of when it does matter which parent gave the child the autosomal allele.

Genomic Imprinting

Genomic (genetic) imprinting refers to differences in gene expression that depend on whether the disease allele is inherited from the mother or the father. For example, when deletion of a 2–4 Mb portion of chromosome 15 is inherited from the father, the child is born

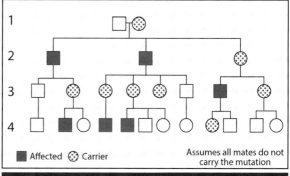

Figure 22-7: X-Linked Recessive Inheritance

■ Affected ⊗ Carrier   Assumes all mates do not carry the mutation with Prader-Willi syndrome. This syndrome presents with severe hypotonia, initial poor feeding and FTT with progression to hyperphagia, short stature, severe obesity, hypogonadism, and intellectual disability. Thus, the deletion of all paternally active genes from this part of the chromosome results in Prader-Willi syndrome.

When the same deletion is inherited from the mother, the child is born with Angelman syndrome. Children with Angelman syndrome appear normal at birth but, over time, develop seizures, intellectual disability, microcephaly, ataxia, hand-flapping behaviors, outbursts of laughter, and a characteristic "puppet-like" gait. Thus, deletion of all the maternally active genes from this part of the chromosome results in Angelman syndrome. The old phrase, "the happy puppet," used to describe children with Angelman syndrome, can be offensive and should not be used.

But it isn't so simple. Genomic imprinting explains only 70% of the cases of Angelman and Prader-Willi syndromes, which leads us to ask: What about the other 30%?

Uniparental Disomy

Uniparental disomy occurs if both copies of a chromosome—or a piece of a chromosome—are inherited from only 1 parent. Thus, considering our case above, if a child inherits two copies of the maternal chromosome 15 (without any deletions), the child lacks the paternally active genes and develops Prader-Willi syndrome. On the other hand, if the child gets both copies from the father, the child lacks maternally active genes and develops Angelman syndrome. Uniparental disomy arises because of nondisjunction of chromosomes during meiosis in the gametes, which results in trisomy (with subsequent loss of 1 chromosome) or monosomy (with subsequent duplication of the chromosome). In both cases, the resulting disomic cell line then has 2 chromosomes originating from only 1 parent. Another condition, which can be caused by uniparental disomy or imprinting defects, is Beckwith-Wiedemann syndrome (refer to Syndromes with Growth Abnormalities in Table 22-4 at the end of this section, and see Endocrinology, Book 3).

Mitochondrial Disorders

Mitochondria have the only genetic material outside of the nucleus. However, the mitochondrial genome is haploid (contains only 1 copy of each gene), not diploid like in the nucleus. Mitochondrial inheritance is unique because the ovum, not the sperm, transmits all the mitochondria to their zygote; therefore, a mother carrying a mitochondrial DNA (mtDNA) mutation passes it on to all her offspring, whereas the father carrying the mutation passes it to none of his offspring (Figure 22-8).

Each mitochondrion contains 2–10 copies of the mtDNA genome, and each cell has hundreds to thousands of mitochondria. At cell division, mtDNA replicates and randomly separates into the daughter cells. If there is an mtDNA mutation, then this results in different mitochondria carrying different amounts of normal and mutated (disease-causing) mtDNA. Also, each cell contains different amounts of normal and mutated mtDNA. This leads to an extremely complex type of mosaicism (heteroplasmy) in which the mutation load can vary from mitochondrion to mitochondrion, from cell to cell, and from tissue to tissue. Homoplasmy occurs when all the mtDNA in an individual is the same.

You can see why mitochondrial disorders are so confusing and so highly variable! Common presentations for mitochondrial disorders include metabolic encephalopathy, cardiac failure, liver failure, and/or lactic acidosis. Although mtDNA disorders are not common, they account for many cases of cerebrovascular accidents, deafness, and diabetes in children.

A few disorders that are caused by mutations in the mitochondrial genome (also see Metabolic Disorders, Book 5):

- **M**yoclonic **e**pilepsy and **r**agged-**r**ed **f**ibers (**MERRF**) is associated with progressive myoclonic epilepsy, myopathy, dementia, and hearing loss.
- **M**itochondrial **e**ncephalopathy, **l**actic **a**cidosis, and **s**troke-like episodes (**MELAS**) presents anytime from toddlerhood to adulthood.
- **Leigh syndrome** presents with basal ganglia defects, hypotonia, and optic atrophy in infancy or early childhood.

GENETICS

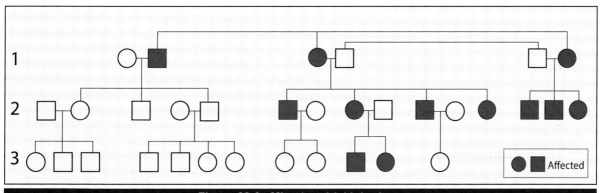

Figure 22-8: Mitochondrial Inheritance

- **Kearns-Sayre syndrome** presents with ophthalmoplegia, retinitis pigmentosa, myopathy, and cardiac conduction defects.
- **Pearson syndrome** presents with anemia, neutropenia, pancreatic dysfunction, and myopathy in infants. Patients who survive beyond infancy (most die in infancy) go on to develop Kearns-Sayre syndrome.

Trinucleotide Repeat Diseases

Overview

A **DNA triplet** is defined as a series of 3 bases in DNA or RNA coding for a specific amino acid. They frequently occur in repeated sequences, 10–20 at a time. Although normally these repeated sequences ("repeats") are steadily transmitted, sometimes they "expand," copying themselves over and over during DNA replication—occasionally causing 100–1,000+ sequential repeats. This "triplet-repeat expansion" leads to several diseases, including Friedreich ataxia and Huntington disease.

Fragile X Syndrome (CGG Repeat)

Fragile X syndrome is the most common inherited intellectual disability syndrome, occurring in 1/1,650 males. Originally, a "fragile site" on chromosome Xq27.3 was identified by cytogenetic analysis in a folate-deficient medium. Although X-linked, its inheritance pattern displays unusual features that are not seen in other X-linked conditions because it has a trinucleotide repeat that can expand unpredictably, leading to different versions of the disorder in different generations and increasing severity with transmission (anticipation).

Fragile X is caused by an unstable CGG (cytosine-guanine-guanine) repeat in the 5′ untranslated region of the fragile X intellectual disability (*FMR1*) gene on the X chromosome.

- Normal: 6–50 repeats
- Premutation: ~ 50 to 55–200 repeats
- Full mutation: > 200 repeats

Diagnosis is made by DNA testing for defects in the *FMR1* gene with either Southern blot analysis or polymerase chain reaction (PCR) analysis.

Full mutation blocks transcription and results in methylation of the CpG (cytosine and guanine separated by a phosphate) island.

Full Mutation (> 200 repeats; common clinical findings in males):

- Intellectual disability
- Large head
- Long face with large ears
- Large hands and feet
- Macroorchidism after puberty
- Hyperextensible joints

Note: About 30% of female heterozygote "carriers" of the full mutation can have this phenotype (except the big testes).

Premutation (~ 50 to 55–200 CGG repeats; 3 distinct clinical disorders):

1) Mild cognitive and/or behavioral deficits on the fragile X spectrum (male and female)
2) Premature ovarian failure (female)
3) **FXTAS** (**f**ragile **X**-associated **t**remor/**a**taxia **s**yndrome):
   - Neurodegenerative disorder of older adult permutation carriers (male and female)
   - Less common in females
   - Mostly in male carriers, usually > 50 years of age for onset
   - > 30% of male carriers develop symptoms
   - Significant variability in progression of symptoms
   - Clinical criteria: intention tremor and gait ataxia, parkinsonism

Note the findings that are unique to females with premutation:

- Increased risk of emotional problems: mild form of anxiety and perseverative thinking, depression, interpersonal sensitivity
- Premature ovarian failure in ~ 20% of cases
- Ovarian dysfunction in 20% of cases
- Mild decrease in FMR1 protein
- Risk of expansion when passed down to offspring

Myotonic Dystrophy (CTG Repeat)

Myotonic dystrophy is another triplet-repeat disease and has these clinical features:

- Autosomal dominant, with variable age of onset and variable severity
- Myotonia with progressive weakness and wasting; involvement of facial and jaw muscles (e.g., ptosis, atrophy of sternocleidomastoid muscles); myotonia on grip testing. (These are the individuals who grip your hand to shake it but have difficulty letting go because their muscles cannot relax out of the grip easily.)
- Other involved organ systems:
  - Eye—cataract
  - Endocrine—testicular atrophy, diabetes mellitus
  - Brain—intellectual disability
  - Skin—premature balding
  - Cardiac—conduction abnormalities
- Congenital myotonic dystrophy: results in marked hypotonia, intellectual disability (60–70% of cases), neonatal respiratory distress, feeding difficulties, and talipes—and can cause neonatal death

Etiology: Mutation affects the CTG (cytosine-thymine-guanine) repeat in the 3′ untranslated region of the myotonin kinase gene on chromosome 19. A normal individual has 5–35 repeats; affected individuals with mutations have ≥ 50 to several thousand repeats.

Severity varies with the number of repeats. **Anticipation** (worsening of genetic disease in subsequent generations) is seen due to expansion with transmission. **Parent of origin effect**: The repeat is more likely to severely expand when passed from the mother; therefore, the most severely affected babies typically inherit the expansion from their mothers.

MULTIFACTORIAL INHERITANCE

PREVIEW | REVIEW

- What factors suggest multifactorial inheritance has occurred?

Most genetic disorders are due to multiple genetic and environmental factors, not to a "single gene" mutation. Multifactorial inheritance is the most common cause of isolated major anomalies observed in the newborn. Examples include neural tube defects, heart defects, schizophrenia, Type 2 diabetes mellitus, cleft palate, and clubfoot. Many of these are present at birth, but some, such as DM and autism, often do not manifest for years. As a general rule, empiric risks of recurrence for most isolated major anomalies are typically in the range of 2–6%.

In general, a multifactorial disease occurs when enough "bad" factors overcome the "good" factors. Some refer to these bad factors as "liability" factors. In other words, enough liability factors must be present to exceed a threshold to result in the disease. For some diseases, this threshold varies depending on the gender.

A good example is pyloric stenosis. Pyloric stenosis normally occurs in about 1/1,200 females and about 1/300 males. This indicates that the "threshold" for this disease is much higher in females than males. In other words, for a female to get pyloric stenosis, she would need to have an unusually high number of liability factors present, especially compared to the case for a male. So, when a female does, in fact, get pyloric stenosis, it means she has more of these "bad" factors, and the consequence is that her offspring are much more likely to have this disorder—even more likely than the offspring of an affected male (who presumably would have pyloric stenosis with fewer liability factors present in the first place). Knowing this, let's consider a woman with a history of pyloric stenosis as a child. Are her boys or her girls more likely to be affected? Boys! Why? Because it takes fewer liability factors—"fewer hoops to jump through"—for males to develop the disease. When the mother is transmitting enough of these factors (remember, we said this is a mother with a history of pyloric stenosis), her son is more likely than her daughter to reach the threshold.

Key features of multifactorial inheritance:

- No discernable pattern.
- Recurrence risk increases as the number of affected individuals in the family increases; e.g., the recurrence risk of a disorder is estimated at 2% if 1 sibling has the disorder, but it increases to 12% if 2 siblings have the disorder. (Remember: In contrast to multifactorial inheritance, the subsequent risk does not change with single gene disorders; the genetic roulette wheel does not remember what has previously occurred.)
- Recurrence risk is higher if the affected individual is a member of the less commonly affected sex. (See the above pyloric stenosis scenario.) This also holds true for infantile autism, in which males are 4× more likely than females to be affected. If a girl in the family has autism, it is twice as likely to recur in a sibling as when a boy is the one with the autism.
- Recurrence risk is higher if the affected individual has a more severe form/case.
- Recurrence risk drops dramatically as the degree of relationship decreases from the affected individual. For example, if a woman has clubfoot, her 1st degree relative has ~ 2.5% risk of clubfoot, but this drops to 0.5% for a 2nd degree relative and to 0.2% for a 3rd degree relative. (The general population has a risk of 0.1%.)
- Recurrence risk correlates with the prevalence in the general population. However, in single gene disorders, the recurrence risk is independent of the general population: If 1 parent is heterozygous for a very rare AD disorder and the other parent is unaffected, the risk is 50% that their child will get the disorder. The risk of siblings having inherited multifactorial disease is lower than the risk for having single gene mutations. However, the risk for siblings inheriting multifactorial disease is greater than that for the general population.
- Environmental factors can play a role; e.g., folic acid supplementation both prior to and through early pregnancy has been proven to prevent neural tube defects and possibly reduce the risk of other birth defects.

TWINS FACTS

PREVIEW | REVIEW

- Are dizygotic twins more likely, less likely, or equally likely to have genetic traits similar to those of a nontwin sibling?
- Name 4 diseases or abnormalities that are more likely to be concordant in monozygotic than dizygotic twins.

Remember: There are monozygotic (identical) and dizygotic (fraternal) twins. Monozygotic twins share 100% of their genes. Dizygotic twins are caused by the fertilization of 2 different egg cells by 2 different sperm cells. Therefore, they share 50% of their genes. From a straightforward genetic perspective, dizygotic twins are no more similar than nontwin siblings.

GENETICS

Traits that are strongly influenced by genes show higher levels of concordance in monozygotic twins than in dizygotic twins; for example:

- Autism (60% concordance in monozygotic twins vs. 0% in dizygotic twins)
- Cleft lip/palate (38% vs. 8%)
- Clubfoot (32% vs. 3%)
- Spina bifida (72% vs. 33%)

RISKS OF GENETIC DISEASE AND DIAGNOSTIC TESTING

PREVIEW | REVIEW

- What are some indications that a genetic disorder is likely?
- A positive prenatal quad screen indicates an increased risk of which 4 disorders?
- What diagnostic testing method is used to detect single gene defects?

GENETIC DISEASE RISK FACTORS

Many parents are concerned about genetic diseases and specific risks for their child. Once a child is born with an abnormality, many parents want to know if this is "genetic" and, therefore, whether the abnormality could happen again.

Clues that a genetic disorder is likely:

- Previous family history of genetic disorder
- Positive neonatal screen
- Congenital anomalies
- Developmental abnormalities
- Neurologic disorders
- Death in utero or soon after birth
- Growth abnormalities
- Multiorgan dysfunction

Indications for chromosomal analysis:

- Multiple birth defects
- Developmental delay, intellectual disability, autism
- Growth abnormalities (e.g., short stature)
- Abnormal sexual development
- Recurrent miscarriages

PRENATAL DIAGNOSTIC TESTING

Prenatal **screening tests** tell if a fetus has the possibility of having a genetic disorder. Maternal blood screening (a.k.a. quad screen) is performed between 15 and 18 weeks of gestation. It measures α-fetoprotein, human chorionic gonadotropin, estriol, and inhibin A. The results, measured as a risk ratio, indicate the likelihood of trisomy 21, trisomy 18, neural tube defects, and abdominal wall defects. If this risk ratio is increased, then further diagnostic testing is needed.

Screening for chromosomal disorders also includes cell-free fetal DNA. Remember, this is a screening test with low false-negative and false-positive results.

Diagnostic testing, on the other hand, tells if a fetus actually has the disorder. Some of the modalities used for prenatal diagnostic testing are ultrasound, amniocentesis, chorionic villus sampling (placenta), and umbilical blood sampling. Cells collected from these invasive procedures can be sent for karyotype, gene testing (single genes or short DNA segments), or biochemical testing (protein amounts or activity). This information is limited, however, in that the test does not reveal how severe the symptoms will be in the patient; and, once diagnosed, many genetic disorders have limited treatment options. Some of the heritable disorders that can be diagnosed prenatally include cystic fibrosis, fragile X, hemoglobinopathies, and Down syndrome.

POSTNATAL DIAGNOSTIC TESTING

Postnatal diagnostic testing is performed on the baby's blood, cord blood, products of conception, or solid tissue. Large defects in the chromosome (e.g., aneuploidies, large deletions, translocations) can be detected by karyotyping, FISH, and comparative genomic hybridization (also called chromosomal microarray or SNP array). FISH uses fluorescent-labeled single-stranded DNA probes that hybridize with a target DNA sequence, revealing the defect.

Comparative genomic hybridization compares the DNA of a patient with that of a normal control to detect any abnormalities. It is a 1st line test for nondysmorphic patients with intellectual disability, autism, and multiple congenital anomalies. Be aware that this test looks for missing or extra material but does not detect chromosomal rearrangements or indicate where extra material is located.

Single gene sequencing is typically performed with the Sanger method. Multiple gene panels and whole exome sequencing use next generation sequencing methods. Older methods, such as Southern blots, are still used to detect trinucleotide repeat disorders and methylation disorders.

GENETIC CONDITIONS ORGANIZED BY PRESENTING SYMPTOMS

PREVIEW | REVIEW

- Chromosomal instability syndromes most commonly have what pattern of inheritance?
- Know the inheritance patterns for common genetic syndromes. (See Table 22-4 at the end of this section.)

- Know Pierre Robin sequence.
- What anomalies are seen in children with hemifacial microsomia?
- What type of head growth is seen with early fusion of the sagittal sutures? Coronal and sphenofrontal sutures? Metopic sutures?
- What is positional plagiocephaly?
- Describe the findings in achondroplasia.
- What skull structural abnormality can occur in infants with achondroplasia?
- What is the most commonly affected bone in Caffey disease?
- Describe a child with osteogenesis imperfecta Type 1.
- Which type of osteogenesis imperfecta is the most severe and usually results in death in infancy?
- Which type of osteogenesis imperfecta has the highest risk of neurologic complications?
- What are the classic scleral findings in osteogenesis imperfecta Type 4?
- What causes most deaths in Marfan syndrome?
- Describe the classic findings in a patient with Marfan syndrome.
- Describe the typical findings in classic Ehlers-Danlos syndrome.
- What are the classic skin findings in neurofibromatosis Type 1?
- How frequently is neurofibromatosis Type 1 due to a new mutation?
- Describe how neurofibromatosis Type 2 differs from neurofibromatosis Type 1.
- What abnormalities do vestibular schwannomas cause in neurofibromatosis Type 2?
- Describe the skin findings in tuberous sclerosis.
- What cardiac tumors are common in infants with tuberous sclerosis?
- What tumors are commonly seen in patients with von Hippel-Lindau syndrome?
- Noonan syndrome has what kind of inheritance pattern?
- What is the most common heart defect seen in Noonan syndrome?
- Beckwith-Wiedemann syndrome has what kind of inheritance pattern?
- What are the features of Beckwith-Wiedemann syndrome?

CHROMOSOMAL INSTABILITY SYNDROMES

Chromosomal instability syndromes refer to a group of disorders that are largely autosomal recessive and have an increased frequency of chromosomal breaks. These include ataxia-telangiectasia, Bloom syndrome, Fanconi syndrome, and xeroderma pigmentosum. At the end of this section is a set of tables listing common congenital anomaly syndromes, including those caused by chromosomal instability; see Table 22-4, starting on page 22-26.

ANOMALIES OF THE HEAD

Cleft Lip / Palate Disorders

Overview

Cleft lip and/or cleft palate is one of the most common craniofacial malformations you will see in your practice. The incidence varies from 1/250 to 1/3,000, depending on the culture and race being reviewed. Native Americans have the highest rates, and African Americans have the lowest rates.

Most cases of cleft lip/palate are sporadic. But there can be recurrence in families, and hereditary factors have been documented. If the first-born child has a cleft lip/palate, the risk of the next sibling having it is 3–4%. If either parent had one as a child, the risk increases further. There are nearly 300 syndromes associated with cleft lip/palate—make sure you know all 300 very well. (Just kidding!)

There is evidence suggesting that maternal folate deficiency contributes to this disorder. More studies are underway.

Airway management and feeding difficulties are the usual problems at birth. These children are at risk for recurrent otitis media and persistent middle-ear effusions.

Generally, surgically repair the lip within the first 5 months of life, and repair a cleft palate at 6–12 months of age.

Sequence refers to a pattern of anomalies that result from a single identifiable event in development.

The following 2 sequences are important to know!

Pierre Robin Sequence

Pierre Robin sequence presents with a primary embryologic defect of mandibular hypoplasia. This leads to a displacement of the tongue, which in turn interrupts the closure of the lateral palatine ridges and results in a U-shaped cleft palate. Patients have glossoptosis (displacement of the tongue into the airway), micrognathia, retrognathia, respiratory distress, and feeding problems. Respiratory compromise can lead to pulmonary hypertension. Macroglossia is not part of the syndrome.

GENETICS

Amniotic Band Sequence

Amniotic band sequence can present with disruptive clefts of the face and palate resulting from amniotic bands adhering to this area. Bands can also form in other parts of the fetal body. Other defects can include constriction rings of the limbs and/or digits and amputations (Image 22-10).

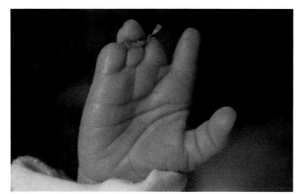

Image 22-10: Amniotic band sequence defects

Hemifacial Microsomia

Findings

The 2nd most common craniofacial malformation is the association of:

• external ear anomalies
  ◦ microtia—smallness of the auricle of the ear with a blind or absent external auditory meatus;
  ◦ anotia—congenital absence of 1 or both auricles of the ears;
  ◦ canal atresia; and/or
  ◦ preauricular tags
• with maxillary and/or mandibular hypoplasia.

The malformations can occur as isolated events or be part of a malformation syndrome. Cervical vertebral anomalies occur in nearly 33% with hemifacial microsomia, and cardiac anomalies occur frequently as well.

Also be aware that renal anomalies occur in about 15% of individuals with these ear malformations, so consider a renal ultrasound for further evaluation.

Goldenhar syndrome (see below) and hemifacial microsomia are considered to be the same disorder, but use the term "Goldenhar syndrome" only if epibulbar dermoids are present.

Goldenhar Syndrome

A child with Goldenhar syndrome (a.k.a. oculo-auriculovertebral spectrum) has all the findings of hemifacial microsomia mentioned above. The patient presents with hemifacial microsomia, epibulbar lipo-dermoids (lateral-inferior, fibrous-fatty masses on the globe), vertebral defects, cardiac anomalies (VSD or outflow tract malformations), and renal anomalies. Preauricular and facial tags and conductive hearing loss are common. This syndrome typically occurs as a

"sporadic" finding, but some researchers propose AD inheritance in certain families. The cause is unknown, but some cases are reported to be due to vascular interruption during embryonic development.

Other Facial Anomaly Syndromes

Branchio-Oto-Renal (BOR) Syndrome

BOR syndrome presents with branchial cleft fistulas or cysts, preauricular pits, cochlear and stapes malformation, mixed sensory and conductive hearing loss, and renal dysplasia/aplasia. Occasionally, patients have pulmonary hypoplasia. It is inherited as an AD disorder.

Treacher-Collins Syndrome (Mandibulofacial Dysostosis)

Treacher-Collins syndrome is another AD disorder and presents with micrognathia (mandibular and maxillary hypoplasia), zygomatic arch clefts, and various forms of ear malformations (e.g., microtia, anotia, atresia). Other characteristic findings include down-sloping palpebral fissures and colobomata (defects) of the lower eyelids. Conductive hearing loss is a frequent occurrence.

Craniosynostosis

Craniosynostosis is the early, pathologic fusion of calvarial sutures. Craniosynostosis occurs sporadically in 1/2,000 live births; 1/25,000 cases are hereditary. The most common, single-suture fusion is sagittal synostosis. The others, in descending order, are coronal > metopic > lambdoid. Isolated lambdoid is very rare, occurring in only 2–3% of cases. Sagittal synostosis is more common in males by a ratio of 5:1.

What head shapes form from the different early fusions?

• Sagittal sutures: result in excessive anterior/posterior growth with a resulting long, narrow head shape with frontal and occipital prominence, known as **scaphocephaly** or **dolichocephaly**.
• Coronal and sphenofrontal sutures: result in unilateral flattening of the forehead, elevation of the ipsilateral orbit and eyebrow, and a prominent ear on the affected side, known as **frontal plagiocephaly**; more common in girls.
• Metopic sutures: result in keel-shaped forehead and hypotelorism, known as **trigonocephaly**.
• Coronal, sphenofrontal, and frontoethmoidal sutures: cause a cone-shaped head, known as **turricephaly**.

Syndromic hereditary forms exist, including Apert and Crouzon syndromes, which are discussed briefly under Craniofacial Syndromes in Table 22-4, starting on page 22-26. Many of these forms can be distinguished from each other by specific hand malformations. Surgical intervention is required to correct the risk of intracranial hypertension, as well as to repair facial asymmetry and make the shape of the head more normal.

There is more on craniosynostosis in Neonatology, Book 1.

Plagiocephaly

See Growth & Development, Book 1, for more information on plagiocephaly.

Positional plagiocephaly is the postnatal flattening of the skull that is caused by the infant's preference of sleeping/resting position. Infants with torticollis frequently have flattening of the occipitoparietal area. It is sometimes severe enough to cause ipsilateral frontal prominence or anterior displacement of the ipsilateral ear.

Plagiocephaly can look like lambdoid synostosis, but you can differentiate one from another by physical examination and, if necessary, skull CT; lambdoid synostosis shows sclerosis of the lambdoid suture. Know that lambdoid synostosis is rare, whereas positional plagiocephaly is common.

Things to look for in positional plagiocephaly:

- Anterior displacement of the ipsilateral ear (posterior/inferior for lambdoid)
- Ipsilateral frontal prominence (absent in lambdoid); most easily noted when looking down at the child from above the head
- Absent contralateral occipitoparietal prominence (present in lambdoid)
- No lambdoid ridge or submastoid prominence (present in lambdoid)
- Stops progressing after 7 months because children generally can roll over and move their head more (Lambdoid continues to progress after 7 months.)

Positional plagiocephaly has become more common since the implementation of the Safe to Sleep recommendations to help prevent SIDS. Positional plagiocephaly improves with tummy time. Special helmets for sleeping are available in severe cases.

SKELETAL DYSPLASIAS

Achondroplasia

Achondroplasia, the most common skeletal dysplasia, occurs in 1/20,000 live births and consists of:

- Disproportionately short stature with rhizomelic shortening (short lengths of the most proximal, or "root," segment of the upper arms and legs compared to the distal segments)
- Lumbar lordosis
- Trident hands
- Macrocephaly
- Characteristic craniofacial findings, including a flat nasal bridge, prominent forehead (frontal bossing), and midfacial hypoplasia (Image 22-11)

Achondroplasia is an AD disorder in which most individuals have a *de novo* mutation of *FGFR3* (fibroblast growth factor receptor 3) on chromosome 4p16.3; the mutation rate increases with advancing paternal age. This gain-of-function mutation results in decreased endochondral ossification, chondrocyte proliferation, and cartilage matrix production.

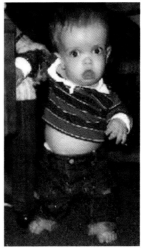
Image 22-11: Achondroplasia

The hands have a "trident" appearance—hands are short and fingers are quite broad, with digits 3 and 4 splayed more distally than proximally. These children are on the growth curve at birth, but by 2–3 months of age, their length has fallen to < 5th percentile. Note that children with achondroplasia typically do not have malformations apart from those mentioned above, and they are of normal intellect.

These children are at increased risk for serous otitis media, motor milestone delay, bowing of the legs, and orthodontic problems. Adults are at risk for obesity and, more seriously, spinal stenosis. Most males have final heights of 46–57 inches and females of 44–54 inches.

Foramen magnum stenosis and/or craniocervical junction abnormalities can occur in infancy and cause compression of the upper cord—resulting in apnea, quadriparesis, growth delay, and hydrocephalus. In 2012, the AAP reaffirmed its 2005 recommendations to measure the size and shape of the fontanelle and monitor the occipitofrontal circumference (with growth curves standardized for achondroplasia) at every pediatric visit. A detailed neurological examination is important; if there are any concerns, neuroimaging and polysomnography are recommended.

Confirm diagnosis with characteristic x-ray findings: squared-off iliac wings, flat and irregular acetabulum roofs, thick femoral necks, and "ice-cream-scoop shaped" femoral heads, as well as the rhizomelic shortening mentioned above.

Thanatophoric Dysplasias

Thanatophoric dysplasias Types 1 and 2 also involve mutations of *FGFR3*, but most cases are lethal. Both are AD and almost always due to *de novo* mutations. Death is either due to compression of the cervicomedullary region of the foramen magnum or due to pulmonary hypoplasia.

Those affected have macrocephaly with very short limbs. X-ray is diagnostic, showing platyspondyly (flatness of the bodies of the vertebrae), flared metaphyses of the long bones, and short iliac bones. Individuals with Type 1 have bowed femurs, whereas those with Type 2 exhibit straight femurs. Also, the Type 2 infants have a "cloverleaf" skull, which is a severe form of craniosynostosis due to premature closure of the sagittal, coronal, and lambdoid sutures.

GENETICS

Infantile Cortical Hyperostosis (Caffey Disease)

Infantile cortical hyperostosis (a.k.a. Caffey disease), transmitted as an AD trait with incomplete penetrance, is characterized by extreme irritability, fever, anorexia, and soft tissue swelling caused by subperiosteal cortical thickening of underlying bone. Soft tissue swelling is painful and indurated but without suppuration and only minimally warm and red. Typically, changes in the bones begin prior to 6 months of age and resolve by 24 months of age. Affected infants are extremely irritable and often febrile. The mandible is involved in > 95% of cases and is the most commonly affected bone. Other frequently involved bones include the clavicles, ribs, long bones, and scapulae.

Mandibular involvement is most helpful in differentiating Caffey disease from nonaccidental trauma. Always consider nonaccidental trauma during any encounter with a pediatric patient where you see periosteal elevation on imaging studies. Typical radiographic abnormalities in Caffey disease include layers of cortical diaphyseal periosteal new bone formation and cortical thickening. Laboratory findings include leukocytosis, elevated erythrocyte sedimentation rate, and increased levels of alkaline phosphatase.

BONE FRAGILITY DISORDERS — OSTEOGENESIS IMPERFECTA

All Types

Osteogenesis imperfecta (OI) refers to a disorder characterized by osseous fragility, short stature, and skeletal findings that vary based on the type. The 4 most common recognized forms of osteogenesis imperfecta are caused by abnormal structure of Type 1 collagen. None of these forms causes retinal hemorrhage or subdural hematomas, which distinguishes osteogenesis imperfecta from abuse.

Osteogenesis Imperfecta Type 1

Osteogenesis imperfecta Type 1 is an AD disease that is also known as "brittle bone disease." It is the mildest and most common type of osteogenesis imperfecta, caused by a decrease in synthesis of Type 1 collagen. Common characteristics include:

↑synthesis of type I collagen

- Multiple fractures (Most occur before puberty and mimic child abuse.)
- Blue sclerae
- Delayed fontanelle closure
- Hyperextensible joints
- Hearing loss
- Decreased stature (usually low normal or near normal)
- Dentinogenesis imperfecta: a disorder of tooth development with discolored, weak teeth

Fractures rarely occur at birth but are frequent in childhood, especially with even minor trauma. By adolescence, fracture frequency diminishes. X-rays show mild osteopenia of the long bones and wormian bones (multiple small bones found in the cranial sutures). Other associated manifestations of scoliosis and hearing loss appear in the patient's 20s and 30s.

Osteogenesis Imperfecta Type 2

Osteogenesis imperfecta Type 2, the most severe form, results in death during the newborn period due to respiratory insufficiency. These children have numerous fractures and severe bone deformity. The skull is very soft, and the limbs are short and bowed. X-ray shows long bones with a "crumpled appearance," and the ribs are beaded due to callus formation. Almost all cases are due to *de novo* AD mutation of the *COL1A1* gene, which does not allow normal formation of Type 1 collagen.

Osteogenesis Imperfecta Type 3

Osteogenesis imperfecta Type 3 presents in the newborn with numerous fractures. This is also called the "progressively deforming" type. Short stature is severe, and many cannot ambulate because they can't bear their own weight. Blue sclerae occur at birth but lighten with age—unlike those in Type 1, which stay dark blue. Most cases are due to a point mutation of the *COL1A1* gene that is similar to the Type 2 mutation. Neurologic complications are most common with Type 3, including hydrocephalus and basilar skull invagination.

Osteogenesis Imperfecta Type 4 →tibial bowing

Osteogenesis imperfecta Type 4 is a milder form, like Type 1. The sclerae are typically white or near-white. Fontanelle closure is delayed, and fractures are often present at birth. These individuals have shorter-than-average stature. Tibial bowing is the hallmark of Type 4. This type is due to AD collagen 1 mutations or due to AR mutations in genes that assist in collagen processing.

Note: The nomenclature continues to evolve for these 4 OI types. It is difficult to predict how quickly the terms make it into standard exam questions. These types of OI are now referred to as follows:

- OI Type 1: classic nondeforming OI with blue sclerae
- OI Type 2: perinatally lethal OI
- OI Type 3: progressively deforming OI
- OI Type 4: common variable OI with normal sclerae

CONNECTIVE TISSUE DISORDERS

Marfan Syndrome

Marfan syndrome is an AD disorder that affects 1/5,000 individuals. Boys and girls are affected equally. The affected organ systems include the eyes, circulatory system, skeleton, skin, lungs, and dura. Most deaths occur due to cardiovascular complications, namely aortic root dilatation and rupture.

The major criteria in Table 22-1 and the scoring system in Table 22-2 on page 22-22 are frequently the main clinical clues in a patient with Marfan syndrome. Look for the child with tall stature, high-arched palate, upward lens dislocation, joint hypermobility (Image 22-12), pectus carinatum or pectus excavatum (Image 22-13), spontaneous pneumothorax, and mitral valve prolapse.

Diagnosis is made by clinical findings known as the **Ghent criteria.** Diagnosis is made if there are any 2 of the following major criteria:

1) Ectopia lentis
2) Aortic dilation or dissection
3) Family history

If there is only 1 major finding, then either a mutation in the *FBN1* gene (encodes the protein fibrillin-1) or ≥ 7 (out of 20) systemic points are required to make the diagnosis. The systemic points include the wrist and thumb signs, chest wall deformity, scoliosis, myopia, pneumothorax, and striae.

Always rule out homocystinuria, which has many features similar to Marfan syndrome but carries a significant risk of stroke and other embolic events and has a much different treatment strategy. Homocystinuria features intellectual disability and a downwardly dislocated lens (in Marfan syndrome the lens dislocates upward).

Because cardiovascular complications are the most serious, annual or semiannual echocardiograms to monitor aortic root diameter are the norm. Antihypertensives are used to treat and prevent aortic root dilatation. Evidence for the best medical management (beta-blocker and/or angiotensin receptor blocker) is ongoing, with prospective trials demonstrating that combination therapy offers better protection against aortic root enlargement than single drugs alone. Individuals should avoid weightlifting and strenuous exercise, but regular aerobic exercise is important for heart health (as it is for everyone).

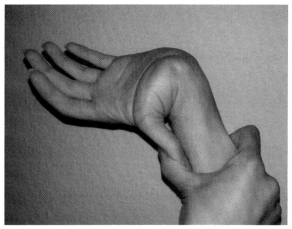

Image 22-12: Marfan syndrome, joint hypermobility

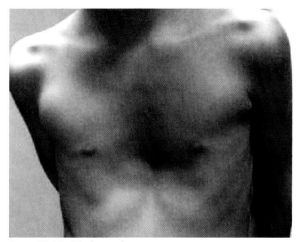

Image 22-13: Marfan syndrome, pectus excavatum

Table 22-1: Revised Ghent Criteria for Marfan Syndrome	
Negative Family History Plus One of the Following Combinations	**Positive Family History in One of the Following Combinations**
Ao (Z ≥ 2) + EL	FHx MFS + EL
Ao (Z ≥ 2) + *FBN1*	FHx MFS + Syst ≥ 7
Ao (Z ≥ 2) + Syst ≥ 7	FHx MFS + Ao (Z ≥ 2 over 20 years old) or FHx MFS + Ao (Z ≥ 3 under 20 years old)
EL + *FBN1* + Ao	FHx MFS + *FBN1*

Major Criteria:
• Ao, aortic dilation or dissection
• EL, ectopia lentis
• *FBN1* mutation
• Syst, systemic features (see Table 22-2 on page 22-22)
• FHx MFS, family history of Marfan syndrome
Z = z-score, which indicates how many standard deviations a data point is from the mean

Points	Features		Points	Features
	**Table 22-2: Scoring System for Systemic Features in Marfan Syndrome**			
3	Wrist and thumb signs	or	1	Wrist or thumb signs
2	Pectus carinatum	or	1	Pectus excavatum or chest asymmetry
2	Hindfoot deformity	or	1	Plain pes planus
2	Pneumothorax			
2	Dural ectasia			
2	Protrusio acetabuli			
1	Skin striae			
1	Myopia > 3 diopters			
1	Mitral valve prolapse			
1	Scoliosis or thoracolumbar kyphosis			
1	Reduced elbow extension			
1	All 3 of the following features: • Reduced upper-to-lower segment ratio • Increased arm span to height ratio (≥ 1.05) • No severe scoliosis			
1	Facial features (≥ 3): • Dolichocephaly • Enophthalmos • Down-slanting palpebral fissures • Malar hypoplasia • Retrognathia			
	**Total Score ≥ 7 indicates systemic involvement**			

Pregnancy greatly increases the risk of accelerated aortic dilatation in women with Marfan syndrome, and pregnant women require extremely close monitoring.

Ehlers-Danlos Syndromes

Ehlers-Danlos syndromes are a group of AD, connective tissue disorders that generally include hyperextensible skin, hypermobile joints, easy bruising, and dystrophic scarring. There are 6 major variants, but the classic type is the one typically found on exams.

The skin findings are classic. Know! Some describe the skin's texture as "wet chamois," a "fine sponge," or "doughy." "Extra" skin is common over the hands, feet, and stomach. The skin is very stretchy and returns to its normal configuration on release, much like a rubber band. The skin is unusually fragile and can split with the slightest trauma, especially at the shins, knees, elbows, and chin. Skin tears generally do not bleed a lot and have a gaping "fish-mouth" appearance. Scarring is abnormal, and scars that appear are typically thin and shiny. Increased bruising occurs, especially in children, as does bleeding from the gums after toothbrushing. All coagulation tests (including PT, PTT, and bleeding time) are normal, except for capillary fragility testing. Wrinkled palms and soles are common, as are pseudotumors at the heels, elbows, and knees from abnormal scarring.

Joint hypermobility is common but does not occur in certain types of Ehlers-Danlos syndromes. Both large and small joints can be involved. Dislocations or subluxations can occur and can be present at birth. Knees and elbows can be extended past 180°, and the fingers can be extended past 90°. Joint mobility decreases with increasing age, and adults can develop arthritis or chronic joint pain.

Mitral valve prolapse and proximal aortic dilatation occur; screen for these with echocardiogram, CT, or MRI.

Aim treatment at prevention with the use of shin guards, high-topped boots, and kneepads. Forbid physical contact sports.

NEUROCUTANEOUS SYNDROMES

Neurofibromatosis Type 1

Neurofibromatosis Type 1 (NF1; formerly known as von Recklinghausen disease) is the most common neurocutaneous disease and affects about 1/3,000 individuals. The most common features are café-au-lait spots and benign cutaneous neurofibromas. Specific diagnosis requires 2 of the 7 criteria. See Table 22-3 for a list of the clinical criteria. Most children meet formal clinical criteria by 10 years of age.

Table 22-3: Clinical Criteria for Neurofibromatosis Type 1
≥ 6 café-au-lait spots of ≥ 5 mm in greatest diameter in prepubertal children and ≥ 15 mm in postpubertal children
≥ 2 neurofibromas of any type or ≥ 1 plexiform neurofibroma
Freckling in the axillary or inguinal areas
Optic glioma
≥ 2 Lisch nodules (iris hamartomas)
Sphenoid dysplasia or thinning of the long bone cortex, with or without pseudarthrosis
1st degree relative (parent, sibling, child) with neurofibromatosis Type 1

Café-au-lait spots (Image 22-14) ordinarily appear in the first 2 years of life, but do not forget that these can also appear with other syndromes, such as McCune-Albright and Russell-Silver syndromes. Axillary freckles appear by adolescence in 75% of cases (Image 22-15). Lisch nodules (benign iris hamartomas) are identified by slit-lamp exam in about 75% of prepubescent children. Optic pathway gliomas occur in 15% of children < 6 years old and sometimes cause visual loss or precocious puberty. Always refer to an ophthalmologist if you suspect NF1.

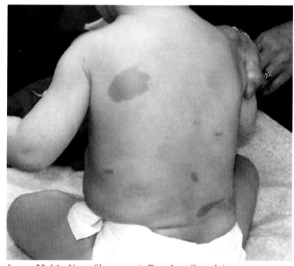

Image 22-14: Neurofibromatosis Type 1, café-au-lait spots

What are **neurofibromas**? They are benign, peripheral nerve sheath tumors that are a collection of Schwann-like cells, fibroblasts, and extracellular matrix. The cutaneous neurofibromas appear at puberty, whereas the plexiform neurofibromas are congenital. Cutaneous neurofibromas can cause discomfort and are cosmetically bothersome, but plexiform neurofibromas have a 10% risk of malignant transformation into malignant peripheral nerve sheath tumors.

Focal areas of T2-weighted signal intensity (FASI) on brain MRI were previously described as unidentified bright objects (UBOs). FASI are believed to represent areas of abnormal myelination. They are most often located in the basal ganglia, along the optic tracts, and in the brainstem, thalamus, and/or cerebellum. They are not associated with a mass effect, malignant potential, or contrast enhancement. Beginning in late adolescence, FASI begin to disappear and are generally absent by 30 years of age.

Bony changes can occur in early childhood years and include sphenoid wing dysplasia, long bone bowing (most commonly of the tibia), and dysplastic scoliosis.

About 50% of affected children have learning disorders, ADHD, and speech disorders. Other features to look for include short stature, macrocephaly, hypertension, constipation, and headaches.

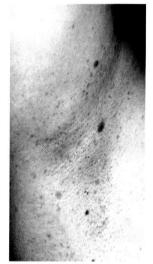

Image 22-15: Axillary freckles

50% of cases are sporadic or *de novo* AD mutations. The phenotypic expression is quite variable from one affected individual to another, even among family members. The *NF1* gene encodes the protein neurofibromin and maps to chromosome 17.

Neurofibromatosis Type 2

Neurofibromatosis Type 2 (NF2) is also an AD disorder. It is characterized by the presence of bilateral vestibular schwannomas (acoustic neuromas). NF1 and NF2 are very distinct and different disorders, with no commonality regarding genetic factors and essentially no clinical overlap. Type 2 is less common than Type 1 and has an incidence of about 1/30,000. The mean age for clinical presentation is 30 years, but children are frequently diagnosed with the disorder. The vestibular schwannomas cause sensorineural hearing loss, tinnitus, imbalance, and facial weakness. Other CNS tumors occur in about 50% of cases and include intracranial meningiomas, spinal schwannomas, cranial nerve schwannomas (most commonly involving CN 5), and ependymomas. Lens opacities or cataracts occur as one of the 1st signs and can be used for screening in children.

Diagnostic criteria: the presence of either bilateral acoustic neuromas alone or a 1st degree relative with NF2 and either unilateral acoustic neuroma, 2 of the previously mentioned CNS tumors, or lenticular opacity. For relatives at risk, do MRI screening to detect vestibular schwannomas small enough to be surgically removed, thereby preserving hearing.

Tuberous Sclerosis

Tuberous sclerosis is an AD disorder that affects 1/6,000 people. There are many features of tuberous sclerosis, but the classic findings are:

- Hypopigmented macules (a.k.a. ash-leaf spots)—the most common presentation in ~ 90% of cases (Image 22-16)
- Shagreen patches—oval-shaped nevoid plaque (skin-colored or occasionally pigmented, smooth or crinkled), appearing on the trunk or lower back

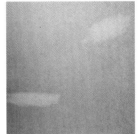

Image 22-16: Hypopigmented macules (a.k.a. ash-leaf spots)

- Facial angiofibromas
- Forehead plaques
- Ungual (nail) and gingival fibromas
- Cortical tubers and subependymal nodules
- Renal angiomyolipomas or renal cysts
- Rhabdomyomas
- Polycystic kidney disease associated with *TSC2* (on chromosome 16)

Tuberous sclerosis has wide variability, both between and within families, much like the variability seen with NF1. Some of the features found in early childhood disappear by adulthood, making diagnosis more difficult. For example, nearly 50% of infants have multiple cardiac rhabdomyomas, but these regress over time. Another associated complication is infantile spasms, which, if they occur, indicate a 50% chance that tuberous sclerosis is present. The hypopigmented macules usually enhance with a Wood's lamp, and this can be helpful in diagnosis.

Tuberous sclerosis is caused by mutations in *TSC1* (found on chromosome 9) or *TSC2* (found on chromosome 16).

The focus of clinical management is controlling seizures and cardiac arrhythmias associated with the cardiac rhabdomyomas. Treat infantile spasms with vigabatrin. Good seizure control improves intellectual outcome.

FAMILIAL CANCER SYNDROMES

Overview

Key features of cancer genetics:

- Genes involved in familial cancer syndromes are also commonly involved in sporadic tumors.

- Gene types involved in oncogenesis include protooncogenes, tumor suppressor genes, and genes involved in DNA repair, apoptosis, and genomic integrity.

Features of cancer syndromes:

- Family history: multiple members in family
- Early age of onset
- Bilateral/Multifocal
- Clustering of specific types
  ◦ Breast and ovarian
  ◦ Retinoblastoma and osteosarcoma
- Multiple tumor types in same person
- Unusual type

Breast and Ovarian Cancer

BRCA1, the first identified breast cancer gene, is localized to chromosome 17q21. It is present in 5% of women and indicates a 50–85% lifetime risk of developing breast cancer, with a 50% chance of occurrence before 50 years of age. This compares to a 12% lifetime risk in the general population. Male breast cancer is rare, but many men with breast cancer carry *BRCA* mutations.

BRCA also is associated with up to a 40% lifetime risk of developing ovarian cancer—and accounts for most patients with familial ovarian cancer, which compares to a 1.5% lifetime risk in the general population. *BRCA1* also increases the risk of colorectal and prostate cancer. *BRCA2* (13q12–13) is associated with a similarly high risk of breast cancer and a 10–20% risk of ovarian cancer. *BRCA2* also increases the risk of melanoma, pancreatic cancer, and prostate cancer. Although only about 5% of breast cancer cases are attributable to a specific genetic abnormality, together the alterations of the *BRCA1* and *BRCA2* genes account for 30–50% of all inherited breast cancer. In patients with a *BRCA* mutation, bilateral mastectomies decrease the incidence of breast cancer by up to 90%. Bilateral oophorectomies decrease the risk of ovarian cancer by up to 90% and can decrease the risk of breast cancer for premenopausal women.

Familial Adenomatous Polyposis

Familial adenomatous polyposis is an AD disorder with a 100% risk of colon cancer (see Gastroenterology, Book 2).

Multiple Endocrine Neoplasia Syndromes

Multiple endocrine neoplasia (MEN) syndromes are a group of rare genetic disorders in which two or more endocrine glands develop tumors or grow excessively. Symptoms vary depending on the glands involved. (See Hyperparathyroidism in Endocrinology, Book 3).

von Hippel-Lindau Syndrome

von Hippel-Lindau (VHL) syndrome is a highly penetrant, AD multisystem cancer disorder that presents with various benign and malignant tumors of the eyes, CNS, kidneys, pancreas, adrenal glands, and reproductive glands. It occurs in about 1/36,000 live births.

It is caused by a mutation in the *VHL* tumor suppressor gene on chromosome 3. Molecular genetic testing of the *VHL* gene detects mutations in nearly 100% of patients.

Diagnosis depends on:

- Finding ≥ 2 hemangioblastomas in the CNS (particularly cerebellum)or retina

or

- Finding 1 single hemangioblastoma plus 1 of the following:
  ◦ Pheochromocytoma
  ◦ Endolymphatic sac tumors
  ◦ Cysts in the kidney/pancreas
  ◦ Renal cell carcinoma
  ◦ Cystadenomas and neuroendocrine tumors of the pancreas

or

- Having a 1st degree relative with VHL and any 1 manifestation listed above

The most classic presentation is a cerebellar hemangioblastoma in adolescence or a retinal angioma by 10 years of age. Renal cysts are common. Renal cell carcinoma presents in the patient's 40s and is the leading cause of mortality in VHL, occurring in nearly 40% of patients.

PTEN Hamartoma Tumor Syndrome

The *PTEN* hamartoma tumor syndrome (PHTS) includes Cowden syndrome (CS) and Bannayan-Riley-Ruvalcaba syndrome (BRRS).

CS is a rare syndrome (1/200,000 in general population) that includes a high risk of benign and malignant hamartomas of the thyroid, breast, and endometrium. Affected patients typically have macrocephaly. Facial papules and trichilemmomas are common. These are often the first presentation of the disease, leading to a late diagnosis—usually in the patient's late 20s. Lifetime risk of cancer:

- Breast cancer—25–50%; most often diagnosed at 38–46 years of age
- Thyroid cancer—10%; typically follicular, rarely papillary, but never medullary thyroid cancer
- Endometrial cancer—approaches 5–10%

BRRS, in contrast to CS, is usually diagnosed around 5 years of age. These patients have macrocephaly, pigmented macules of the glans penis, lipomas, and nonmalignant intestinal hamartomatous polyposis (which can cause obstruction).

The diagnosis of PHTS is made only when a *PTEN* mutation is identified. About 85% of patients diagnosed with CS and 65% of patients diagnosed with BRRS have a detectable *PTEN* gene mutation.

Two-Hit Origin of Cancer

Retinoblastoma is a good model of the "two-hit origin of cancer."

Facts about two-hit origin of cancer:

- Basis for both hereditary and sporadic cancers.
- Involves loss of tumor suppressor function.
- Retinoblastoma as the model; loss of both copies of the *RB1* gene leads to tumor.
  ◦ Sporadic cases—2 somatic mutations in same cell.
  ◦ Hereditary cases—inherited (germline) mutation (1st hit) and 2nd somatic mutation in same cell (2nd hit). Remember that the germline mutation is present in all the patient's cells, so these individuals are at a higher risk of developing bilateral or multifocal retinoblastoma, as well as other tumors (e.g., osteosarcomas), later in life.
- Loss of heterozygosity.
  ◦ Molecular evidence for the existence of a tumor suppressor gene.
  ◦ Involves analysis of DNA polymorphisms near tumor suppressor genes.
  ◦ Test is done on tumor tissue.

CONGENITAL ANOMALY SYNDROMES

Starting on the next page, Table 22-4 describes some congenital anomaly syndromes. Syndromes shown with a pink background are frequently fodder for exams. Review these well—especially if you are taking the initial certification exam.

**THE MEDSTUDY HUB:
YOUR GUIDELINES AND
REVIEW ARTICLES RESOURCE**

For both the review articles and current Pediatrics practice guidelines, visit the MedStudy Hub at

medstudy.com/hub

The Hub contains the only online consolidated list of all Pediatrics guidelines! Guidelines on the Hub are continually updated and linked to the published source. MedStudy maintains the Hub as a free online resource, available to all physicians.

GENETICS

Table 22-4: Some Important Congenital Anomaly Syndromes to Know			
Category	**Syndrome**	**Signs and Symptoms**	**Inheritance Pattern/ Gene Mutation**
Craniofacial Syndromes	Treacher-Collins syndrome	Cleft palate, malar hypoplasia, micrognathia, lower eyelid missing medial lower lid lashes, hearing loss, ear anomalies	AD 100% *TCOF1* mut.
	Waardenburg syndrome I	Partial albinism, white forelock, premature graying, telecanthus (lateral displacement of inner canthi of eyes), heterochromia of iris, cleft lip/palate, cochlear deafness, occasional absent vagina, occasional Hirschsprung disease	AD > 90% *PAX3* mut.
	Stickler syndrome	Pierre Robin sequence (micrognathia, cleft palate, glossoptosis [dorsal displacement of the tongue], airway obstruction, feeding difficulty), high myopia, retinal detachment, midface hypoplasia	AD 70–80% *COL2A1* mut. 10–20% *COL1A1* mut. Some forms are AR and due to other genes.
	Crouzon syndrome	Craniosynostosis with turricephaly, proptosis, hypertelorism, strabismus, maxillary hypoplasia	AD 100% *FGFR2* mut.
	Apert syndrome	Craniosynostosis, brachycephaly, acrocephaly, hypertelorism, proptosis, strabismus, maxillary hypoplasia, narrow palate ("cathedral ceiling"), syndactyly, broad thumbs (most commonly with mitten-hand deformity: complete fusion of 2, 3, or 4 fingers with common nail bed ["single nail"])	AD 100% *FGFR2* mut.
	Cleidocranial dysostosis	Brachycephaly, frontal bossing, wormian bones (abnormal intrasutural bones), delayed eruption of deciduous and permanent teeth, supernumerary and fused teeth, hypoplastic/absent clavicles, joint laxity	AD 60–70% *RUNX2* mut.
Chromosome Instability Syndromes	Ataxia-telangiectasia	Ataxia, telangiectasia, especially of sclera, frequent infections, malignancies, growth failure, worsening CNS function, carriers are at an increased risk of breast cancer	AR > 95% *ATM* mut.
	Bloom syndrome	Intrauterine growth restriction (IUGR), microcephaly, malar hypoplasia, facial telangiectasia, malignancies	AR > 90% *RECQL3* mut.
	Fanconi anemia	Pancytopenia, hypoplastic thumb and radius, hyperpigmentation, abnormal facial features	AR (multiple genes)
	Xeroderma pigmentosa	Photosensitivity, skin atrophy, pigmentary changes, malignancies	AR (multiple genes)
Syndromes with Short Stature	Noonan syndrome	Short stature, congenital heart defects (commonly pulmonary valve stenosis), pectus excavatum, webbed neck, low-set ears, hypertelorism, lymphedema, bleeding diathesis	AD ~ 50% *PTPN11* mut.
	Williams syndrome	Growth delay, intellectual disability, stellate iris, hypoplastic nails, periorbital fullness, anteverted nares, supravalvular aortic stenosis, friendly with "cocktail party personality" (i.e., very social)	7q11.23 microdeletion
	Cornelia de Lange syndrome	IUGR, microcephaly, hirsutism, down-turned mouth, heart defects, microbrachycephaly, micrognathia, low hairline, synophrys, long eyelashes, thin upper lip, low-set ears, micromelia (hands/feet) or phocomelia; 2,3 syndactyly of toes	AD > 50% have a gene mutation (*NIPBL*) Multiple other genes in the cohesion complex make up the rest.
	Dubowitz syndrome	IUGR, telecanthus, ptosis, eczema, hypotrichosis, behavioral and developmental disorders	AR (gene unknown)

Table 22-4: Some Important Congenital Anomaly Syndromes to Know (Continued)			
Category	**Syndrome**	**Signs and Symptoms**	**Inheritance Pattern/ Gene Mutation**
Syndromes with Growth Abnormalities	Prader-Willi syndrome (paternal)	Severe hypotonia at birth, obesity (usually after 2 years of age), short stature, hypogonadism, mild intellectual disability, small hands and feet	15q11–13 deletion (paternal) in 70% of cases Maternal uniparental disomy in 25% of cases
	Angelman syndrome (maternal)	Jerky ataxic movements, microcephaly, characteristic gait, hypotonia, midface hypoplasia, prognathism, seizures, uncontrollable bouts of laughter, severe intellectual disability	15q11–13 deletion (maternal) in 70% of cases *UBE3A* mut. (maternal) in 11% of cases Paternal uniparental disomy in about 5% of cases
	Beckwith-Wiedemann syndrome	Large for gestational age (LGA), generalized overgrowth, macroglossia, ear lobe creases, posterior auricular pits, omphalocele, Wilms tumor, cryptorchidism, hemihypertrophy	AD 11p15.5 deletion Multiple gene muts. (*KCNQIOTI, H19, CKNIC*) Paternal uniparental disomy in about 20% of cases
	Sotos syndrome	LGA, macrocephaly, prominent forehead, hypertelorism, intellectual disability, large hands/feet	AD 80–90% *NSD1* mut. or 5q35 deletion
	Proteus syndrome	Macrodactyly, soft/connective tissue hypertrophy, hemihypertrophy, nevi, lipomas, lymphangiomata, hemangiomata, accelerated growth	Sporadic; due to somatic mosaicism for activating *AKT1* mutations
Syndromes with Limb Abnormalities	Möbius syndrome	Cranial nerve abnormalities, hypoplastic tongue and/or digits, limb deficiency, Poland anomaly (absence of the pectoralis major/minor muscles), ipsilateral breast hypoplasia (absence of 2−4 rib segments)	Sporadic
	Rubinstein-Taybi syndrome	Short stature and limbs, microcephaly, beaked nose, broad thumbs and great toes, congenital heart disease, intellectual disability	AD *CREBBP* mut. 30–50% Microdeletion (detected by FISH) ~ 10% *EP300* mut. 3–8%
Syndromes with Thumb/Radii Defects and Hematologic Abnormalities	Fanconi anemia	(See Chromosome Instability Syndromes, above.)	AR Multiple genes
	Diamond-Blackfan syndrome	Triphalangeal thumb, radial hypoplasia, hypoplastic anemia, congenital heart defects	AD Multiple genes
	Thrombocytopenia with absent radius (TAR) syndrome	Thrombocytopenia, absent radii, normal thumbs, petechiae	AR > 95% *RBMA8* deletions/ duplications ~ 3% *RBMA8* mut.
	Holt-Oram syndrome	Radial ray abnormalities (triphalangeal thumb), ASD and other congenital heart disease in 75% of individuals, no hematological anomalies	AD > 70% *TBX5* mut.

GENETICS

Category	Syndrome	Signs and Symptoms	Inheritance Pattern/ Gene Mutation
Syndromes with Severe Neurologic Manifestations	Sturge-Weber syndrome	Hemangioma in trigeminal nerve distribution, glaucoma, seizures, meningeal hemangiomata	Sporadic
	Rett syndrome	Most affected are females; apparently normal psychomotor development for ~ 6–18 months, followed by rapid regression in language and motor skills; repetitive, stereotypic hand movements replace purposeful hand use (hand wringing); autistic features; episodic apnea and/ or hyperpnea; gait ataxia; tremors; seizures; acquired microcephaly	X-linked dominant. Majority are female; rare in males (but more severe phenotype); almost all (99%) are new mutations. 80% *MeCP2* mut. 8% deletion/duplication
	Prader-Willi and Angelman syndromes	(See Syndromes with Growth Abnormalities, above.)	
	Meckel-Gruber syndrome	Encephalocele (occipital), microcephaly, poly-cystic (dysplastic) kidney, polydactyly, lethal	AR Multiple genes
	Miller-Dieker syndrome	Lissencephaly, microcephaly, micrognathia, ante-verted nares, vertical wrinkles of the forehead	80% *de novo* deletion 17p13.3 20% inherited translocation
	Walker-Warburg (**HARD + E**) syndrome	**H**ydrocephalus, **a**gyria (congenital lack of the convolutional pattern of the cerebral cortex), **r**etinal **d**ysplasia, **e**ncephalocele	AR Multiple genes
Metabolic Syndromes with Congenital Anomalies (Discussed in Metabolic Disorders, Book 5, and/or Endocrinology, Book 3)	Menkes disease	Progressive neurologic deterioration, sparse/bro-ken hair (pili torti), skeletal changes, decreased serum copper and ceruloplasmin	X-linked
	Wilson disease	Kayser-Fleischer rings, abnormal copper metabolism; neurological, liver, or psychological manifestations; low ceruloplasmin but elevated urine copper	AR
	Zellweger syndrome	Hypotonia, flat occiput, epicanthal folds, hepa-tomegaly, camptodactyly (flexion of one or both interphalangeal joints of one or more fingers, usually the little finger), cerebral defects, retinal lesions, renal cysts, peroxisomal defects	AR
	Glutaric acidemia Type II	Hepatomegaly, facial dysmorphism, renal cysts, GU anomalies	AR
	Smith-Lemli-Opitz syndrome	Short stature; microcephaly; ptosis, anteverted nares; syndactyly of toes 2,3; cryptorchidism; hypospadias; intellectual disability; cholesterol metabolism defect	AR
	Kallmann syndrome	Short stature, intellectual disability, hypogonado-tropic hypogonadism, anosmia	X-linked

Table 22-4: Some Important Congenital Anomaly Syndromes to Know (Continued)

Table 22-4: Some Important Congenital Anomaly Syndromes to Know (Continued)			
Category	**Syndrome**	**Signs and Symptoms**	**Inheritance Pattern/Gene Mutation**
Common Associations and Other Miscellaneous Syndromes	VATER/**VACTERL**	**V**ertebral defects, **a**nal atresia, **c**ongenital heart defect, **t**racheo**e**sophageal fistula, **r**enal malformations, **l**imb (radial) dysplasia	Sporadic
	CHARGE	**C**oloboma, congenital **h**eart defects, choanal **a**tresia, growth and intellectual **r**etardation, **G**U anomalies (hypogonadism), **e**ar anomaly, or hearing loss	AD *CHD7* mut.
	McCune-Albright syndrome	Multiple bony fibrous dysplasia, café-au-lait spots, precocious puberty	Sporadic
	Neurofibromatosis Type 1	Café-au-lait spots, axillary freckling, neurofibroma, plexiform neurofibroma, sphenoid bone dysplasia, malignancies (< 5%), optic glioma, Lisch nodules, learning disability, macrocephaly	AD *NF1* mut.
	MURCS	**Mü**llerian duct aplasia, **r**enal aplasia, **c**ervicothoracic **s**omite anomalies	Sporadic
	Opitz syndrome (G/BBB syndrome)	Hypertelorism, telecanthus, high nasal bridge, cleft lip/palate, hypospadias, laryngotracheoesophageal cleft	X-linked dominant/AD
	Alagille syndrome	Bile duct paucity with cholestasis, peripheral pulmonic stenosis, posterior embryotoxon, butterfly vertebrae, characteristic triangular-shaped facies with long nose, broad midnose, and pointed chin	AD 89% *JAG1* mut. 7% *JAG1* deletion (detected by FISH) 1–2% *NOTCH2* mut.

GENETICS

MedStudy

METABOLIC DISORDERS

SECTION EDITOR

Pamela Trapane, MD
Clinical Professor, Stead Family Department
 of Pediatrics
Program Director, Medical Genetics
 Residency Program
Medical Director, Division of Medical Genetics
University of Iowa Hospitals and Clinics
The Sahai Family Professor of Medical
 Education, Carver College of Medicine
Iowa City, IA

MEDICAL EDITOR

Lynn Bullock, MD
Colorado Springs, CO

REVIEWER

Reem Saadeh-Haddad, MD
Assistant Professor
Clinical Geneticist
Department of Pediatrics
MedStar Georgetown University Hospital
Washington, DC

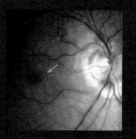

Table of Contents

METABOLIC DISORDERS

METABOLIC DISORDERS OVERVIEW

PREVIEW | REVIEW

- What are the 3 mechanisms that typically cause metabolic disorders?
- How are most inborn errors of metabolism inherited?
- Mitochondrial disorders are inherited from which parent?

METABOLISM REVIEW

Figure 23-1 presents an overview of the metabolic processes discussed in this section. Metabolism encompasses all the enzyme-catalyzed reactions that occur in our body. These reactions can be considered either catabolic or anabolic reactions. **Catabolism** is the breaking down of proteins, carbohydrates, and fats into simple molecules (amino acids, simple carbs, and fatty acids).

These simple molecules can be used for **anabolic** processes, e.g., making required tissue proteins and fats, and for glycogenesis and gluconeogenesis.

These same simple molecules can alternately be further catabolized to make energy needed for anabolic processes.

These interrelated metabolic processes consist of **protein**, **carbohydrate**, and **fat** metabolism.

A genetic defect causing a problem in an enzyme in a metabolic pathway is called an inborn error of metabolism (IEM).

CAUSES OF IEMs

Most IEMs result from a single gene defect causing deficiency in the production or function of a single enzyme or cofactor. Names for the IEMs typically reflect the primary affected metabolite.

IEM signs and symptoms are caused by the resulting upstream or accessory pathway buildup of toxic product or by the insufficient production of a required metabolite. Some disorders combine these effects.

There are many IEMs. Before we jump into them, let's give some structure and priority to what you will be reviewing.

Except for a review of newborn screening (NBS) at the end, the rest of the section is broken up into 3 main topics based on the general mechanism of the defect:

Intoxications (starting on page 23-3) are due to toxic buildup upstream of the affected enzyme. These occur mainly in the protein catabolism pathway, although there

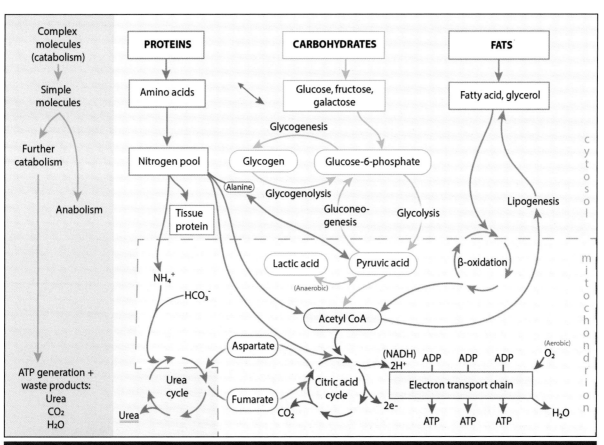

Figure 23-1: Metabolism Summary

are some in the carbohydrate pathway (galactose and fructose disorders).

Energy utilization defects (starting on page 23-12) cause problems with converting food into energy or problems with utilizing normal sources of stored energy (i.e., glycogen and fat). So, it makes sense that these disorders involve:

- defects in fatty acid oxidation,
- glycogen storage diseases, and
- defects in mitochondrial DNA mutations.

The last one makes sense if you remember that all chemical energy production required by the cell occurs in the mitochondria. In fact, virtually all the processes below the dashed line in Figure 23-1 on page 23-1 occur within the mitochondria (except some urea cycle reactions occur in the cytosol).

Complex-molecule defects (starting on page 23-20) occur when the deficiency in a particular enzyme results in abnormal or unregulated synthesis of complex molecules. These complex molecules include mucopolysaccharides, mucolipids, glycoproteins, and sphingolipids. There are also disorders of peroxisomes, mineral absorption and metabolism, porphyrin production (porphyrias), purine metabolism, and lipoproteins and lipids.

The following conditions are the must-know topics in this section. Go circle these now!

Intoxications:

- Disorders of amino acid metabolism
  - Classic phenylketonuria (PKU; page 23-5)
  - Maple syrup urine disease (MSUD; page 23-6)
  - Glutaric acidemia Type 1 (page 23-7)
  - Homocystinuria (page 23-7)
- Urea cycle disorders (page 23-7)
  - Carbamoyl phosphate synthetase 1 (CPS1) deficiency
  - Ornithine transcarbamylase (OTC) deficiency
- Organic acidemias
  - Isovaleric acidemia (page 23-9)
- Sugar intolerances
  - Galactosemia (page 23-10)
  - Hereditary fructose intolerance (aldolase B deficiency; page 23-11)

Energy utilization defects:

- Defects in fat metabolism
  - Medium-chain acyl-coenzyme A (CoA) dehydrogenase (MCAD) deficiency (page 23-15)
- Glycogen storage diseases (GSDs; the most prevalent ones are AR)
  - Type 1 GSD (von Gierke disease; page 23-15)
  - Type 2 GSD (Pompe disease; page 23-17)

Complex-molecule defects:

- Mucopolysaccharidoses (MPS; all AR except MPS Type 2 = X-linked recessive)
  - MPS Type 1 (Hurler syndrome; page 23-21)
  - MPS Type 2 (Hunter syndrome; page 23-21)
- Sphingolipidoses
  - Gaucher disease (page 23-23)
  - Niemann-Pick disease (page 23-24)
  - Tay-Sachs disease (page 23-25)
  - Fabry disease (page 23-25)
- Peroxisomal disorders
  - Zellweger syndrome (page 23-26)
- Disorders of minerals
  - Menkes disease (a.k.a. kinky hair disease; page 23-26)
- Purine disorders
  - Lesch-Nyhan disease (page 23-29)

Notice that the previous disorders are all autosomal recessive (AR) except MPS Type 2.

INHERITANCE PATTERNS

When faced with a critically ill child, it is crucial to identify an IEM vs. infection vs. nutritional disorder vs. exogenous intoxication. However, most of us find this extremely challenging. In the early 1900s, when inborn errors of metabolism were first described by Archibald Garrod, there were only 4 diagnoses. Today, there are > 400!

Here are a few orienting points on inheritance of IEMs:

- Most IEMs have autosomal recessive inheritance.
- Next most common are those that are X-linked.
- Only a few are autosomal dominant (AD) disorders.
- Many of the described diseases are caused by mutations in the mitochondrial genome.

IEMs are rare, with most occurring in < 1/15,000 births, but altogether they account for ~ 20% of diseases in sick, full-term newborns!

Certain populations have a markedly higher prevalence of individual disorders. If an exam question specifically mentions a patient's ethnicity or genetic background, it is probably a clue to consider an IEM! Example: Compared with the general population, Ashkenazi Jews are more typically carriers of gene mutations causing Tay-Sachs disease or Type 1 Gaucher disease. The incidence of Type 1 Gaucher disease is nearly 1/900 in the Ashkenazi population (vs. 1/40,000 in the non-Jewish population). The incidence of Tay-Sachs disease is 1/4,000 in the Ashkenazi population vs. 1/100,000 in the non-Ashkenazi population.

For discussion of inheritance types, please refer to Genetics, Book 5. We briefly discuss mitochondrial inheritance now due to its relevance and complexity.

MITOCHONDRIAL INHERITANCE

As mentioned, mitochondria supply the chemical energy for the cell. It might surprise you that each cell contains from hundreds to ~ 2,000 mitochondria!

Mitochondria are coded for by nuclear genes from both parents, but, unlike any other animal organelle, mitochondria contain their own genome, termed mitochondrial DNA (mtDNA). Disorders in mitochondria can arise from mutations of nuclear DNA (usually AR), but they can also arise from a defect in the mtDNA, which comes solely from the mother. This mtDNA is a circular DNA strand with only 37 genes. Most are related to the oxidative phosphorylation (in the electron transport chain). A few genes are involved with forming tissue proteins.

Due to this maternal transmission pattern, women who have a genetic mutation in the mitochondria pass it to all their children, whereas men never pass it on.

Heteroplasmy describes mitochondria having > 1 genome. Each mitochondrion contains 2–10 copies of the mtDNA. But this is only the start! Because of the random nature of distributing these strands during cell division and because the mitochondria themselves are randomly distributed during cell division, we can end up with cells with a wide variation in the number of affected mitochondria. For this same reason, each oocyte (egg) from the mother has varying numbers of affected mitochondria. And, getting to the point of this paragraph, this is why, even though all of the mother's children may inherit the mtDNA defect, the expression can vary widely between siblings. This variability in expression can make family history unreliable.

IEM — INTOXICATIONS

PREVIEW | REVIEW

- Disorders of intoxication present in what 3 forms?

- When should you suspect an IEM in an infant with acute encephalopathy? Why are these infants generally normal at birth?

- How does chronic encephalopathy present?

- What are the most useful diagnostic tests for disorders of amino acid metabolism?

- What is PKU?

- How do patients with PKU present?

- Which subset of children with hyperphenylalaninemia presents with severe neurologic disease, even with dietary treatment that maintains normal phenylalanine levels? What is the treatment for these children, since dietary restriction does not work?

- What is tyrosinemia?

- Which disease is NTBC used to treat?

- What is alkaptonuria? What happens to the urine in children with this disorder?

- Describe the symptoms of MSUD.

- Name the 3 branched-chain amino acids.

- How do you diagnose MSUD?

- Differentiate the lens findings in Marfan syndrome vs. homocystinuria.

- What molecule is the problem in all urea cycle disorders?

- How are almost all urea cycle disorders inherited? Which one is not inherited in this manner? How is it inherited?

- You are presented with an infant with elevated ammonia, no liver abnormalities, and no ketoacidosis. Which type of defect should you consider?

- What is the importance of a citrulline level?

- What is the importance of ordering a urinary orotic acid level?

- An infant with encephalopathy presents with a smell of sweaty feet. What is a possible diagnosis?

- How does PA present in early infancy?

- What is the triad of symptoms associated with carboxylase deficiency?

- Describe galactosemia.

- What is a common screening test for galactosemia?

- What is the only manifestation of galactokinase deficiency?

- What is the significance of fructokinase deficiency?

- How might aldolase B deficiency present?

INTOXICATION OVERVIEW

IEM intoxications are caused by upstream or accessory pathway buildup of toxic chemicals (see Table 23-1 on page 23-4):

1) Disorders of **amino acid metabolism**
2) **Urea cycle** disorders
3) **Organic acidemias**
4) **Sugar intolerance**

We'll go over these one by one, but first, let's look at how IEM intoxications present.

Table 23-1: IEMs — Intoxications

Disorder	Initial Laboratory Testing
Amino acid disorders (e.g., MSUD)	Plasma amino and urine organic acids High anion gap metabolic acidosis with ketonuria
Urea cycle defects (e.g., OTC deficiency)	Plasma ammonia markedly increased Minimal metabolic acidosis Respiratory alkalosis
Organic acidemias (e.g., isovaleric acidemia)	High anion gap metabolic acidosis with ketonuria Plasma ammonia mildly to moderately increased Hypoglycemia Increased glycine Abnormal urine organic acid Plasma amino acids
Sugar intolerances (e.g., galactosemia, fructose)	Newborn screening enzymatic testing Urine organic acids Liver enzyme analysis

INTOXICATION PRESENTATIONS

Overview

There are many causes of IEM intoxications, but their clinical presentations can be characterized as:

• acute encephalopathy,
• chronic encephalopathy, or
• acid-base disturbances.

Acute Encephalopathy

Suspect IEM intoxication if acute encephalopathy occurs without warning in previously normal neonates or young infants—and progresses rapidly.

Symptoms can include:

• Unexplained seizures
• Coma
• Lethargy
• Hypertonia
• Hypotonia

Because of the acute onset, focal neurologic deficits are usually not present.

Most of these infants are normal at birth, following uneventful pregnancies. However, once the infant disengages from the maternal circulation, extra substrates start to build up due to the infant's own metabolic impairment, and large increases in brain-diffusible molecules (i.e., small molecules such as glucose, ammonia, and amino and organic acids) cause toxic effects on the brain.

After a symptom-free interval, the infant begins to have feeding problems, lethargy, irritability, and vomiting. The toxic effect is usually much more pronounced when the infant/child is under stress or in an increased catabolic state (such as with viral/bacterial illness or fasting), or, in some types, with an increase in protein ingestion.

Generally, 4 categories of "small-molecule defects" present with acute encephalopathy. Table 23-1 outlines key things to look for in exam questions. We discuss each in more detail later in this section.

Once you identify these infants, work quickly to prevent further damage. The key strategy in the acute phase is to:

1) stop catabolism by providing adequate calories and
2) dilute toxins and promote excretion with generous hydration.

Intravenous fluids (typically 10% dextrose in 0.45% saline, with 20 mEq/L of potassium [if urine output is adequate]) are run at 1.5× maintenance—or sometimes even faster. Sodium bicarbonate is used only if the serum bicarbonate level is < 15 mEq/L—and then only with great care. Perform hemodialysis or hemofiltration in severe cases to remove the toxic small molecules. Once you identify the specific problem, proceed with appropriate therapy (i.e., dietary restriction, disease-specific medications).

Chronic Encephalopathy

Chronic encephalopathy presents in a slowly progressive manner as toxic metabolites build up. The symptoms are not immediately life-threatening; however, this usually changes over time as more and more damage occurs.

The most common examples are **PKU** and **homocystinuria**. Both cause symptoms after a period of exposure. With PKU, the buildup of phenylalanine eventually kills brain cells, causing loss of developmental milestones and, eventually, permanent brain damage. Homocystinuria causes problems after exposure to high levels of homocysteine and subsequent damage to the blood vessels, resulting in clots and stroke.

Acid-Base Disturbances

Overview

IEM intoxications can present as an acid-base disturbance. Acid-base abnormalities are generally due to either accumulation of fixed anions or loss of bicarbonate (which is almost always due to renal tubular dysfunction).

Accumulation of Fixed Anions

In the case of accumulation of fixed anions, the plasma chloride concentration is normal and the anion gap is increased (> 10 mEq/L). These disorders become more pronounced with increased catabolic states, such as after surgery, during illness, or with dietary changes involving increased protein intake. The child usually presents with feeding difficulties and failure to thrive (FTT). This category of disease includes organic acidurias, ketoacidosis, and lactic acidosis +/– pyruvate elevations.

Loss of Bicarbonate

Kidney injury results in renal loss of bicarbonate. Only a few metabolic disorders involve proximal renal tubular dysfunction with bicarbonate loss.

DISORDERS OF AMINO ACID METABOLISM

Overview

The most valuable diagnostic tests for amino acid metabolism disorders are examination of plasma amino acids and urine organic acids. You need to do both. These disorders are typically single-gene deficiencies. Systemic manifestations are typical because of the large amount of small-molecule metabolites in the circulation, frequently resulting in intellectual disability. These disorders fall into the intoxication classification of disorders. Presentation can be either acute or chronic, depending on the disorder.

Phenylalanine-Tyrosine Disorders

Classic Phenylketonuria (PKU)

PKU is an AR disorder in which phenylalanine cannot be converted to tyrosine. The enzyme defect is in phenylalanine hydroxylase (PAH). This results in high levels of phenylalanine (Phe) in the blood and large amounts of phenylpyruvic acid in the urine. PKU occurs in 1/10,000 to 1/20,000 births.

Clinical findings vary, depending on when treatment is initiated and on the degree of metabolic control. Phe in high amounts is toxic to the CNS. Those who remain untreated have severe intellectual disability with IQs of < 30. The damage becomes irreversible by 8 weeks of age. PKU infants appear normal at birth, but early symptoms occur in > 50% of those affected. The most common presentations in infants include vomiting, irritability, an eczematoid rash, and a peculiar odor— "mousy," "wolflike," or musty in character—that is due to the phenylacetic acid in the urine. Nearly all of those affected are fair haired and fair skinned, compared to their unaffected relatives. EEGs are abnormal.

Diagnosis, made by demonstrating an elevated serum concentration of Phe, must occur in the neonatal period to prevent serious consequences. In the U.S., universal NBS for PKU in the 1st few days of life occurs in all 50 states. The next step following a positive screen is a quantitative analysis of the concentrations of Phe and tyrosine.

Most patients identified by the screening test are false positives due to delayed maturation of amino acid–metabolizing enzymes and very high tyrosine concentrations.

Therapy is straightforward: Limit the dietary intake of Phe for life. All infants should be supervised by a dietician familiar with PKU, and Phe levels need to be frequently monitored to determine how much dietary restriction is necessary. You must give Phe for normal growth and development, even in PKU infants. Even after infancy, CNS damage occurs if the Phe levels get too high. Tyrosine is an essential amino acid in PKU patients due to their inability to convert Phe to tyrosine.

Maternal PKU refers to the teratogenic effects of elevated Phe on the developing fetus in a mother with untreated PKU. Infants do not actually have PKU, but they can have growth deficiency, microcephaly, intellectual disability, and congenital heart defects—very similar to fetal alcohol syndrome. This is managed by strict dietary control of Phe in the mother.

Hyperphenylalaninemia

Patients with hyperphenylalaninemia are without classic PKU but have elevated levels of Phe in the blood. Most of these infants have a milder deficiency of the PAH enzyme and can tolerate higher amounts of Phe.

A subset of these patients, however, has a defect in the synthesis or recycling of biopterin. These patients have neurologic symptoms that progress despite dietary treatment that maintains normal Phe levels. They have a defect in either the synthesis of tetrahydrobiopterin, a cofactor for PAH, or they have a defect in the enzymes that regenerate tetrahydrobiopterin from dihydrobiopterin. Both of these result in diminished conversion of Phe to tyrosine. Tetrahydrobiopterin is also a cofactor for the hydroxylation of tryptophan and tyrosine, so you get interference in the synthesis of important compounds such as serotonin, dopa, and norepinephrine.

Clinically, these infants present with severe neurologic disease with marked hypotonia, spasticity, and posturing. Drooling is common, and psychomotor developmental delay is marked.

Treatment includes Phe restriction and supplementation of biopterin and biogenic amine precursor (i.e., 5-hydroxytryptophan and dopa).

Tyrosinemia ↑ tyrosine

Tyrosinemia refers to a group of disorders in which blood tyrosine levels are elevated. The most common form, particularly in premature infants, is a transient tyrosinemia due to delayed maturation of tyrosine-metabolizing enzymes. Tyrosinemia can also occur in scurvy and liver diseases. We discuss the 3 inborn errors of tyrosine metabolism; they all are autosomal recessive.

Hereditary tyrosinemia Type I (a.k.a. hepatorenal tyrosinemia) is due to a deficiency of fumarylacetoacetate hydroxylase, which is the final step in tyrosine metabolism. It is common in the

[handwritten margin notes: FTT, hepatoblastoma, RTA, Rickets]

French-Canadian population. The severe symptoms result from accumulation of succinylacetone; although tyrosine itself has some toxicity, this is mild compared with succinylacetone.

Infants are affected early, and most have a rapid course to death; some, however, progress more slowly. FTT, hepatomegaly with hepatic adenomas that progress to hepatoblastomas, and liver failure are the most common presentations. These infants are not intellectually disabled. They have renal tubular acidosis resembling Fanconi syndrome, as well as x-ray findings of rickets.

You can diagnose this type by finding elevated levels of tyrosine in the plasma, but the definitive diagnostic finding is succinylacetone in the urine.

Nitisinone (NTBC [based on chemical formula]) is the treatment for tyrosinemia Type I. This blocks tyrosine metabolism before the fumarylacetoacetate hydrolase enzyme, which prevents the accumulation of toxic metabolites (i.e., succinylacetone). Because NTBC blocks tyrosine breakdown, tyrosine levels are elevated, causing symptoms like tyrosinemia Type II if not treated. Patients must be on a diet low in tyrosine and Phe.

Tyrosinemia Type II (Richner-Hanhart syndrome; oculocutaneous tyrosinemia) is a deficiency of tyrosine aminotransferase, which is the 1st step of tyrosine metabolism. Patients present with corneal ulcers or dendritic keratitis, along with red papular or keratotic lesions on their palms and soles; 50% have intellectual disability. They do not have the liver toxicity seen in Type I disease since they do not build up succinylacetone. The eye and skin lesions are from deposition of tyrosine itself. Treat with a diet low in tyrosine, but even this is not always curative.

Tyrosinemia Type III is very rare. It is due to deficiency of 4-hydroxyphenylpyruvate dioxygenase, and patients can have intellectual disability. Patients respond well to a diet low in tyrosine.

Alkaptonuria

Alkaptonuria is due to deficiency in homogentisate 1,2-dioxygenase, which is the 3rd step in tyrosine metabolism. This causes an accumulation of homogentisic acid; however, blood levels of tyrosine are not elevated. Excretion of dark-colored urine is the classic finding in alkaptonuria.

This is an interesting syndrome. Fresh urine is normal, but, as it "sits" and alkalinizes, the oxidation of homogentisic acid proceeds and a dark-brown/black pigment forms. Staining of diapers is sometimes noted by parents of affected infants.

Most children tend to be asymptomatic. Often the disorder is first suspected in adulthood, when their routine urinalysis sample turns brown while sitting at the nursing station for a prolonged time. By the time they are in their 30s, adults start to have pigment deposition in the ears and sclerae. This is called ochronosis. Later,

ochronosis arthritis can occur, which is the major medical complication of the disorder. Some patients also have aortic root dilatation or valvular involvement, but, overall, the prognosis is good and lifespan is normal.

Infantile Parkinsonism

Infantile parkinsonism is an AR deficiency of tyrosine hydroxylase and causes severe parkinsonism in infants. A less severe form of the disease is known as Segawa syndrome (dopa-responsive dystonia). Patients present between 1 and 9 years of age with dystonic posture or movement of 1 limb. Intelligence is normal. There is also an AD variant.

Maple Syrup Urine Disease *[handwritten: Pleu, val, iso]*

If you have a newborn with the odor of maple syrup, think of maple syrup urine disease (MSUD). The defect in MSUD is in the oxidative decarboxylation of ketoacids (the ketoacids are what smell sweet), which are formed by catabolism of the branched-chain amino acids (BCAAs).

Note that this disorder comes after catabolism of BCAAs into ketones (problems with catabolism of BCAAs are discussed under Organic Acidemias on page 23-9). Even so, MSUD is often discussed as one of the organic acidemias, many of which also involve defects in BCAA metabolism.

AR mutations can occur in 4 different genes and cause MSUD. The incidence is ~ 1/150,000. It occurs more frequently in populations with consanguinity, such as the Pennsylvanian Mennonites.

Classic MSUD presents with CNS disease early in infancy, and the urine (or hair or skin) smells like maple syrup. Infants are well at birth but start having symptoms by 3–5 days of life, with rapid progression to death in 2–4 weeks without treatment. Babies have feeding difficulties, irregular respirations, or loss of the Moro reflex. Severe seizures, opisthotonos (head, neck, and back held in abnormal position), and rigidity are typical presenting signs. Death follows decerebrate rigidity from cerebral edema.

Milder forms of the disease have intermittent, branched-chain aminoaciduria, characterized by ataxia and repeated episodes of lethargy, progressing to coma but without intellectual disability. Stressors, such as infection, frequently induce this form.

These patients have a high anion gap metabolic acidosis with ketonuria. Diagnose by finding increased amounts of the 3 BCAAs—**leucine**, **isoleucine**, and **valine**—in the plasma and urine. Finding **alloisoleucine**, an abnormal amino acid, is diagnostic for MSUD.

Therapy: Aim for dietary control of leucine, isoleucine, and valine. If therapy is started early, before damage has occurred, normal IQ is possible. There is a very rare form of MSUD that responds very well to thiamine.

Glutaric Acidemia Type 1

Glutaric acidemia Type 1 is an AR enzyme defect (glutaryl-CoA dehydrogenase) in the catabolic pathway of lysine, hydroxylysine, and tryptophan; it is the only clinically relevant disorder in the lysine-hydroxylysine-tryptophan group of disorders.

These infants present with macrocephaly at birth but generally have normal development until they have a febrile illness or metabolic stressor, at which time they suddenly develop hypotonia and dystonia. CT/MRI shows frontal and cortical atrophy at birth, with increased extraaxial space, and, after symptoms of dystonia develop, degeneration of the caudate nucleus and putamen occurs. Striatal degeneration occurs in some during the 1st few years of life if they have a metabolic decompensation.

This is the 1 metabolic disease that can cause subdural hematomas and retinal hemorrhages, which can be mistaken for child abuse. Increased extra-axial space causes stretching of the bridging veins, making them susceptible to hematomas.

Diagnosis: Urine organic acids test shows increased excretion of glutaric and 3-hydroxyglutaric acids. Carnitine levels are usually low.

Treat with L-carnitine, riboflavin, and a special diet—and rapid implementation of IV fluids containing glucose when ill, particularly with febrile illnesses. This regimen helps prevent symptoms and striatal degeneration if given early, before symptoms develop.

Around 10% of patients never have problems, and around 10% of patients have problems despite good therapy.

Homocystinuria

Homocystinuria is a heterogeneous group of disorders caused by 6 types of genetic defects that disrupt the inter-related pathways of methionine metabolism. Originally, the term was used specifically to indicate disease due to a defect in the cystathionine β-synthase enzyme. This is an AR disorder. All diseases in this group cause elevated levels of homocysteine.

Clinically, patients with cystathionine β-synthase deficiency have marfanoid habitus, developmental delay, lens dislocation, and an increased risk of thromboembolism in both arteries and veins. These symptoms can present within the first 10 years of life, and the risk of embolic events persists throughout adult life. Clotting studies are normal, but elevated homocysteine levels cause increased platelet stickiness. Intellectual disability is fairly common. The joints are limited in mobility (not hypermobile as in Marfan syndrome) and are osteoporotic.

Suspect homocystinuria in a child with subluxation/dislocation of the ocular lens. Lenticular subluxation is usually downward and medial. Memory aid: Think of

downward (downward = low IQ), as opposed to Marfan syndrome, which is upward (upward = normal IQ).

Initial testing for diagnosis includes amino acid screening of plasma and urine to check for excess homocysteine, methionine, or homocysteine levels. Confirmatory testing demonstrates a decreased level of activity of cystathionine β-synthase in fibroblasts. NBS specifically tests for methionine levels.

Treatment: Large doses of pyridoxine (vitamin B_6) cause a decrease in the total plasma homocysteine levels (in the vitamin-responsive form). Generally, affected individuals also require a diet low in methionine (which gets broken down into homocysteine). These patients need to be followed by a metabolic specialist over time. Betaine is another therapy that helps to convert homocysteine back into methionine, which can then be used for other purposes in the body.

Glycine and Oxalate Abnormalities — Nonketotic Hyperglycemia

This is an AR inborn error of metabolism in which large amounts of glycine build up in body fluids without detectable accumulation of organic acids. The highest levels of glycine are in the CNS. This presents as intractable seizures in the neonatal period or as hiccups *in utero* in the classic form. It can present as seizures and hypotonia in the milder, later-onset form of the disease. Severe intellectual disability is typical in those who survive.

Diagnosis is made by an increased ratio of CSF glycine to serum glycine. Prenatal diagnosis is possible by biochemical analysis of chorionic villus biopsy. Sodium benzoate seems to reduce CSF glycine levels and decrease seizures. Dextromethorphan has also been used with some success.

UREA CYCLE DISORDERS

The urea cycle converts nitrogen waste to urea, which is water soluble and safely excreted by the kidney. Nitrogen waste comes from catabolism of proteins as ammonium (NH_4^+) and from muscle breakdown.

The urea cycle (Figure 23-2 on page 23-8) occurs in the liver and the periportal hepatocytes, in a series of reactions distributed between the mitochondria and the cytosol.

Before we get started on the enzymes, know that the bad effects of not breaking down NH_4^+ are increases in ammonia (NH_3) and glycine, both of which easily pass the blood-brain barrier and have a very toxic effect on the brain. Brain edema occurs quickly, and ammonia levels between 100 and 200 μmol/L cause lethargy, vomiting, and confusion. Higher levels result in coma.

During normal metabolism, ammonium (NH_4^+) initially becomes part of glycine, glutamine, and carbamoyl phosphate via different enzymes. A cyclic

METABOLIC DISORDERS

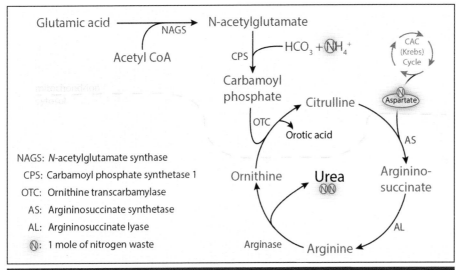

Figure 23-2: The Urea Cycle

cascade of reactions follows the formation of **carbamoyl phosphate**—it is converted to **citrulline**, which then combines with nitrogen-containing aspartate to become **argininosuccinate**, then **arginine**, and, finally, **urea**. Note that of 2 moles of nitrogen in urea, 1 mole comes from ammonium and another from aspartate—which is supplied by the citric acid cycle (CAC; a.k.a. Krebs cycle).

Any of the enzymes in the urea cycle can be defective due to IEMs. Let's look at these:

1) *N*-acetylglutamate synthetase (**NAGS**) deficiency

2) Carbamoyl phosphate synthetase 1 (**CPS1**) deficiency—severe disorder

3) Ornithine transcarbamylase (**OTC**) deficiency—most common; X-linked; severe disorder

4) Argininosuccinate synthetase (**AS**) deficiency (a.k.a. citrullinemia)

5) Argininosuccinate lyase (**AL**) deficiency—accumulation of argininosuccinic acid with argininosuccinic aciduria

6) **Arginase** deficiency (a.k.a. argininemia)

All of the urea cycle disorders have autosomal recessive inheritance, except for OTC deficiency, which has X-linked inheritance (and is also the most common!).

Does it matter where the defect is in the cycle? Yes! Usually, the more upstream the defect is, the higher the ammonia levels and more severe the symptoms.

Review Figure 23-2. The most severe urea cycle defects are **CPS1 deficiency** and **OTC deficiency**. These infants are typically born healthy and at term (because the mom can filter out the excess ammonia easily during pregnancy). But by 5 days of age, in the classic form of the disease, the elevated ammonia levels result in clinical symptoms of lethargy, hypotonia, vomiting, and poor feeding. These infants progress rapidly to coma and death if the hyperammonemia is not quickly identified and treated.

With either CPS1 or OTC deficiency, plasma ammonia levels can be > 1,000 μmol/L (normal < 35 μmol/L). In addition to elevated ammonia levels, a key diagnostic clue is that these infants usually have a respiratory alkalosis, not a metabolic acidosis, as would be expected with sepsis or other metabolic disorders.

Late-onset urea cycle defects do occur and typically are partial enzyme deficiencies, precipitated by infection or some other stressor. Symptoms include loss of appetite, lethargy, vomiting, and behavioral changes. Some females with OTC deficiency experience later onset; their symptoms can be precipitated by pregnancy and childbirth. Also, be aware that valproate and haloperidol can unmask partial urea cycle defects.

Diagnosis: Once you clinically suspect the child has a urea cycle defect, order ammonia level, quantitative plasma, and urinary organic acids to establish the specific defect in urea synthesis.

Table 23-2 lists specific laboratory findings seen with the urea cycle disorders. As you read the following, consult both the table and Figure 23-2; it all makes sense!

• Glutamine, alanine, and asparagine are elevated—because they are storage forms for nitrogen, which cannot be excreted.

• Citrulline is absent or very low in proximal disorders such as OTC and CPS1 defects—because citrulline is the direct product of these reactions.

• Orotic acid is a byproduct of the OTC-catalyzed reaction and is a very sensitive indicator of OTC deficiency. It helps differentiate between OTC and CPS1 deficiency.

• Plasma arginine concentration is low in all urea cycle defects except for argininemia (i.e., arginase deficiency). Without replacement, affected individuals have hair fragility and rash.

Acute treatment centers on volume replacement with D10W, restricting dietary protein, minimizing catabolism and enhancing anabolism, replacing deficient amino acids, and pushing alternate pathways to eliminate nitrogen waste.

Pushing these alternative pathways is done with an IV solution of **sodium benzoate–sodium phenylacetate**.

The alternate pathways for nitrogen removal use sodium benzoate, which is conjugated in the liver with

Table 23-2: Metabolite Levels in Urea Cycle Disorders					
	Glutamine, Alanine, Asparagine	Citrulline	Orotic Acid (Urine)	NH₃	Arginine
NAGS/CPS1	High	Absent or low	Low	Very high	Low
OTC			Very high		
AS		Very high	High	High	
AL					
Arginase		Normal	Normal	Normal	Very high

glycine to make hippuric acid and sodium phenylacetate, Sodium phenylacetate conjugates with glutamine to form phenylacetylglutamine. The hippuric acid and phenylacetylglutamine are easily excreted in the urine.

But if the plasma ammonia level is > 200 μmol/L and/or the infant is in a coma, hemodialysis is the best method to clear the ammonia.

Chronic management involves a high-caloric, protein-restricted diet with additional amino acids as needed. More and more patients with infantile-onset disease are having liver transplants with improved long-term outcomes.

ORGANIC ACIDEMIAS

Overview

Organic acidemias (a.k.a. organic acidurias) are a group of rare inherited disorders caused by a defect in specific enzymes that process proteins, especially BCAAs.

An organic acid is a chemical compound with ≥ 1 carboxyl groups (COOH) in its structure. The kidneys clear most organic acids, so it is easiest to examine the urine for these disorders—which is why these disorders are also called organic acidurias.

Organic acidemias are characterized by a high anion gap metabolic acidosis (HAGMA) with normal chloride and hyperammonemia. They are, for the most part, AR disorders.

Note that maple syrup urine disease is sometimes considered an organic acidemia, but it also belongs in the amino acid metabolism disorders. It causes a ketonuria and elevated BCAAs (leucine, isoleucine, and valine) in the urine.

All organic acidemias have overlap in complications, including bone marrow suppression and pancreatitis.

Isovaleric Acidemia sweaty feet

Isovaleric acidemia (IVA) is an AR disorder and a defect in the 3rd step of **leucine metabolism**.

If you have a newborn with the odor of sweaty feet, think of IVA, especially if the infant has encephalopathy. The enzyme defect is in isovaleryl-CoA dehydrogenase. These patients cannot convert isovaleryl-CoA to 3-methylcrotonyl-CoA, so they have increased levels of isovaleryl-CoA.

IVA can present in the newborn period with an acute episode of severe HAGMA and moderate ketosis with vomiting, which can lead to coma and death, but more typically it presents later, in infancy or childhood, and is precipitated by an infection or increased protein intake. A chronic intermittent form with pancytopenia and acidosis occurs in infants who survive the acute episode.

Diagnose IVA with urine organic acids. Prenatal diagnosis is possible.

Treatment in the acute setting is aimed at the acidosis, which usually responds to IV glucose and bicarbonate. Center long-term treatment on restricting leucine intake and prescribing carnitine and/or glycine to increase conversion of isovaleryl-CoA to isovalerylglycine, which is excreted easily.

3-Methylcrotonyl-CoA Carboxylase Deficiency

3-methylcrotonyl-CoA carboxylase (a.k.a. 3MCC, or BMCC) deficiency, an AR disorder, is a defect in the 4th step of **leucine metabolism**. The biotin-containing enzyme, 3-methylcrotonyl-CoA carboxylase, is missing and 3-methylcrotonyl-CoA is not converted to 3-methylglutaconyl-CoA.

Patients present between 1 and 3 years of age with acute metabolic acidosis, hypoglycemia, and carnitine deficiency—typically during a stressful event (e.g., an infection). The majority of affected individuals never have any decompensation or symptoms related to the enzyme defect.

Diagnose with urine organic acid analysis, which shows increased excretion of 3-methylcrotonylglycine and 3-hydroxyisovaleric acid.

Acute treatment consists of IV glucose, fluids, and electrolytes. Long-term therapy consists of oral carnitine to correct carnitine deficiency, if present, and biotin to enhance enzymatic function.

Although the majority of patients with this disorder identified by NBS most likely will not have problems, this disease can be serious. Because we can't tell who is likely to get sick, we treat them all.

METABOLIC DISORDERS

Propionic Acidemia

Propionic acidemia (PA) is an AR disorder due to a deficiency in propionyl-CoA carboxylase, a biotin-containing enzyme that converts propionyl-CoA to D-methylmalonyl-CoA. Propionyl-CoA is an intermediary in the oxidation of **v**aline, **m**ethionine, **i**soleucine, and **t**hreonine. A mnemonic to remember these amino acids is **VoMIT**—which is what kids with PA do when they get sick. The vomiting can be so severe that babies with PA get worked up for pyloric stenosis.

In the early neonatal period, PA can present as severe ketoacidosis with or without hyperammonemia. The infant will have encephalopathy, vomiting, and bone marrow depression. A milder presentation is ketoacidosis precipitated by infection or vomiting. Other major problems include malnutrition with FTT, recurrent infections, cardiomyopathy, and pancreatitis.

Diagnose by examining urine organic acids. Look for large amounts of 3-hydroxypropionic and methylcitric acids. Abnormal ketone bodies are common, too.

Treatment is dietary restriction of protein (usually < 1 g/kg/day). To decrease intake of the amino acids that are prone to produce more propionyl-CoA, non-toxic amino acids are supplemented in a special formula. Carnitine is helpful in increasing excretion of propionyl-CoA.

Multiple Carboxylase Deficiency alopecia

Biotin is the cofactor for 4 essential carboxylases that are important in the metabolism of dietary **fats**, **carbohydrates**, and **proteins**. There are 2 disorders associated with **biotin** deficiency or inability to incorporate biotin:

1) **Biotinidase deficiency**. Biotinidase extracts biotin from food and recycles biotin from carboxylase enzymes. It has variable severity, and symptoms can appear from several days to years after birth.

2) **Holocarboxylase synthetase deficiency**. This enzyme incorporates biotin into the carboxylase enzymes. This deficiency has neonatal onset.

In both disorders, the absence of functional carboxylases results in the inability to properly metabolize propionyl-CoA, 3-methylcrotonyl-CoA, acetyl-CoA, and pyruvate. This leads to the classic triad of carboxylase deficiency: encephalopathy, alopecia, and skin rash. Seizures, hearing loss, and blindness can also be complications of untreated disease.

Biotinidase deficiency typically presents later than holocarboxylase deficiency and has a perioral dermatitis that looks like acrodermatitis enteropathica.

Diagnose by analyzing urine organic acid and finding increased 3-methylcrotonylglycine and 3-hydroxyisovaleric acid with lactic acids. Multiple carboxylase deficiency can also be found on newborn screening for biotinidase deficiency (and is included

in most states). Holocarboxylase deficiency should be detected with the expanded newborn panels.

Treatment is quite effective with free biotin in doses of 5–20 mg/day. This usually reverses all disease manifestations.

Methylmalonic Acidemias

There are a group of inherited disorders that cause methylmalonic acidemias (MMA; a.k.a. methylmalonic aciduria). All ultimately inhibit methylmalonyl-CoA mutase function. These either affect mutase activity or interfere with the formation of **cobalamin** (vitamin B_{12}).

Those affecting mutase activity are **mut(0)**—no activity—and **mut(–)**—residual but low activity.

Those affecting cobalamin formation are termed **cblA**, **cblB**, **cblC**, **cblD**, **cblF**, **cblH**, and **cblJ**.

Clinically, these patients present early with hyperammonemia, ketoacidosis, and thrombocytopenia—or later with chronic ketotic hyperglycinemia, vomiting, and FTT. A late-onset complication is renal failure of uncertain origin, and cardiomyopathy can also occur.

Diagnose with organic acid analysis of urine, which shows increased methylmalonic acid and abnormal ketone bodies, as with PA. Homocystinuria is also present if the patient has the enzyme deficit in the pathway that blocks the synthesis of methyl-B_{12}, resulting in increased methylmalonic acid and increased levels of homocysteine.

Treatment relies on restricting dietary protein. Carnitine is useful. Liver and kidney transplantation can be beneficial. If the patient has both methylmalonic aciduria and homocystinuria, treat with betaine (which provides another methyl donor for the conversion of homocysteine to methionine) and IM vitamin B_{12}.

SUGAR INTOLERANCES

Galactose Metabolism Disorders

Overview

Inadequate metabolism of galactose can be caused by 3 different enzymes necessary for converting galactose to glucose:

1) Galactose-1-phosphate uridyltransferase (GALT)
2) Galactokinase
3) Uridine diphosphate galactose 4-epimerase (UDP-galactose 4-epimerase, or GALE)

Galactosemia

Lactose in dairy products is hydrolyzed by lactase in the intestine into glucose and galactose. Galactose is quickly converted to more glucose. Galactosemia is deficiency of the enzyme GALT, causing galactose to be metabolized poorly or not at all. Galactose and its derivative molecules then build up in cells and tissues, especially the liver, kidneys, and brain.

Classic galactosemia is usually what we think about when we say "galactosemia." It is an AR disorder occurring in 1/60,000 births where there is a mutation of both copies of the *GALT* gene resulting in no detectable GALT activity. These patients have 2 copies of severely affected genes (shown as G/G). **Clinical galactosemia** results from similar, but not as severe, damage to both copies of the *GALT* gene (G/G); detectable, but insufficient, GALT function remains. Remember, because this is an autosomal recessive disorder, both genes must be affected to have any enzyme deficiency.

In untreated classic or clinical galactosemia, infants present clinically in the first few days of life after their first lactose meal with some combination of:

- Jaundice
- Hepatosplenomegaly
- Cataracts
- Irritability
- Hypoglycemia
- Cirrhosis
- Intellectual disability
- Vomiting
- Seizures
- Lethargy
- Poor weight gain
- Vitreous hemorrhage
- Ascites

Those affected are at increased risk for *E. coli* sepsis, which usually precedes the diagnosis of galactosemia.

The **Duarte variant** is a damaged gene that codes for a partially functional GALT. It is the most common galactosemic gene mutation, with 12% of those with Caucasian ancestry and 3% of those with Asian ancestry being carriers. Individuals who are Duarte-variant homozygous (D/D) have about 50% of normal red cell enzyme activity but do not have symptoms. Individuals who are compound heterozygous (D/G) have only 25% of activity, with elevated galactose-1-phosphate levels. These patients are usually asymptomatic, but most practitioners restrict lactose intake if the RBC galactose-1-phosphate levels are elevated.

Suspect this disorder in patients with galactosemia symptoms or when you discover a reducing substance in urine while the patient is drinking breast milk, cow's milk, or formula containing lactose. Reducing substances in the urine is usually done by labs as a reflex test when the urine shows no glucose, but this is neither sensitive nor specific enough to confirm or rule out the diagnosis. Definitive diagnosis requires deficient activity of GALT in RBCs or other tissues, while also showing an increased concentration of galactose-1-phosphatase.

NBS for galactosemia is widespread in the U.S. Many states use a fluorescent spot test (Beutler test) for GALT activity, whereas other states examine galactose-1-phosphate levels; note that the Duarte variant is often not picked up by the latter test.

For classic or clinical galactosemia, elimination of lactose and galactose from the diet reverses growth failure and renal/hepatic problems. Even cataracts regress. Give soy-based formula instead. Unfortunately, for unclear reasons, long-term complications are typical, even with treatment, including ovarian failure, amenorrhea, developmental delay, and learning disabilities that worsen with age. Speech disorders are also very common.

Galactokinase Deficiency

Cataracts alone typically characterize this disorder. Otherwise, the infant is asymptomatic. Treatment is dietary restriction of galactose.

Uridine Diphosphate Galactose 4-Epimerase (UDP-Galactose 4-Epimerase) Deficiency

The accumulated metabolites are extremely analogous to those seen in galactosemia, but there is also an increase in cellular UDP-galactose. This deficiency may not be detected on an NBS.

There are 2 forms of this disease:

1) **Benign** form: Individuals are healthy, and no treatment is necessary. The only evidence is seen in RBCs.

2) **Generalized** form: This clinically resembles galactosemia, with the additional symptoms of hypotonia and nerve deafness. Treatment with dietary restriction of galactose is effective. The GALT activity is normal, unlike in classic galactosemia.

Fructose Metabolism Disorders

Benign Fructosuria (Fructokinase Deficiency)

This is benign, requires no treatment, and has no clinical manifestations. It is an incidental finding when you discover fructose during a urine screen for reducing substances.

Hereditary Fructose Intolerance (Aldolase B Deficiency)

This is a severe disease of infancy and appears when the infant ingests fructose-containing food. The enzyme, which is deficient in these patients, normally causes the hydrolysis of fructose 1-phosphate and fructose 1,6-bisphosphate into 3 sugars: dihydroxyacetone phosphate, glyceraldehyde 3-phosphate, and glyceraldehyde. With the enzymatic deficiency, the accumulation of fructose 1-phosphate leads to severe toxic symptoms in patients who ingest fructose.

The incidence is estimated to be approximately 1/23,000.

Those affected are completely healthy until they ingest fructose or sucrose (table sugar, which consists of fructose and glucose). Usually, the culprit is juice or sweetened cereal. It can look much like galactosemia, but onset is generally later when exposed to fructose, as opposed to the 1st week or so of life, when patients are exposed to lactose.

METABOLIC DISORDERS

Symptoms after introduction of fructose or sucrose into the diet include jaundice, hepatomegaly, vomiting, lethargy, seizures, and irritability. Laboratory results will show prolonged clotting time, low albumin, elevated bilirubin and transaminases, and proximal tubular dysfunction. If fructose intake continues, severe hypoglycemia occurs, followed by liver and kidney failure and death. Sugar ingestion causes hypoglycemia!

Suspect this deficiency if you find fructose as a urinary reducing substance during a symptomatic episode.

A definitive diagnosis depends on assaying fructose 1,6-bisphosphate aldolase B activity in the liver. Genetic testing is also available and can make biopsy unnecessary in some patients.

Treatment consists of complete dietary elimination of all sources of fructose and of its progenitors, sucrose and sorbitol. Due to unsuspected sources of these sugars, an expert nutritionist is mandatory. Treatment reverses the liver and kidney damage, and it improves growth. With treatment, intellectual disability is very uncommon. Symptoms improve with age, especially as those affected develop an aversion to sweets (and have lovely teeth because of it).

IEM — ENERGY UTILIZATION DEFECTS

PREVIEW | REVIEW

- What events exacerbate energy defect disorders?
- What are some of the ways a patient with an energy utilization defect can present?
- Where does fatty acid oxidation occur? Why is this important?
- What is the most common disorder affecting mitochondrial fatty acid oxidation and ketogenesis?
- How do most patients present with disorders of fatty acid oxidation?
- What are the laboratory tests you would order to detect disorders in fatty acid oxidation?
- Which medical problems occur in patients with LCHAD that do not develop in those with VLCAD or MCAD?
- How is MCAD diagnosed?
- Describe glucose-6-phosphatase deficiency. Which organs are most commonly affected?
- How do patients with Type 1 GSD present?
- Which laboratory findings are common in patients with Type 1 GSD?
- How is Type 1 GSD diagnosed?
- What causes Type 4 GSD?
- How does a child with Type 4 GSD present?
- How does a child with Fanconi-Bickel syndrome present?
- What is different about Type 0 GSD?
- What is the metabolic disorder in Pompe disease?
- Which laboratory tests are elevated in Type 2 GSD?
- How does a child with Type 5 GSD present?
- Which laboratory test is elevated at rest and increases after exercise in patients with McArdle disease?
- Describe fructose 1,6-diphosphatase deficiency.
- True or false? All mtDNA disorders are inherited from the father.
- What is the triad of symptoms associated with Kearns-Sayre syndrome?
- In MELAS, which symptom typically occurs long before a stroke?

OVERVIEW

These disorders have symptoms related to the inability to use energy due to disruption of normal metabolic pathways (see Figure 23-1 on page 23-1). Our bodies derive energy in a specific order during fasting:

1) Blood glucose
2) Breakdown of stored glycogen
3) Fatty acid oxidation (a.k.a. β-oxidation) in the fatty acid spiral
4) Breakdown of amino acids for glucose synthesis

Disorders of energy metabolism can occur with a breakdown in any of the above metabolic processes or elsewhere in the adenosine triphosphate (ATP) pathway. Examples of these disorders are:

- Fatty acid oxidation defects
- Glycogen storage diseases (defects in making or breaking down glycogen)
- Mitochondrial disorders (Krebs cycle and mitochondrial respiratory chain disorders)

PRESENTATION

Fasting or illness with increased energy needs can exacerbate an energy defect metabolic disorder and bring on decompensation. There may or may not be hypoglycemia. Patients can present with FTT, hypotonia, cardiac dysfunction, lactic acidosis, or weakness and fatigue.

The presentation is determined by the effect on the cells. If muscle is affected, such as with mitochondrial defects, then weakness is noted. If the body is unable to utilize the oxidative phosphorylation pathway, lactic acid builds up. See Table 23-3 for a listing of findings.

Table 23-3: Presentation of Various Disorders of Energy Metabolism

Fatty acid (β-) oxidation defects	Hypoketotic hypoglycemia Hypotonia Cardiomyopathy SIDS Reye-like syndrome
Glycogen storage diseases	Hepatomegaly Hypoglycemia Lactic acidosis FTT
Mitochondrial disorders	Lactic acidosis Seizures Cardiomyopathy Hypotonia/Myopathy +/– hypoglycemia

DEFECTS IN FAT METABOLISM

Overview

Remember: Fatty acid oxidation (β-oxidation) occurs in the mitochondria, and this process provides the main energy source for heart and skeletal muscle (Figure 23-3). Also, β-oxidation generates acetyl-CoA, which enters the Krebs cycle and thus provides energy to other tissues when the supply of glucose is gone. Fatty acids are initially conjugated to carnitine. Then carnitine is transported across the mitochondrial membrane and released into the mitochondrial matrix as an acyl-CoA before it can be catabolized in the β-oxidation spiral.

Diseases that limit β-oxidation do so by:

• Decreasing carnitine uptake by cells
• Inhibiting fatty acids from entering mitochondria
• Blocking β-oxidation

If β-oxidation is impaired, there is limited energy available for the heart and skeletal muscles at rest; it also limits the ability of the brain to cope with low-glucose settings. Thus, a child with a defect in β-oxidation is the poster child for disorders of energy metabolism. These are nearly all AR disorders.

There are 12 known disorders affecting mitochondrial β-oxidation and ketogenesis (with medium-chain acyl-CoA dehydrogenase [MCAD] deficiency being the most common). Age of onset varies from birth to adulthood. The most common clinical presentations involve the hepatic, skeletal, muscular, and cardiac systems. Neonates can present with arrhythmias, hypoglycemia, or with sudden death. (Makes sense, doesn't it? The heart cannot function correctly because of the lack of energy and hypoglycemia.) Sometimes they have renal cystic dysplasia. Older children can have arrhythmias or cardiomyopathy. Muscle weakness is typical, as is exercise-induced rhabdomyolysis. Patients with these disorders are susceptible to metabolic decompensation in times of stress (e.g., prolonged fasting, infection, surgery).

Evaluation involves these main laboratory studies:

• Routine lab measurements—i.e., CBC, electrolytes, liver function studies, ammonia, lactate, creatine phosphokinase (CPK), urine ketones
• Free carnitine and acylcarnitine levels in the blood
• Gas chromatography and mass spectrometry analysis of organic acids
• Analysis of plasma acylcarnitine and urine acylglycines by specialized techniques

Definitive diagnosis of these disorders requires measurement of specific enzyme activity or mutation analysis.

Treat the acute presentation with IV D10½NS or D10NS and possibly L-carnitine. Long-term therapy revolves around keeping the glucose from getting low, especially important when the patient is stressed by illness or decreased intake (including the period of fasting while sleeping at night) and catabolism.

We'll now discuss some of the more clinically relevant (and quizzable) disorders.

Carnitine Uptake Defect (Primary Carnitine Deficiency)

This AR defect occurs in the plasma membrane of the cell. This disorder is caused by a deficiency of the carnitine transporter in the kidneys, where free carnitine is recycled for use by the body. When this transporter is not functioning, free carnitine is lost in the urine, resulting in low levels of free carnitine in the serum. Patients present in early infancy or later childhood with cardiomyopathy or recurrent episodes of encephalopathy and

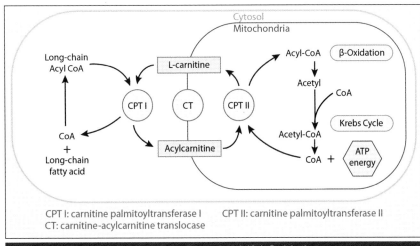

Figure 23-3: Fatty Acid (β-) Oxidation

CPT I: carnitine palmitoyltransferase I   CPT II: carnitine palmitoyltransferase II
CT: carnitine-acylcarnitine translocase

METABOLIC DISORDERS

hypoketotic hypoglycemia. If the skeletal muscles are involved, weakness is prominent. Conduction defects and arrhythmias are rare with this disorder, in contrast to other disorders.

Diagnose by finding very low levels of carnitine in tissues. In serum, it may be undetectable or < 1 μmol/L. However, keep in mind that losses from fatty acid oxygenation defects or organic acidurias can also cause fairly severe carnitine deficiency or secondary deficiency. Treat with L-carnitine, which results in dramatic improvement. Administer orally for chronic maintenance; administer IV for emergencies.

Defects of Fatty Acid Entry into Mitochondria

Short-chain and medium-chain fatty acids can enter mitochondria directly, but CoA esters that are longer than 12 carbons require transport with carnitine palmitoyltransferase I and II (CPT I and CPT II) and by carnitine-acylcarnitine translocase (CT). AR disorders occur and cause defects in these enzymes.

All transporter defects can present in infancy with fasting-induced hypoglycemia, liver failure, and cardiomyopathy. However, they can all have later phenotypes as well.

CPT I deficiency presents in early childhood with hypoketotic hypoglycemia, hepatomegaly, and liver malfunction. Patients can also have nervous system dysfunction and seizures. Symptoms can be triggered by periods of fasting or illness.

The most common phenotype of CPT II deficiency is a myopathic, or "muscular," type that occurs in young adults. Here, the patient has exercise-induced muscle pain and rhabdomyolysis.

The other phenotype of CPT II is extremely rare, occurs only in infants/children, and is a hepatocardiomuscular form. If it occurs early, the infants die in 1–2 weeks with complete liver and heart failure. Those presenting later with the rare phenotype of CPT II have hypoketotic hypoglycemia, cardiomyopathy, and muscle disease.

CT deficiency presents in the newborn with hyperammonemia, conduction defects, and high CPK. Prognosis is good if the infant survives the early initial insult.

Diagnosis: For CPT I, serum carnitine levels are normal or elevated (key: no other disorder elevates carnitine—elevated carnitine is otherwise seen only in excessive supplementation), and the serum acylcarnitine profile is normal. In CPT II and CT deficiency, serum carnitine levels are very low with elevated C_{16} esters (an abnormal acylcarnitine profile).

Treat acute cases with IV glucose and aggressive hydration. Avoidance of fasting alleviates symptoms. Give carnitine if serum carnitine levels are low. Medium-chain triglyceride (MCT) oil, which can enter the mitochondria without these enzymes, provides an alternative energy source as well.

Defects in β-Oxidation

Overview

Once acyl-CoA is in the mitochondria, it enters the β-oxidation cycle. Here, a series of reactions occurs, and defects/deficiencies of the enzymes can cause problems. Different enzymes cleave different lengths of carbon chains.

3 main AR conditions are discussed in this group:

1) Defects in very-long-chain acyl-CoA dehydrogenase (VLCAD)
2) Defects in long-chain 3-hydroxyacyl-CoA dehydrogenase (LCHAD)
3) Defects in medium-chain acyl-CoA dehydrogenase (MCAD)

Very-Long-Chain Acyl-CoA Dehydrogenase (VLCAD) Deficiency

VLCAD deficiency presents in infancy as arrhythmias with severe cardiomyopathy and sudden death. It occasionally is found in older infants and children with hepatic, cardiac, or muscular abnormalities.

Diagnose by finding elevated saturated and unsaturated C_{14-18} esters. Free carnitine is usually low.

Treatment includes frequent meals with a high-carbohydrate diet and avoidance of fasting, especially for infants. If an acute episode occurs, give IV glucose and fluids. You can use MCTs because their oxidation does not involve VLCAD.

Long-Chain 3-Hydroxyacyl-CoA Dehydrogenase (LCHAD) Deficiency

LCHAD is the long-chain–specific enzyme, and it acts on all acyl groups longer than 8 carbons. LCHAD deficiency can stand alone or be combined with 2 other enzymes: long-chain enoyl-CoA hydratase and β-ketothiolase. Patients with the stand-alone deficiency usually present in infancy with fasting-induced hypoketotic hypoglycemia, although some will have cardiomyopathy or, later in adulthood, exercise-induced rhabdomyolysis. Sometimes a clue in the history is the pregnancy. Was it complicated with acute fatty liver or **HELLP (h**emolysis, **e**levated **l**iver function tests, and **l**ow **p**latelets) syndrome?

Patients with LCHAD deficiency frequently develop cholestatic liver disease and have retinopathy with hypopigmentation or focal pigment aggregations later in life. Note: These are not seen in MCAD or VLCAD deficiency!

Therapy is similar to that for VLCAD and MCAD. Frequent meals, without prolonged fasting, are recommended, especially for infants. You also can use MCT oil and carnitine. Oral docosahexaenoic acid may reverse retinopathy if it occurs.

Medium-Chain Acyl-CoA Dehydrogenase (MCAD) Deficiency

Medium-chain triglycerides (MCTs) are triglycerides whose fatty acids have an aliphatic tail of 6–12 carbon atoms. MCAD deficiency, the most common β-oxidation defect, typically presents in the first 2 years of life. The infant/child will have fasting-induced lethargy and hypoglycemia. Seizures and coma are typical. MCAD deficiency—as well as the majority of other fatty acid oxidation disorders—has been implicated in some cases of Reye syndrome and SIDS. In an acute episode, elevated liver transaminases and CPK with hypoglycemia occur. Liver biopsy shows microvesicular steatosis.

Diagnose MCAD deficiency by finding elevated C_8 and C_{10} esters. Free serum carnitine is low sometimes but not consistently.

Acute treatment is IV glucose and bicarbonate. Restrict MCTs from the diet because there is no acyl-CoA dehydrogenase to break them down and the resultant buildup of these chains is toxic to the cells.

As preventive maintenance, avoid fasting when healthy; however, during illness, rapid intervention is most important. If carnitine is low, oral replacement can be helpful, but evidence of benefit is lacking.

In the U.S., the majority of states mandate screening for MCAD deficiency because it responds so well to treatment. Prior to NBS, 25% of infants died with the 1st metabolic crisis.

Glutaric Acidemia Type 2 (Multiple Acyl-CoA Dehydrogenase Deficiency)

Glutaric acidemia Type 2 is caused by AR defects in electron-transfer flavoprotein (ETF) and ETF-ubiquinone oxidoreductase. These enzymes transfer electrons from acyl-CoA dehydrogenases involved in fatty acid and amino acid oxidation from flavin adenine dinucleotide (FAD) coenzymes into the respiratory chain.

The neonate typically presents with severe hypoglycemia, metabolic acidosis, hyperammonemia, and the odor of sweaty feet, as with IVA (isovaleric acidemia). Frequently, the patient has cardiomyopathy, facial dysmorphism, and severe renal cystic dysplasia.

Diagnose by finding glutarylcarnitine, isovalerylcarnitine, and straight-chain C_4, C_8, C_{10}, and C_{12} esters. Serum carnitine is low, and ketones are absent. Patients with absolute deficiency die in the first few weeks, usually due to conduction defects. Those with incomplete defects survive into adulthood.

Treatment relies on avoidance of fasting and sometimes requires continuous intragastric feeds. Carnitine is useful. You cannot use MCTs because all of the acyl-CoA dehydrogenases are deficient.

GLYCOGEN STORAGE DISEASES

Mono- and Polysaccharides

Glycogen storage diseases (GSDs) are disorders of carbohydrate metabolism essentially involving 3 monosaccharides (glucose, galactose, and fructose) and 1 polysaccharide (glycogen):

- **Glucose** is the main source of energy. When metabolized, glucose makes ATP via glycolysis (glucose is converted to pyruvate) or mitochondrial oxidative phosphorylation (pyruvate is converted to carbon dioxide and water). Eating, gluconeogenesis, and breakdown of storage glycogen maintain glucose levels.
- **Galactose** is derived from lactose (galactose + glucose), which is in milk and milk products.
- **Fructose** is found in the diet (fruits and vegetables) and is also derived from sucrose (fructose + glucose).
- **Glycogen** is the storage form of glucose. Defects in glycogen metabolism usually lead to buildup of glycogen in tissues, resulting in GSDs.

Most Common GSDs

Most of these diseases are inherited as AR traits (except for phosphoglycerate kinase deficiency and 1 form of phosphorylase kinase deficiency, both of which are X-linked disorders). The frequency of all forms of GSD is about 1/20,000.

The most common GSDs are:

- **Type 1 GSD** (von Gierke disease; see below)—This is due to either decreased glucose-6-phosphatase or translocase deficiency and is not to be confused with glucose-6-phosphate dehydrogenase (G6PD) deficiency, a completely different disease.
- **Type 2 GSD** (Pompe disease; page 23-17)—This does not present as an energy metabolic defect but is a lysosomal storage disease that has excess glycogen storage.
- **Type 3 GSD** (debrancher deficiency).
- **Type 9 GSD** (liver phosphorylase kinase deficiency).

The most common adult disorder is myophosphorylase deficiency (Type 5, or McArdle disease).

We subdivide these glycogen storage diseases into those that mainly affect the liver vs. those that mainly affect muscle tissues.

GSDs Presenting with Hypoglycemia and Hepatomegaly

Type 1 GSD (von Gierke Disease)

Type 1 GSD is due to a defect in glucose-6-phosphatase in the liver, kidney, and intestinal mucosa.

There are 2 subtypes:

1) **Type 1a**—defect in the glucose-6-phosphatase enzyme
2) **Type 1b**—defect in the translocase that transports glucose-6-phosphatase across the cell membrane

Both subtypes cause the same deficit, which is failure to convert glucose-6-phosphatase to glucose in the liver. The affected individual has excess storage of glycogen in the tissues and suffers from severe and rapid fasting hypoglycemia.

Clinically, these patients present at about 3–4 months of age with FTT, hypoglycemic seizures, and/or hepatomegaly—at a time when babies start to eat less often and parents are trying to get them to sleep through the night. The kids have "doll-like faces with fat cheeks," thin extremities, short stature, and a large protuberant abdomen due to the hepatomegaly. The kidneys are also hypertrophied, but the spleen and heart are normal in size.

Types 1a and 1b are similar, except that 1b has associated recurrent bacterial infections due to neutropenia and impaired neutrophil function. Oral and intestinal mucosa ulcers also occur with Type 1b.

In the long term, the liver is the most commonly affected organ, but other organ systems are also affected. Gout usually appears in puberty because of the elevated uric acid. Puberty itself is usually delayed, but sexual development is otherwise normal. Pancreatitis can occur because of the elevated lipids. Note that the triglyceride levels remain elevated even with regular feeding/ dietary maintenance.

By 20–30 years of age, most patients develop hepatic adenomas that can bleed and occasionally become malignant. Pulmonary hypertension and osteoporosis can occur. Proteinuria occurs in all patients > 20 years of age. Hypertension, kidney stones, and abnormal creatinine clearance are common. With advanced disease, focal segmental glomerulonephritis develops.

Diagnose by looking for hypoglycemia, lactic acidosis, hyperuricemia, and hyperlipidemia (increased VLDL, LDL, and apolipoproteins B, C, and E). Note: Even though these patients have hepatomegaly, the liver transaminases are usually normal. The plasma can appear milky because of the hypertriglyceridemia. Also, if you give glucagon or epinephrine, blood glucose levels do not rise, but lactate does. Gene-based mutation analysis provides the definitive diagnosis. Liver biopsy is generally not required.

Aim treatment at preventing hypoglycemia with continuous gastric feeds and oral administration of uncooked cornstarch when the patient is old enough for pancreatic enzymes to break it down (> 1 year of age). Fructose and galactose cannot be converted to free glucose, so restrict these in the diet. Use allopurinol to lower uric acid levels. Granulocyte colony-stimulating factor (G-CSF) has been used to correct the neutropenia of Type 1b–affected individuals. Some patients have difficulty with bleeding, especially during surgery, because they have platelet dysfunction. You can correct this with a constant infusion of glucose for 24–48 hours prior to surgery.

Type 3 GSD

Type 3 GSD is also known as debrancher deficiency or limit dextrinosis.

Type 3 is due to a deficiency of glycogen-debranching enzyme. This enzyme (along with phosphorylase) is responsible for complete degradation of glycogen. When the enzyme is deficient, an unusual type of glycogen is formed that resembles limit dextrin (i.e., fragments remaining after exhaustive hydrolysis of glycogen). Type 3 is AR and has an increased incidence in non-Ashkenazi Jews of North African descent.

Patients with Type 3 GSD present with:

• Hepatomegaly
• Hypoglycemia
• Short stature
• Skeletal myopathy
• Cardiomyopathy

In 85% of patients, it presents with both liver and muscle abnormalities; this is known as Type 3a GSD. In the other 15%, it involves only the liver and is known as Type 3b GSD.

It is difficult to clinically distinguish between Type 3 and Type 1, but usually the kidneys are not enlarged in Type 3. In Type 3, the hepatomegaly and hepatic symptoms typically improve after puberty, although some patients—particularly those of Japanese ancestry— go on to develop cirrhosis. Unlike Type 1, the liver in Type 3 is fibrotic. Fasting ketosis is prominent in Type 3, and, unlike Type 1, lactate and uric acid are normal.

In Type 3a, muscle weakness is a less prominent issue in children, but it becomes the main feature in adults. In females, polycystic ovaries frequently occur, but infertility is not an issue.

In Type 3a, deficient debranching enzyme activity can be demonstrated in the liver, skeletal muscle, and heart. In Type 3b, only the liver is involved. DNA testing provides definitive diagnosis without the need for liver or muscle biopsy.

Diet is less stringent in Type 3 than in Type 1. Frequent high-carbohydrate meals are generally effective in preventing hypoglycemia. Also, patients do not need to restrict fructose and galactose, as do those with Type 1.

With Type 3b, liver symptoms usually improve with age and disappear after puberty. However, cirrhosis can occur later in life. In Type 3a, muscle weakness/atrophy worsens in adulthood.

Type 4 GSD (Andersen Disease)

Type 4 GSD is also known as branching enzyme deficiency or amylopectinosis.

Deficiency of branching enzyme causes accumulation of an abnormal glycogen that has decreased solubility; its structure resembles amylopectin. It is a rare AR disorder.

There are many clinical presentations for this disorder, but the most common is cirrhosis of the liver with hepatomegaly and FTT in the first 18 months of life. The cirrhosis is so severe that death usually occurs by 5 years of age. The abnormal accumulation of the amylopectin-like material is widespread in the liver, heart, skin, brain, nerves, and intestine. There is also a neuromuscular form of this disorder.

Treatment is supportive, and there is no specific therapy.

Type 6 GSD (Hers Disease)

Type 6 GSD is also known as liver phosphorylase deficiency.

This is very rare, and it appears that patients with liver phosphorylase deficiency have a benign course. Those affected have hepatomegaly and growth retardation in childhood, but these resolve before or at puberty. Usually, no specific therapy is required.

Type 9 GSD

Type 9 GSD is also known as liver phosphorylase kinase deficiency.

4 of the defects that cause phosphorylase kinase deficiency and resulting problems are:

1) **X-linked liver** phosphorylase kinase deficiency: This is a very common liver glycogenosis. It typically presents within the first 5 years of life with hepatomegaly and growth retardation, but these conditions resolve by adulthood. Hypoglycemia is mild, if present at all. By adulthood, most individuals are completely asymptomatic, even though they have persistent deficiency. However, they occasionally go on to develop cirrhosis and possibly require liver transplant.

2) **Autosomal liver and muscle** phosphorylase kinase deficiency: This is an AR form occurring in the liver and muscles. Its presentation is very similar to that of the X-linked form. Some also have muscle hypotonia.

3) **Autosomal liver** phosphorylase kinase deficiency: This is the AR form of the X-linked disease mentioned above and involves only the liver. It is not benign like the X-linked form; many of these patients develop cirrhosis.

4) **Muscle-specific** phosphorylase kinase deficiency: This is the other X-linked disorder, and it causes cramps and myoglobinuria with exercise or progressive muscle weakness/atrophy. The enzyme is deficient only in muscle, not in the liver or the blood.

Type 11 GSD (Fanconi-Bickel Syndrome)

Type 11 GSD is also known as hepatic glycogenesis with renal Fanconi syndrome.

This is rare and occurs as an AR defect in the glucose transporter 2 (*GLUT2*) gene, which transports glucose in and out of the hepatic, pancreatic, intestinal, and renal epithelial cells. Patients have proximal renal tubular dysfunction and accumulation of glycogen in the liver and kidney. There are < 100 cases reported worldwide. Look for parents who are consanguineous.

Children present at < 1 year of age with FTT, rickets, and a large, protuberant abdomen due to the hepatomegaly. Liver transaminases are normal, however. Oral galactose and glucose-tolerance tests show impaired tolerance. Diagnosis is by tissue biopsy; treatment is not very helpful, with growth retardation as the primary manifestation (e.g., poor height attainment).

Type 0 GSD

Type 0 GSD is also known as glycogen synthase deficiency. It is an AR condition.

This is not actually a GSD per se because the enzyme deficiency leads to a decrease in glycogen stores. Infants present with early morning drowsiness and fatigue and sometimes seizures with hypoglycemia and hyperketonemia. There is no hepatomegaly. Genetic testing is available to confirm diagnosis. Diagnosis can also be established by enzyme testing from liver biopsy. Treatment is symptomatic, involving frequent feedings rich in protein and a nighttime snack of uncooked cornstarch to prevent hypoglycemia. Most patients do well and survive into adulthood.

GSDs Presenting with Muscle Disorders

Overview

These disorders can be further separated based on whether there is also cardiac involvement. Type 2 (Pompe disease) is the main disorder in the skeletal and/or cardiac category. Those without cardiac involvement are Type 5 (McArdle disease) and Type 7 (Tarui disease).

Type 2 GSD (Pompe Disease)

Type 2 GSD is another AR condition. It is classified as both a GSD and a lysosomal storage disorder. It is due to a deficiency in the lysosomal acid α-1,4-glucosidase (a.k.a. acid maltase), which is responsible for breaking down glycogen in lysosomal vacuoles.

It does not fall into an energy metabolism defect category. Symptoms are due to the buildup of complex molecules, not primarily from energy problems. It is a lysosomal storage defect with excess storage of glycogen. It is different from the other GSDs in that the glycogen accumulates in the lysosomes and not in the cytoplasm.

METABOLIC DISORDERS

Pompe disease has a wide variety of phenotypic presentations:

- **Infantile-onset form**: This is the most severe and presents with cardiomegaly, hypotonia, and death before 1 year of age. The infant is normal at birth but soon develops generalized muscle weakness, hypotonia, macroglossia, hepatomegaly, FTT, and heart failure due to hypertrophic cardiomyopathy. ECG shows a high-voltage QRS and a shortened PR interval.
- **Juvenile/Late-childhood form**: Slowly progressive skeletomuscular manifestations occur without cardiac involvement. Patients present with slowed developmental milestones, such as delayed walking. Swallowing difficulties, proximal muscle weakness, and respiratory muscle depression then follow. Death may occur before these individuals reach their 20s.
- **Adult form**: This presents in those 20–70 years of age as a slowly progressive myopathy without cardiac involvement. Clinically, patients have progressive proximal muscle weakness, including in the trunk. Lower extremities are more severely affected than the upper extremities. The pelvic girdle and diaphragm are most seriously affected. Initially, the adult might present with increased sleepiness, morning headache, and exertional dyspnea.

Diagnosis: Look for elevated CPK, aspartate aminotransferase (AST), and lactate dehydrogenase (LDH), especially in the infantile form. Muscle biopsy shows vacuoles full of glycogen on staining. There are reduced or absent levels of acid glucosidase activity in muscle or skin fibroblasts.

Treatment: Enzyme replacement therapy (ERT) is available. In the juvenile and adult forms, institute a high-protein diet. Nocturnal ventilatory support may be necessary, which improves daytime symptoms.

Type 5 GSD (McArdle Disease)

Type 5 GSD is an AR disorder due to deficiency of muscle phosphorylase. This deficiency reduces ATP (adenosine triphosphate) generation by glycogenolysis and results in glycogen accumulation in the muscle.

Symptoms are usually not present until patients reach their 20s or 30s, although many can remember symptoms from childhood, including exercise-induced muscle cramps and exercise intolerance. The exercise can be either brief and intense (such as sprinting) or sustained and less intense (such as walking up a hill). Many patients report a "second-wind" phenomenon: if they rest, they can resume the exercise. 50% report burgundy-colored urine after exercise, which is from myoglobinuria due to rhabdomyolysis.

CPK is elevated at rest and increases after exercise. Exercise also increases ammonia and uric acid in the blood.

What suggests the diagnosis? No increase occurs in blood lactate level, but instead an increased ammonia level is found when the patient exercises. This suggests a defect in the conversion of glycogen or glucose to lactate. Enzymatic assays on muscle tissue or DNA analysis for the myophosphorylase gene provide definitive diagnosis.

Treatment is geared toward avoiding strenuous exercise to prevent rhabdomyolysis. Gradual aerobic training or oral fructose/glucose intake can improve exercise tolerance.

Type 7 GSD (Tarui Disease)

Type 7 GSD is an AR disorder mainly reported in Ashkenazi Jews and people of Japanese descent.

It is due to deficiency of muscle phosphofructokinase. The lack of muscle phosphofructokinase causes fructose 6-phosphate to become fructose 1,6-diphosphate.

The symptoms—early onset of fatigue and pain with exercise—are similar to Type 5.

However, Type 7 differs from Type 5 in the following ways:

- Usually present in childhood.
- Hemolysis occurs.
- Increased uric acid levels that are worsened by exercise.
- An amylopectin-like glycogen is deposited in muscle fibers.
- Exercise intolerance is much worse after a carbohydrate-loaded meal; glucose can't be used by the muscle, and the presence of the glucose inhibits the ability of the lipolysis to provide the muscle with energy via fatty acids and ketones.

Remember: With Type 5, glucose consumption before exercise helps.

Diagnosis: Find the defect in affected tissues through biochemical or histochemical means.

Aim treatment toward preventing strenuous exercise.

Gluconeogenesis

Fructose 1,6-diphosphatase deficiency is a defect in gluconeogenesis. Patients have severe episodes of metabolic acidosis, hypoglycemia, hyperventilation, seizures, and coma. Decrease in oral intake during an illness or gastroenteritis precipitates events. This contrasts with hereditary fructose intolerance, in which renal and liver functions are normal. Diagnose by finding the enzyme deficiency in liver or intestinal biopsy. Treat with IV glucose. For the long-term, patients must avoid fasting and eliminate fructose and sucrose from the diet. Cornstarch is helpful for preventing hypoglycemia.

MITOCHONDRIAL DNA MUTATIONS

Overview

Cellular respiration (oxidative phosphorylation) occurs in the mitochondria using a series of enzymes to convert carbohydrates and fatty acids into ATP. All disorders of mitochondrial DNA (mtDNA) are maternally inherited, but not all mitochondrial disorders are caused by mtDNA mutations. The majority are due to recessive mutations in the nuclear DNA, but they can also be AD or X-linked. By definition, these are energy metabolism (i.e., cellular respiration) defects.

The diseases below are based on phenotype. Note: Different mutations can cause the same phenotype, and similar mutations can cause different phenotypes!

Kearns-Sayre and Chronic Progressive External Ophthalmoplegia (CPEO) Syndromes

The following triad classifies these syndromes: ptosis, ophthalmoplegia, and ragged-red fiber myopathy. This triad is very specific for the presence of an mtDNA mutation.

Kearns-Sayre syndrome is the most severe and can begin in infancy, childhood, or adolescence. In addition to the triad, multisystem disease is common, particularly including:

• Cardiomyopathies
• Diabetes mellitus
• Cerebellar ataxia
• Deafness

Some present in infancy with a variant called Pearson syndrome, which has pancytopenia and pancreatitis (think Ps).

CPEO-plus is a disorder of intermediate severity that begins in adolescence or adulthood and has variable systemic involvement, including the eyelids and eye muscles.

Isolated CPEO is the mildest variant, but clinical signs/symptoms worsen with age. These individuals can progress to CPEO-plus or Kearns-Sayre syndrome.

These 3 variants are usually due to a rearrangement of mtDNA. Most of the mutations are spontaneous events during oogenesis or early embryogenesis and are not inherited. They can also occur as nuclear DNA mutations and be transmitted in an AD or AR fashion.

Myoclonic Epilepsy and Ragged-Red Fiber (MERRF) Disease

MERRF usually begins anytime from late childhood to adulthood. The 3 typical traits seen in this disorder are:

1) Epilepsy
2) Cerebellar ataxia
3) Ragged-red fiber myopathy

Myoclonic jerks occur at rest and increase in frequency and amplitude with movement. Most of these are due to an A-to-G mutation of a nucleotide in the transfer RNA (tRNA) used by mtDNA.

Mitochondrial Encephalopathy, Lactic Acidosis, and Stroke-Like Episodes (MELAS)

MELAS can appear at any age, but most cases present before 45 years of age and are known as "stroke of the young." The stroke can be associated with migraines, seizures, or both. It can be difficult to distinguish MELAS from other causes of stroke, especially now that we are seeing more young people with atherosclerotic disease. Look for myopathy, ataxia, cardiomyopathy, deafness, and diabetes mellitus presenting before the stroke. Cerebellar ataxia most commonly occurs long before the stroke. The gene mutation is an A-to-G mutation in tRNA and is maternally inherited.

Note: As many as 1% of patients with adult-onset diabetes mellitus have the mutation, which brings an increased risk of stroke. Think of an oxidative phosphorylation disease in any young person with diabetes mellitus and stroke.

Leigh Syndrome

Consider Leigh syndrome (a.k.a. subacute necrotizing encephalopathy) when you see severe neurological findings (mental and movement), respiratory dysfunction, and ataxia with bilateral hyperintense signals on T2-weighted MRI of the basal ganglia, cerebellum, or brainstem. It typically occurs during infancy/early childhood. Mitochondrial DNA mutations are usually responsible, although nuclear DNA mutations can also be causative, and it can have AR transmission. Besides the findings listed above, patients can have cardiomyopathy, sensory and motor neuropathies, and muscle weakness.

Mitochondrial DNA Depletion Disorders

There is a quantitative reduction in the amount of mtDNA.

These disorders present in neonates and infants with:

• Mitochondrial myopathy
• Hypotonia
• Liver dysfunction
• CPEO
• Severe lactic acidosis

Diagnose by Southern blot analysis, which shows greatly reduced numbers of mtDNA copies in affected tissues.

METABOLIC DISORDERS

IEM — COMPLEX-MOLECULE DEFECTS

PREVIEW | REVIEW

- True or false? Most infants with MPS are normal at birth.

- What are the common features of Hurler syndrome?

- Which 2 things distinguish Hurler syndrome from Hunter syndrome?

- Describe Sanfilippo syndrome.

- What is Morquio syndrome?

- What should you consider when a child presents with Hurler syndrome–like characteristics and hyperplastic gums?

- What are sphingolipidoses?

- What is Gaucher disease Type 1, and how does it present?

- Which type of Gaucher disease does not have CNS involvement?

- How effective is mutation screening for Gaucher disease in Ashkenazi Jews?

- How does NPD Type C present?

- What is the classic eye finding in Tay-Sachs disease?

- Describe a child with Tay-Sachs disease.

- How is Fabry disease inherited?

- What happens in children with Fabry disease when they are excessively overheated, as in exercise?

- What is the function of the peroxisome?

- Name the physical features of a patient with Zellweger syndrome.

- What metal has impaired utilization in Menkes disease?

- What are the common findings in hepatic porphyrias?

- Which drugs can trigger AIP attacks?

- How do children with PCT present?

- Which therapy results in remission of PCT?

- How does an individual with X-linked sideroblastic anemia present?

- How does a child with EPP present?

- How can a child with adenylate deaminase deficiency present?

- Describe Lesch-Nyhan disease.

- What do you look for in homozygous children with FH?

- Which disease should you suspect in a child whose father and 3 uncles all have tendon xanthomas?

- If you draw blood from a child with excessive chylomicronemia, spin it down, and leave the plasma in a test tube overnight, what will you see in the morning? Which complaints would you expect from an affected child?

- What is Smith-Lemli-Opitz syndrome?

MUCOPOLYSACCHARIDOSES, MUCOLIPIDOSES, AND GLYCOPROTEINOSES

Overview

These are complex-molecule defects because symptoms result from lysosomal storage of large complex molecules. All of these disorders are progressive, and most are fatal. Most of these are usually known by their eponym (e.g., MPS 1H = Hurler's).

Infants are normal at birth, and the phenotypic characteristics of the disease appear over time as storage material accumulates. Exceptions are mucolipidosis Type 2 (inclusion-cell [I-cell] disease) and GM1 (monosialotetrahexosylganglioside) gangliosidosis, which present in infancy.

Remember: This is where Pompe disease fits in, but it was initially classified as a GSD and has not yet been reclassified.

See Table 23-4.

Table 23-4: Complex-Molecule Defects	
Category	**Examples**
Lysosomal storage diseases	MPS Gaucher disease Niemann-Pick disease Types A, B, and C Tay-Sachs disease Fabry disease Neuronal ceroid lipofuscinosis
Peroxisomal diseases	Zellweger syndrome spectrum X-ALD Refsum disease Mevalonate kinase Rhizomelic chondrodysplasia punctata
Intracellular trafficking and processing defects	Menkes disease (kinky hair disease; copper defect) Wilson disease (copper defect) Hemochromatosis (iron defect) α_1-Antitrypsin deficiency Congenital disorders of glycosylation
Inborn errors of cholesterol synthesis	Smith-Lemli-Opitz syndrome Hypercholesterolemia (AD) Apolipoprotein E deficiency Tangier disease Desmosterolosis

Mucopolysaccharidoses

Overview

Mucopolysaccharidoses result from defects in the catabolism of glycosaminoglycans by various lysosomal hydrolase enzymes. Lysosomes are cytoplasmic organelles that have enzymes, which phagocytose (degrade) the micromolecules (mucopolysaccharides, glycoproteins, and various lipids). Depending on the specific mucopolysaccharidosis (MPS) disorder, there is accumulation of dermatan sulfate, heparan sulfate, or keratan sulfate in target organs.

Presentation is usually in 1 of 3 forms:

1) Dysmorphic/Coarse features: MPS 1H, MPS 2, MPS 6
2) Learning difficulties, behavior problems, and dementia: MPS 3
3) Severe bone dysplasia: MPS 4

Screen urine first for glycosaminoglycans, but inaccurate/false-negative results are common. WBC and plasma lysosomal enzyme studies can be helpful. Radiographs demonstrating dysostosis multiplex (skeletal abnormalities) are diagnostic. ERT is available for some of these disorders.

Mucopolysaccharidosis Type 1 (Hurler Syndrome)

MPS 1 is AR and due to a defect in the gene coding for α-L-iduronidase. Disease presentations vary widely. MPS 1 subtypes represent a spectrum and include Hurler syndrome, Hurler-Scheie syndrome (not discussed here), and Scheie syndrome.

Those severely affected have Hurler syndrome (MPS 1H) and are frequently diagnosed within the first 2 years of life. They have coarsened facial features, with midface hypoplasia, large tongues, and corneal clouding. Early on, they have frequent URIs and may have inguinal/umbilical hernias. Head circumference is typically larger than the 95th percentile, and communicating hydrocephalus is common. They have severe intellectual disability. Obstructive sleep apnea is also typical, with surgical treatment often needed. Skeletal growth is usually normal during the 1st year, but severe growth retardation soon develops. These kids are at high risk for atlantoaxial subluxation. Evidence of hepatosplenomegaly and cardiac disease is seen systemically. Deafness is common.

Prognosis is generally related to the cardiac involvement, which can be severe and may predict early cardiomyopathy and death. Older children frequently have mitral and atrial valvular involvement. Early coronary artery disease is common.

Less severely affected individuals are often not diagnosed until early adulthood. Usually, they present with bone abnormalities (e.g., spondylolisthesis of L5/S1, degenerative bone loss) or eye problems (e.g., corneal clouding, retinal disease). There is a variant called Scheie syndrome (MPS 1S) in which patients have normal intelligence and life span; carpal tunnel syndrome is characteristic in this form.

Treatment of choice is ERT for those with milder forms and later onset of symptoms. Hematopoietic stem cell transplant (HSCT) is successful in infants/children < 18 months of age to prevent intellectual deterioration—and provides a good chance for long-term survival. However, complex spinal surgery is still required because the HSCT does not correct the skeletal abnormalities. It appears that HSCT is useful only for MPS Types 1H and 6. (Type 6 is very rare and not discussed here.)

Mucopolysaccharidosis Type 2 (Hunter Syndrome)

MPS 2 is X-linked recessive and is due to a defect in the gene that encodes for iduronate-2-sulfatase on the X chromosome. Therefore, only males display the trait (except for the rare affected female patient who has Turner syndrome, a chromosomal translocation, or nonrandom X inactivation).

Clinically, these patients can present with a very wide range of findings. If children are severely affected, it can look like a milder form of MPS 1 because most live into their midteens. In milder forms of MPS 2, normal life span is possible, as is the ability to reproduce and have normal intelligence. When compared, MPS 2 is distinct from MPS 1 in 2 ways:

1) MPS 2 is inherited as X-linked recessive (the only one that is X-linked).
2) Corneal clouding does not occur. (Remember that you have to be able to see well to hunt: Hunter's = no corneal clouding.)

In those severely affected, diagnosis is usually made by 2 years of age.

Typical findings are:

- Learning difficulties (with challenging behavior, ADHD, or seizures)
- Middle ear disease
- Hernias
- Coarse facial appearance
- Diarrhea
- Joint stiffness
- Hepatosplenomegaly

A nodular rash around the scapulae and the extensor surfaces is pathognomonic (but rare in children). Atlantoaxial instability, as seen in MPS 1, is unusual in MPS 2. However, you can see cervical cord compression leading to cervical myelopathy. Adults with MPS 2 have upper respiratory obstruction and sleep apnea.

Cardiomyopathy is rare in younger patients, but uncomplicated valvular lesions are relatively common. Over time valvular heart leaflets become dysfunctional owing to glycosaminoglycan accumulation. Accumulation also results in thickened myocardium that eventually leads to coronary artery compromise and myocardial disease.

Treat with ERT, which replaces the protein the body does not make in affected individuals. ERT improves most symptoms, including movement, stiff joints, breathing, growth, and facial features. Treatment, however, does not reverse or prevent CNS disease.

Mucopolysaccharidosis Type 3 (Sanfilippo Syndrome)

There are 4 described variants of MPS 3 (A, B, C, and D); Type 3A is the most common. Each variant is AR and due to mutations in different enzymes. All variants are unable to break down heparin sulfate. The disease is usually diagnosed at ~ 4–5 years of age, with severe CNS involvement and mild somatic disease. This disproportionate CNS involvement is unique among the mucopolysaccharidoses. It typically follows a classic triphasic pattern:

- Phase 1: Developmental delay with recurrent URIs, diarrhea, and sleep disturbance occurs before 1 year of age.
- Phase 2: Severe, challenging behavior with hyperactivity and aggression. These children have no concept of danger to themselves and must be watched continuously. Family life is completely uprooted. Major tranquilizers are usually required to sedate the child and modify the aggressive behavior. Precocious puberty is common, as well as progressive loss of motor skills.
- Phase 3: Swallowing dysfunction develops with further deterioration to a vegetative state by the midteens. Death occurs by the 20s.

Mucopolysaccharidosis Type 4 (Morquio Syndrome)

MPS 4 is due to a deficiency of galactose-6-sulfatase, resulting in defective degradation of keratan sulfate. MPS 4 characteristics include short-trunk dwarfism, fine corneal deposits, and skeletal (spondyloepiphyseal) dysplasia distinct from other types of MPS, along with normal intelligence.

These patients present during the 1st year of life with severe skeletal dysplasia but are not dysmorphic. Vertebral platyspondylisis is typical.

Adults with the severe form are < 3½ feet in height and have:

- Fixed hip flexion
- Genu valgum
- Pes planus
- Sternal protrusion
- Short neck

Odontoid dysplasia is universal and can be life-threatening. Most of the bone deformities cannot be corrected, and most patients eventually require motorized wheelchairs. Dental decay is also common.

Mucolipidoses

Mucolipidosis Type I (Cherry-Red Spot Myoclonus Syndrome)

Mucolipidosis (ML) I includes a wide range of presentations—from hydrops fetalis in infancy to juvenile sialidosis, myoclonus/ataxia, and a macular cherry-red spot. Most commonly, it presents between these 2 extremes, with a mild Hurler-like phenotype and a cherry-red spot. Death occurs in the late teens.

Mucolipidosis Type II (I-Cell Disease)

ML II presents as a defect in the posttranslational modification of lysosomal enzymes, in which a target sequence (mannose-6-phosphate) fails to attach to the enzyme. This causes the lysosomal enzymes to be "lost" in the extracellular spaces because they can't be directed to the lysosomes. Without the lysosomal enzymes, the lysosomes can't break down a variety of substrates. As the substrates accumulate in the lysosomes, they become toxic to the cell and inhibit cellular function. ML II causes severe clinical and radiologic abnormalities—and looks like Hurler syndrome in terms of physical findings. Periosteal new bone formation is prominent. Hyperplastic gums are the clue to look for (so, Hurler syndrome–like characteristics with hyperplastic gums). Unlike with the other disorders in this group, the head circumference is usually small. Death usually occurs in early childhood due to infection or cardiac failure.

Mucolipidosis Type III (Pseudo-Hurler Polydystrophy)

This is usually a milder disorder with later onset of clinical symptoms, between 2 and 4 years of age, with survival into the 60s. Approximately 50% of patients have some learning disabilities or intellectual disability. The main problem is orthopedic, with severe joint stiffness. Patients cannot raise their arms above their heads, and they also have progressive hip dysplasia. Carpal tunnel syndrome and cardiac valvular lesions are typical. Patients share many features with MPS 1 and 4 but have no mucopolysacchariduria.

Glycoproteinoses

Note

There are numerous rare disorders due to these deficiencies. Only the most common or most tested on exams are listed here.

Mannosidosis

This is usually due to α-mannosidase deficiency. It can present as Hurler-like early in infancy or as a more chronic form later in life. Immunologic abnormalities are most common, and URIs are prevalent.

Others

Salla disease and infantile sialic acid storage disease (ISSD) are both forms of sialic acid storage disease. They are very rare and are found mainly in those of Finnish descent. ISSD is severe, and affected infants present with hydrops fetalis, severe infections, and FTT. Salla disease is less severe and presents mainly with learning difficulties.

SPHINGOLIPIDOSES

Overview

Sphingolipidoses are characterized by defects in the lysosomal breakdown of sphingolipids. Again, these are disorders of complex molecules. When the deficient enzymes can't break down the lipids effectively, there is a buildup of ceramide, which is the lipophilic core. There is also a buildup of 1 of 2 hydrophilic compounds: either oligosaccharide (comprising the glycosphingolipids) or phosphorylcholine (which is sphingomyelin).

The glycosphingolipids can be divided into 3 groups:

1) Globosides (RBC membranes and kidney)

2) Gangliosides (gray matter of the brain in synaptic terminals)

3) Galactocerebrosides (cerebral white matter)

Thus, if you know which "-side" is involved, you can figure out where the problem will occur! The glycosphingolipids (globosides, gangliosides, and galactocerebrosides) and sphingomyelin are mainly components of cell membranes. Remember that each of these conditions has a range of ages for onset, from neonatal to adult, depending on the level of enzyme activity. Generally, the more enzyme activity, the later the age of onset.

Gaucher Disease

Type 1

Gaucher disease Type 1 is the most common lysosomal storage disease, affecting 1/900 Ashkenazi Jews (carrier rate in this group is 1/15). It is due to a deficiency of lysosomal glucocerebrosidase and results in an increased accumulation of glucocerebroside in the reticuloendothelial system. This is a non-CNS disease with only visceral involvement.

Splenomegaly is the most common presentation and is usually found incidentally on a routine physical examination. Abdominal protuberance is common. The hypersplenism predisposes to significant thrombocytopenia, which can result in severe bleeding. Younger children may complain of "growing pains" in the lower extremities, especially at night, and there may be bone infiltration with Gaucher cells (i.e., large macrophages laden with cerebrosides). Growth retardation is typical in those with severe disease.

At examination, look for an anemic-like complexion with increased pigmentation of the skin. Generally, though, these children look well, considering the extent of splenomegaly they have.

Diagnosis: Bone marrow studies show Gaucher storage cells. Confirm diagnosis by finding a deficiency of β-glucosidase in leukocytes or cultured skin fibroblasts.

Treatment: The best treatment is ERT. Splenectomy is contraindicated because it causes increased storage in the lysosomes in the bone, resulting in worsened bone disease. Bone crises usually require narcotics. ERT is standard, with biweekly infusions of glucocerebrosidase. This reverses the hematologic and early skeletal complications of the disease.

Type 2 (Acute Neuronopathy)

Type 2 is also due to a deficiency of lysosomal glucocerebrosidase. This causes increased accumulation of glucocerebroside both in the reticuloendothelial system and the brain. Infants are usually normal initially; however, by 2–4 months of age, they start having feeding difficulties and FTT. They develop strabismus, difficulty swallowing, and opisthotonic posturing. They have huge livers and spleens, but their liver function tests are typically only mildly affected. In a few infants, a macular cherry-red spot is visible bilaterally.

A characteristic lab result is an increased plasma tartrate-resistant acid phosphatase. Bone marrow aspiration shows classic Gaucher storage cells—large, mononucleated histiocytes with cytoplasm containing basophilic material that looks like wrinkled tissue paper. Unlike the later-presenting forms of Gaucher disease, skeletal involvement is minimal.

You can confirm diagnosis by finding a deficiency of β-glucosidase in the leukocytes or cultured fibroblasts. Treatment for Type 2 is supportive. Bone marrow transplant is not helpful. Most of these infants die before 2 years of age due to FTT or pneumonia.

Type 3 (Subacute Neuronopathy)

Type 3 is also due to a deficiency of lysosomal glucocerebrosidase. Previously, it was thought to be uncommon and occurring only in those of Swedish descent. Now we know it crosses all ethnic groups. There are 2 main groups for presentation:

1) **Type 3a** has more prominent neurologic findings with little visceral involvement.

2) **Type 3b** has prominent, severe visceral involvement.

Type 3a presents in early-to-middle childhood with myoclonus, dementia, and ataxia. Look for isolated, supranuclear, horizontal-gaze palsy. You'll see blinking, superimposed upward looping of the eyes, and head thrusting. Tonic-clonic seizures are typical later, along with spasticity. Hepatosplenomegaly is common but is not as severe as in Type 3b. Patients generally die before 30 years of age.

Type 3b cases appear as though they have severe Type 1 disease at ~ 2–3 years of age (described previously on page 23-23). The degree of hepatosplenomegaly is impressive and rapidly progressive compared to Type 1. Hepatocellular dysfunction is prominent with FTT, ascites, nosebleeds, and easy bruising. Portal hypertension and esophageal varices are common. The progression in the viscera is so rapid that neurologic manifestations are usually masked or never develop. The main finding of neurologic significance can be oculomotor apraxia: Eye movements are not well executed.

Bone marrow shows the Gaucher cells. Confirm diagnosis by looking for deficiency of β-glucosidase in leukocytes or cultured skin fibroblasts. Bone marrow transplant is very effective in reversing the visceral and hematologic problems. We do not yet know the impact of bone marrow transplant on neurologic deterioration.

Type 4

These infants present with severe Gaucher disease and have thick, shiny, collodion-like skin. They have multiple congenital anomalies, hepatosplenomegaly, hypertonic and hyperreflexic movements, neck retraction, and a poor sucking mechanism. Nonimmune hydrops can be severe. They usually die within days or weeks.

Gaucher Disease Summary

Points to remember about the types of Gaucher disease:

• Type 1 is the most common and does not have CNS involvement.
• Type 2 has the earliest onset, with neurologic symptoms as well as bleeding tendency.
• Type 3 has neurologic symptoms that are later in onset and more chronic than in Type 2.
• Type 4 is the most severe type; neonate dies within days to weeks.
• All forms include hepatosplenomegaly, bone lesions, and some lung disease.
• Diagnosis: 97% of mutations in Ashkenazi Jews, as compared to ~ 75% in the non-Jewish population, can be detected by screening for the 5 most common mutations.
• Note: ERT does not work for the neurologic disease of Gaucher Types 2 and 3!

Niemann-Pick Disease

Type A

Type A is a very rare form of Niemann-Pick disease (NPD), occurring mainly in Ashkenazi Jews. Its degenerative and neurovisceral manifestations result from a deficiency of acid sphingomyelinase.

It initially causes vomiting, diarrhea, and FTT. Hepatosplenomegaly is prominent by 3 months of age.

Neurologic problems occur at ~ 5–10 months of age with hypotonia, progressive loss of motor skills, and reduction in spontaneous movements. 50% of those affected have macular cherry-red spots, but usually these do not appear until after the occurrence of advanced neurologic disease. Patients develop interstitial lung disease and frequent lung infections. Respiratory failure is a common cause of death, usually by 2–3 years of age.

Diagnose by finding low levels of sphingomyelinase in leukocytes or cultured fibroblasts. Treatment is supportive.

Type B

NPD Type B is due to incomplete deficiency of acid sphingomyelinase, and it is also most common in Ashkenazi Jews. It is the same as NPD Type A but has more residual enzyme activity; therefore, it is less severe than Type A—with later onset, longer survival, and little-to-no CNS involvement.

Clinically, it looks and presents just like Type 1 Gaucher disease, with isolated hepatosplenomegaly. Bone marrow studies show the foamy storage histocytes, as seen in NPD Type A; however, in Type B, the marrow also contains sea-blue histiocytes. Treatment is supportive, but severe disease appears to respond to bone marrow transplant.

Type C

Type C is the most common form of NPD and occurs in 250–500 children (1/150,000) each year in the U.S. The defect is not a lysosomal enzyme disorder, but instead is likely due to routing of cholesterol esters within and through the lysosome. Cholesterol accumulates within the lysosomes of the reticuloendothelial system. It is categorized with the lysosomal deficiency disorders because it was classified before we had the molecular genetic know-how to classify it correctly, but it does appear to cause secondary buildup of GM2 (disialotetrahexosylganglioside) gangliosidosis.

Most cases occur between 3 and 5 years of age with signs of ataxia and hepatosplenomegaly. In older children, the 6- to 12-year range, presentation usually includes poor school performance and impaired fine motor skills. Organomegaly generally occurs but is not present in up to 10% of cases. Cataplexy (e.g., sudden loss of motor movement after an emotional scare) and narcolepsy (i.e., uncontrolled attacks of sleep during the day) are common. On physical examination, the most common finding is supranuclear, vertical-gaze palsy (downward, upward, or both). Voluntary, vertical eye movement is lost, but reflex "doll's eye" movements are preserved. Dysphagia is common and, if progressive, results in the need for a feeding tube. Death in the teenage years is common.

Another possible phenotype is isolated organo-megaly. This is being further examined and is likely underdiagnosed.

Diagnosis: Demonstrate intralysosomal accumulation of unesterified cholesterol in cultured fibroblasts.

Treatment is supportive, but limited data suggests that substrate reduction therapy may be beneficial for some patients with Type C.

Tay-Sachs Disease *cherry red spot*

Tay-Sachs disease is an AR disorder that causes mutations in the *HEXA* gene, resulting in disruption of the enzyme β-hexosaminidase A. This enzyme breaks down the glycolipid GM2 ganglioside. As a result of the enzymatic defect, GM2 ganglioside builds to toxic levels in the neurons, especially in the brain and spinal cord, causing progressive destruction of the neurons. Symptoms include blindness, deafness, and paralysis. Increasingly toxic levels can result in death.

Diagnosis is made by demonstrating low hexosaminidase A activity in blood or tissue and is confirmed by DNA analysis.

There are 2 forms:

1) The **infantile form** usually begins within the 1st few months of life and is due to β-hexosaminidase α-subunit deficiency. The 1st symptom, usually at 3–6 months of age, is frequently an enhanced startle reflex to noise or light and quick extension of the arms and legs with clonic movements. Unlike the Moro reflex, this does not diminish with repeated stimuli. Motor skills are progressively lost. Axial hypotonia, extremity hypertonia, and hyperreflexia are common. In > 90% of infants, a macular cherry-red spot (Image 23-1) occurs bilater-

ally. This is due to storage of lipids that causes white discoloration everywhere in the retina except the fovea, which remains the normal red color of the retina. Macrocephaly is common. Auditory stimuli cause seizures. Visceral organs are normal. By 2–3 years of age, the child has decerebrate rigidity and is blind and unable to respond to stimuli. Autonomic dysfunction also occurs. Frequently, the child dies by 4–5 years of age.

2) The **juvenile/adult form** occurs in Ashkenazi Jews and has an indolent presentation. Early in childhood, the children are labeled "clumsy and awkward." The 1st sign may be an intention tremor (usually by 10 years of age). School problems can occur early on with dysarthria. By adolescence, proximal muscle weakness occurs with fasciculations and atrophy. Psychiatric symptoms are common and include anxiety, depression, and suicide. Usually, with appropriate help, patients with this form can continue to ambulate until their 60s.

Fabry Disease *X-linked*

Fabry disease is the only sphingolipidosis transmitted as an X-linked recessive disease; thus, it mainly affects boys. However, some heterozygous girls develop similar pain crises. Boys present at puberty with complaints of severe, episodic neuropathic pain in the hands and feet. Fever and increased erythrocyte sedimentation rate (ESR) are common with the pain crises. Heat exposure, especially during physical exertion, initiates the pain crises, and the patient does not sweat or sweats very little (hypohidrosis).

Usually, by the mid-to-late teenage years, the affected boys develop angiokeratomata—tiny, red-to-dark blue, papular lesions on the buttocks, scrotum, penis, buccal mucosa, and in the umbilicus. They are individual, ectatic blood vessels covered with a few layers of skin. The lesions are without other symptoms, except they tend to bleed if traumatized.

Corneal opacities are common but do not interfere with vision. Renal disease, coronary artery disease, and stroke occur in early adulthood even in some manifesting heterozygous females. Autonomic nervous system dysfunction occurs and can present as chronic diarrhea, constipation, and the hypohidrosis described above. Cerebrovascular complications include hemiparesis, vertigo, diplopia, nystagmus, headache, ataxia, and memory loss.

Diagnosis: Urine shows casts and Maltese crosses (birefringent lipid globules). Confirm by finding deficiency of lysosomal α-galactosidase in plasma, leukocytes, or cultured skin fibroblasts.

Treatment: Painful peripheral neuropathy appears to respond to carbamazepine or gabapentin. IV infusion of purified α-galactosidase seems to also relieve pain. ERT is clinically available and approved by the FDA; however, no consistent recommendations currently exist for its use in females and children. Renal transplant is required for end-stage renal disease.

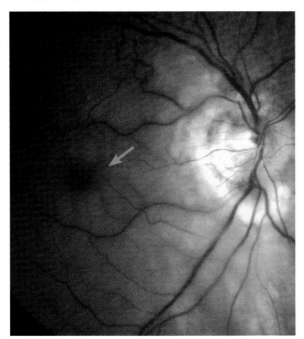

Image 23-1: Tay-Sachs cherry-red spot

METABOLIC DISORDERS

Sphingolipidoses Pearls

Know!

- All disorders are AR, except for Fabry disease (X-linked).
- ERT is available for Gaucher's and Fabry's.
- ERT is effective in preventing/reversing the hematologic and early skeletal complications of Gaucher's (all types), but it does not affect the neurologic problems of Types 2 and 3.
- Gaucher's and Fabry's are included on some U.S. states' NBS.
- See Table 23-5 to help you remember which sphingolipidoses involve the CNS.

Table 23-5: Sphingolipidoses — CNS or Not?

CNS Diseases	
CNS only	Tay-Sachs
CNS with hepatosplenomegaly	Gaucher Types 2 and 3 NPD Types A and C
CNS with vascular and pulmonary involvement	NPD Type A
Non-CNS Diseases	
Predominantly hepatosplenomegaly	Gaucher Type 1 NPD Type B
Peripheral nervous system +/– skin lesions and cardiac, renal, vascular, or pulmonary involvement	Fabry disease

PEROXISOMAL DISORDERS

Overview

First, what are peroxisomes? These are organelles that have a single membrane and are found in just about all cells except RBCs. Peroxisomes contain > 50 different enzymes, including a group of important enzymes that catalyze β-oxidation of fatty acids. These enzymes differ from the mitochondrial enzymes that break down fatty acids. The peroxisomal enzymes oxidize very-long- and long-chain fatty acids, whereas the mitochondrial enzymes oxidize the long-, medium-, and short-chain fatty acids. Another difference is that in peroxisomal oxidation, the 1st step is the production of hydrogen peroxide (H_2O_2), which is later eliminated by another enzyme in the peroxisomal cascade.

Generally, there are 2 classes of peroxisomal disorders:

1) Peroxisomal biogenesis disorders, which involve a deficiency of multiple peroxisome functions
2) Single-function disorders, in which only 1 peroxisomal function is missing

The peroxisomal biogenesis disorders are all AR, and their combined frequency for the 12+ disorders is about 1/50,000. Zellweger syndrome is the classic one usually described. The single-function peroxisome disorders are much less typical and can be AR or X-linked in inheritance. The most commonly described is X-linked adrenoleukodystrophy (X-ALD).

Zellweger Syndrome Spectrum

These are at the severe end of the spectrum for disorders of peroxisome function; this includes **infantile Refsum disease** and **neonatal adrenoleukodystrophy**. Onset of symptoms ranges from birth to 1–2 years of age with loss of skills and a progressive course. These infants have characteristic facies with high forehead, epicanthal folds, broad-based nasal bridge, anteverted nares, and micrognathia. Other prominent findings include a large anterior fontanelle, cataracts, pigmented retinopathy, hearing loss, and vision loss. Liver function is abnormal and jaundice occurs. Calcific stippling (discrete, precise calcifications) of the patella and epiphyses of the long bones is common. Most die before 1 year of age.

Confirm diagnosis by demonstrating elevated serum levels of very-long-chain fatty acids, phytanic acid, and pipecolic acid.

X-Linked Adrenoleukodystrophy

There are multiple clinical presentations for boys with X-ALD. Most severe is the childhood cerebral form. It rapidly progresses with central demyelination and begins between 3 and 10 years of age. The childhood cerebral form occurs in > 33% of those affected and eventually progresses to death within 5–10 years of diagnosis. Almost all these boys have adrenal insufficiency. Another phenotype is adrenomyeloneuropathy. It doesn't show up until the 30s or 40s and presents with distal axonopathy of the spinal cord, causing gait disturbance and urinary sphincter dysfunction; ~ 66% have adrenal insufficiency, and nearly 40% have cerebral effects. Diagnosis is aided by looking for elevated plasma very-long-chain fatty acid levels, particularly C26:0.

DISORDERS OF MINERAL METABOLISM OR ABSORPTION

Menkes Disease (Kinky Hair Disease)

This is a very rare X-linked recessive disease (therefore, only present in males) due to a mutation in the Menkes gene (*ATP7A*), which causes impaired uptake of copper. It occurs in about 1/50,000 to 1/250,000 births.

Males usually present in the neonatal period with premature delivery, temperature instability, hypothermia, hypotonia, and hypoglycemia. They have characteristic facies: pudgy cheeks and sagging jowls and lips. Hair and eyebrows are sparse with little pigment and are easily broken. We call it kinky hair disease because of the characteristic look of the hair. Under the microscope, the hair has pili torti—a flattened shaft with clusters of narrow twists at irregular intervals. By 2–3 months of age, infants have progressive neurologic deterioration, along with seizures and loss of milestones, if they ever made any developmental gains. Collagen and bone formation are abnormal. This is one of the few genetic diseases that can have subdural hematomas and retinal hemorrhages not due to child abuse. It usually progresses, with death at ~ 2 years of age.

Copper measurements are high in intestinal biopsies but low in liver biopsies. When considering the diagnosis in an infant, you cannot rely on copper and ceruloplasmin levels because they are normally low. You need to measure dopamine-ß-hydroxylase; partial deficiency of this enzyme is a hallmark of Menkes disease.

Wilson Disease

Wilson disease is an AR disorder of copper metabolism that results in excessive copper accumulation in tissues. (See Gastroenterology, Book 2.)

Hereditary Hemochromatosis

Hereditary hemochromatosis is most commonly due to a mutation in the *HFE* gene that causes increased iron absorption from the intestines. (See Gastroenterology, Book 2.)

PORPHYRIAS

Overview

These disorders are caused by an enzyme defect in the heme synthesis pathway. They are classified based on hepatic or erythropoietic overproduction and accumulation of the porphyrin precursor or the porphyrins. Generally, those of a hepatic nature present with neuropathy, mental disturbances, and abdominal pain; the erythropoietic group has cutaneous photosensitivity.

Hepatic Porphyrias

Acute Intermittent Porphyria (AIP)

AIP is an AD disorder seen most commonly in Scandinavians and the British, occurring in about 1/20,000 births. It is due to a deficiency (usually about 50% of normal) of porphobilinogen (PBG) deaminase (a.k.a. hydroxymethylbilane [HMB] synthase or uroporphyrinogen I synthetase). Phenotypic expression is variable. Most heterozygous children are asymptomatic, unless some factor increases the production of pyrogens. The factors are varied and include endogenous and exogenous gonadal steroids, drugs, alcohol, and low-calorie diets.

The most common drugs that precipitate AIP attacks (and are frequently found on exam questions):

- Barbiturates (e.g., phenobarbital)
- Sulfonamide antibiotics
- Antiseizure medications (e.g., carbamazepine, valproic acid)
- Griseofulvin
- Synthetic estrogens (birth control pills)

Note: Aspirin, phenothiazines, glucocorticoids, insulin, and acetaminophen are not likely to cause problems.

Abdominal pain is the most common symptom, along with ileus, abdominal distention, and decreased bowel sounds. Abdominal tenderness and fever are absent because AIP is not inflammatory; it affects only the nerves. Patients may also complain of nausea and vomiting with pain in the limbs, neck, or chest. Dysuria and urinary retention also occur.

Peripheral neuropathy is caused by axonal degeneration and initially affects motor neurons, particularly those of the proximal shoulder and arm muscles. Sensory changes are less prominent than the motor dysfunction. Progressive weakness without effective treatment can lead to respiratory and bulbar paralysis. Mental symptoms are common, including anxiety, insomnia, depression, and paranoia during acute attacks.

Seizures can occur as part of the disease course. Compounding the problem, most antiseizure medications induce AIP attacks. Typically, seizures are treated with benzodiazepines (especially clonazepam) or levetiracetam. Hyponatremia is another cause of seizures and must also be treated; it occurs when neuronal degeneration affects the hypothalamus, resulting in syndrome of inappropriate antidiuretic hormone secretion (SIADH).

After an attack of AIP, the abdominal pain resolves in a few hours. The muscle weakness improves over several days but can take years to return to normal.

Initial screening consists of testing urine for elevated PBG. Diagnosis of AIP: Measurement of PBG deaminase activity of approximately 50% in RBCs; you also can screen asymptomatic family members. A normal PBG level in the stool rules out AIP.

Treat acute attacks of AIP with narcotic analgesics for the abdominal pain, and give phenothiazines for nausea and vomiting. IV glucose (300 g/day) can be helpful with continuous parenteral infusion if the patient cannot maintain oral intake. IV heme is probably the most effective therapy if given early. Infuse 4 g of heme (usually as heme albumin or heme arginate) daily for 4 days, as soon as an attack begins. Some women have cyclical attacks, which can be prevented with a luteinizing hormone–releasing hormone analog.

Porphyria Cutanea Tarda (PCT)

PCT is the most common of the porphyrias and is caused by a deficiency of the hepatic synthetic enzyme uroporphyrinogen decarboxylase (UROD). There are 4 types:

- Type I—sporadic
- Types II and III—familial
- Type IV—occurs after exposure to halogenated, aromatic hydrocarbons

Type I has normal UROD levels in RBCs. Type II is UROD deficient in RBCs and other tissues. Type III is UROD deficient only in the liver. Type IV occurs in normal individuals and results from a decrease in UROD enzymes in the liver on exposure to hydrocarbons.

Blistering skin lesions are the predominant clinical feature in PCT. Patients present with cutaneous photosensitivity and develop fluid-filled vesicles and bullae on the sun-exposed areas of the face, the dorsa of the hands and feet, the forearms, and the legs. Milia can precede or follow the vesicles. Hypertrichosis and hyperpigmentation are also typical.

Excess alcohol, iron, and estrogen can contribute to the development of hepatic UROD deficiency. Drugs also have been implicated, including accidental exposure to the fungicide hexachlorobenzene, dioxin, and chlorophenols.

Patients usually have liver damage and are predisposed to develop hepatocellular carcinoma. There is also an association between PCT and hepatitis C.

Diagnosis: increased porphyrin levels in liver, plasma, urine, and stool. Types II and III can be diagnosed by finding decreased UROD activity in RBCs.

Treatment is aimed at preventing exposure to the offending agent. Usually, phlebotomy to reduce hepatic iron can achieve complete response. A unit of blood (450 mL) can be removed every 1–2 weeks. Remission typically occurs after 5 or 6 phlebotomies. After remission, some stay well whereas others require repeated phlebotomies. You can also treat PCT with chloroquine or hydroxychloroquine; these combine with excess porphyrins and enhance excretion. Give only small doses (125 mg) because larger doses may precipitate an acute attack.

Erythropoietic Porphyrias

X-Linked Sideroblastic Anemia

This is due to deficient activity of the erythroid form of aminolevulinic acid (ALA) synthase and results in ineffective erythropoiesis and weakness. Infant boys develop refractory hemolytic anemia, pallor, and weakness. Secondary hypersplenism is typical. Blood smears show hypochromic, microcytic anemia with anisocytosis, poikilocytosis, and polychromasia (cells of many different sizes, irregular shapes, and different colors, respectively). WBCs and platelets are normal. Hemoglobin is reduced; MCV and MCHC are both decreased.

Bone marrow studies show a hypercellular marrow with megaloblastic erythropoiesis. Sideroblasts are usually seen. Urinary porphyrin and its precursors are normal. Definitive diagnosis is finding the mutations in the erythroid ALA synthase gene.

Anemia typically responds to pyridoxine (vitamin B_6). Those who do not respond require transfusions and long-term chelation therapy.

Erythropoietic Protoporphyria (EPP)

EPP is an AR disease that is due to a partial deficiency of ferrochelatase. The inheritance pattern appears to be AD with incomplete penetrance due to the prevalence of a specific mutation in the European population (about 10% of Europeans are unaffected carriers of the *IVS3-48T>C* mutation). Protoporphyrin accumulates abnormally in erythroid cells and plasma and is excreted in bile and feces. This is the most common porphyria in children.

Skin photosensitivity is the major clinical feature and begins in childhood. It is different from the other porphyrias in that vesicles are not common—and pigment changes, severe scarring, and hypertrichosis are unusual. It looks more like angioedema, and within minutes of sun exposure, patients have redness, burning, itching, and swelling.

The source of the excess protoporphyrin is the bone marrow reticulocyte. Liver function is usually normal, but chronic liver disease occasionally develops. Gallstones can also occur and contain protoporphyrin.

Diagnostic findings are elevated levels of protoporphyrin in bone marrow, RBCs, plasma, bile, and feces. Urinary levels of porphyrin and its precursors are normal. Ferrochelatase activity is decreased in fibroblasts.

Treatment: Oral β-carotene improves tolerance to sunlight. Hepatic complications are more difficult to treat. Cholestyramine and activated charcoal cause the interruption of protoporphyrin circulation and lead to its excretion in the feces. Splenectomy can be helpful for those with significant splenomegaly. Transfusions and IV hemin help in suppressing protoporphyrin production. A few patients with severe liver dysfunction have received liver transplants.

PURINE DISORDERS

Overview

Purines, made up of carbon and nitrogen, are major components of cellular energy (e.g., adenosine triphosphate [ATP]), cellular signaling (e.g., cyclic adenosine monophosphate [cAMP]), and DNA/RNA production. Defects in the enzymes used to metabolize purines can lead to clinical disorders.

Phosphoribosyl Pyrophosphate Synthetase Superactivity

Phosphoribosyl pyrophosphate synthetase superactivity is a rare X-linked disorder that causes gout. A severe phenotype with gout, neurodevelopmental delay, and sensorineural deafness occurs in young children. Allopurinol treatment is effective.

Adenylate Deaminase Deficiency

This deficiency is caused by an AR trait that occurs in 1–2% of the population. It presents as muscle weakness and cramping following vigorous exercise. Serum creatine kinase may be increased, but there is no myoglobinuria. Muscle biopsy is normal. A specific histochemical stain is necessary for diagnosis, and many with the deficiency are asymptomatic.

Lesch-Nyhan Disease

Lesch-Nyhan disease is an X-linked recessive disorder caused by deficiency of hypoxanthine guanine phosphoribosyltransferase (HGPRT). This enzyme preserves hypoxanthine and guanine and then converts them to nucleotides.

These males are normal at birth but have FTT, hypotonia, emesis, and irritability by 3–6 months of age. Most patients exhibit abnormal posturing by 18 months of age, and by 2–3 years of age, self-mutilation, the most disturbing manifestation, develops. The children bite their lips and fingers. Renal stones and gout occur because of the huge increase in uric acid production.

Diagnose by finding HGPRT deficiency in RBCs and cultured skin fibroblasts.

DISORDERS OF LIPIDS AND LIPOPROTEINS

Note

Screening guidelines are discussed in Cardiology, Book 3.

Hyperlipoproteinemia Disorders

Familial Combined Hyperlipidemia

Familial combined hyperlipidemia is a syndrome in which low-density lipoprotein (LDL) is usually elevated but the LDL receptor activity is normal. The increased LDL is due to overproduction of very low–density lipoprotein (VLDL) and apolipoprotein B (apoB) in the liver. It occurs in ~ 1/100 births. These children can have elevated LDL alone (Type 2a), elevated LDL and triglyceride (Type 2b), or normal LDL and elevated triglyceride (Type 4). This presents in adults with early coronary artery disease, so ask about the child's family history of early heart disease. Corneal arcus (i.e., deposition of lipid in the peripheral corneal stroma) can occur, but xanthomas do not. Management consists of lifestyle

changes in diet and exercise and statin drugs to lower LDL cholesterol.

Familial Hypercholesterolemia

Familial hypercholesterolemia (FH) occurs in 1/200 to 1/500 births. This AD disorder is caused by mutations at the gene locus for LDL receptor protein. Heterozygous children are usually asymptomatic in the 1st decade, but by the 2nd decade, nearly 10–15% develop xanthomas of the Achilles or extensor hand tendons.

Achilles tendonitis or tenosynovitis can be the 1st clue in a teenage patient. Homozygous children develop planar xanthomas (flat, orange-colored skin lesions) from birth to 5 years of age.

Serum cholesterol is usually 600–1,000 mg/dL. Tendon and tuberous xanthomas occur between 5 and 15 years of age. Angina and symptomatic coronary disease occur in the 2nd decade and have been documented in those < 10 years of age.

Untreated FH male heterozygotes have a 100% risk of developing coronary heart disease by 70 years of age, whereas untreated females have a 75% risk. Treatment reduces this risk by normalizing cholesterol.

Look for a child with parents who have tendon xanthomas or with many 1st degree relatives with highly elevated LDL cholesterol levels. Be aware that other conditions (e.g., biliary cirrhosis, congenital biliary atresia, myelomas, Wolman disease) can cause lipid deposition, but other findings are also apparent to help you differentiate among them.

Treatment consists of a combination of lifestyle (diet and exercise) changes, cholesterol-lowering statins, and, in severe cases, LDL apheresis.

Be on the lookout for **sitosterolemia**, a rare inherited plant sterol storage disease. This disorder has tendon xanthomas in the 1st decade but only moderate hypercholesterolemia.

Hyperapobetalipoproteinemia

Hyperapobetalipoproteinemia has a characteristic elevated LDL apoB level with a normal LDL level, while triglycerides can be normal or elevated. It is due to overproduction of VLDL.

Familial Hypertriglyceridemia

These children have normal total cholesterol and LDL levels; however, they have elevated VLDL and triglyceride levels (Type 4 pattern). If the triglyceride level is > 2,000 mg/dL, the patient can present with pancreatitis.

Lipoprotein-Lipase Deficiency

Lipoprotein-lipase enzyme deficiency/defectiveness results in huge increases of chylomicrons with marked hypertriglyceridemia (up to 10,000 mg/dL). Marked chylomicronemia usually indicates that the body cannot clear dietary fat. You can demonstrate this by leaving an affected individual's plasma in a test tube overnight: in the morning, a thick, creamy layer is apparent. VLDL is normal, and LDL and high-density lipoprotein (HDL) are low.

It usually presents before 10 years of age with abdominal pain as the initial complaint; colic, in particular, occurs in infants < 1 year of age. Eruptive xanthomas, hepatosplenomegaly, and retinal deposits can occur; atherosclerosis usually does not.

Hyperlipoproteinemia Type 5

These patients have a marked triglyceride level due to increased chylomicrons and VLDL. Pancreatitis, eruptive xanthomas, and hyperinsulinemia are common. Many of these cases exhibit AD inheritance.

Dysbetalipoproteinemia (Hyperlipoproteinemia Type 3)

Patients with dysbetalipoproteinemia have elevated cholesterol and triglyceride levels. Characteristic for this syndrome is plasma VLDL that is cholesterol enriched and has β, rather than pre-β, electrophoresis. This disease usually doesn't manifest until adulthood, with xanthomas in the creases of the palms and tuberous xanthomas of the elbows, knees, and buttocks. Premature atherosclerosis is common, although tendon xanthomas are not.

Hypolipoproteinemia Disorders

Abetalipoproteinemia (Bassen-Kornzweig Syndrome)

Abetalipoproteinemia is a rare AR disorder that presents in children with fat malabsorption, hypolipidemia, retinitis pigmentosa, cerebellar ataxia, and acanthocytosis. Chylomicrons, VLDL, and LDL are absent from plasma. Cholesterol and triglycerides are low. Clinically, this is important because the fat-soluble vitamins (A, D, E, and K) are dependent and cannot be absorbed or transported properly. However, only vitamin E deficiency is clinically apparent because of other transport mechanisms available. The retinal and nervous system effects are due to vitamin E deficiency.

Diagnosis is by jejunal biopsy, failure to form chylomicrons after a fatty meal, or demonstration of the absence of apoB in plasma.

Smith-Lemli-Opitz Syndrome

Smith-Lemli-Opitz is an AR disorder due to a defect in cholesterol biosynthesis resulting from deficient activity of 7-dehydrocholesterol reductase. It occurs in ~ 1/20,000 to 1/40,000 births. Remember: Cholesterol is very important in embryogenesis. Therefore, if abnormalities occur during this time, expect marked dysmorphology. The clinical findings range from an isolated partial 2-3–toe syndactyly (Image 23-2) with developmental delay to severely malformed fetuses that die *in utero*.

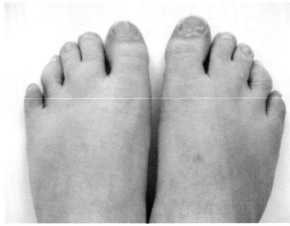

Image 23-2: Partial 2-3–toe syndactyly

The characteristic facial features of the severe form include:

- Microcephaly
- Hypertelorism
- Broad nasal tip
- Cleft palate
- Low-set ears
- Narrow bifrontal diameter
- Ptosis
- Anteverted nostrils
- Micrognathia

In the severe form, the following additional findings are also typical:

- Postaxial polydactyly
- Overlapping fingers
- Abnormal thumbs
- Partial 2-3–toe syndactyly
- Hypospadias
- Ambiguous genitalia

All organ systems can be affected, and intellectual disability is standard. Congenital heart defects are common and should be investigated.

Serum levels of 7-dehydrocholesterol will be elevated, and cholesterol will be normal to low. Remember: The enzyme is deficient, so you get a backup of 7-dehydrocholesterol, and the cholesterol level inversely correlates with severity of disease.

No treatment has proven effective. Treatment with dietary cholesterol and bile-acid supplements to correct serum cholesterol levels may be helpful.

Tangier Disease

Tangier disease is a rare disorder in which plasma HDL is abnormal and deficient. Cholesterol ester is deposited in tissues, resulting in enlarged, orange-yellow tonsils; splenomegaly; and peripheral neuropathy.

NEWBORN SCREENING

PREVIEW | REVIEW

- What is the purpose of the newborn screening?

Since its inception, newborn screening (NBS) has detected progressively more inborn errors of metabolism. What was once known as the PKU test has now expanded to cover about 36 disorders in most U.S. states. It is important to know which disorders can be detected on NBS. NBS is accomplished in most states by tandem mass spectroscopy in newborn screening laboratories.

The goal of the NBS is to detect life-threatening and/or potentially serious disorders that can be treated effectively.

Currently, NBS tests only for IEMs that cause intoxications and/or energy metabolism defects:

- Amino acid defects
- β-oxidation defects
- Galactosemia
- Biotinidase deficiency

Nonmetabolic disorders on NBS are:

- Hemoglobinopathies
- Endocrine disorders such as congenital adrenal hyperplasia and congenital hypothyroidism
- Cystic fibrosis
- Immune deficiencies

Other disorders included on NBS that are not blood based include hearing impairments and congenital heart defects.

NBS does not screen for the liver forms of GSDs or mitochondrial defects.

Historically, NBS did not screen for lysosomal storage disorders. As this group of disorders has become treatable with ERTs or bone marrow transplants, there is a move to include them on the NBS. Some states have implemented screening for Fabry's, Gaucher's, MPS 1H (Hurler's), Pompe's, and Krabbe's (a.k.a. globoid cell leukodystrophy, which is a lysosomal storage disorder that results in globoid cell formation and decreased myelin in the central and peripheral nervous system). Stay tuned, as this list will likely continue to grow.

THE MEDSTUDY HUB: YOUR GUIDELINES AND REVIEW ARTICLES RESOURCE

For both the review articles and current Pediatrics practice guidelines, visit the MedStudy Hub at

medstudy.com/hub

The Hub contains the only online consolidated list of all Pediatrics guidelines! Guidelines on the Hub are continually updated and linked to the published source. MedStudy maintains the Hub as a free online resource, available to all physicians.

METABOLIC DISORDERS

MedStudy

HEMATOLOGY

SECTION EDITOR

Courtney Thornburg, MD
Associate Professor of Pediatrics
University of California—San Diego
La Jolla, CA

MEDICAL EDITOR

Lynn Bullock, MD
Colorado Springs, CO

REVIEWER

Donald W. Coulter, MD
Associate Professor, Pediatrics
University of Nebraska Medical Center
Children's Specialty Physicians
Specialty Pediatric Center
Omaha, NE

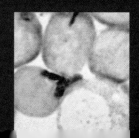

Table of Contents

HEMATOLOGY

DEVELOPMENTAL CHANGES OF RED BLOOD CELLS

PREVIEW | REVIEW

- Describe the changes in location that take place in fetal RBC production.
- What regulates the production of RBCs?
- Where is EPO produced in the fetus? After birth?
- What factors are responsible for the "physiologic anemia of infancy"?
- What is the difference between fetal hemoglobin and adult hemoglobin?
- What happens to the oxygen dissociation curve after birth?

SITES OF BLOOD FORMATION

The anatomic sites for red blood cell (RBC) formation change during embryonic and fetal life. The 1st site of red blood cell formation in the fetus is the yolk sac at 2 weeks of gestation. By the 8th week of gestation, RBC formation shifts to the liver, increases, peaks at 5 months, and then decreases thereafter. The bone marrow takes over at 5 months of gestation and remains the predominant site for RBC production. In extraordinary circumstances, such as myelofibrosis or severe hemolytic anemia, RBC production occurs in extramedullary sites, such as the liver and spleen.

yolk sac → liver → BM

RED BLOOD CELL INDICES

The amount of oxygen delivered to tissues depends on the supply and function of RBCs and hemoglobin. There are laboratory tests that demonstrate this.

The **mean corpuscular volume (MCV)** reflects the size of the RBCs, whereas the **mean corpuscular hemoglobin (MCH)** and the **mean corpuscular hemoglobin concentration (MCHC)** reflect the amount of hemoglobin in RBCs. MCH is the average mass of hemoglobin in each RBC. MCHC is a related value demonstrating the ratio of hemoglobin mass to the volume of RBCs.

Red blood cell distribution width (RDW) measures variability in RBC size. An increased RDW means increased variation in RBC size.

Reticulocytes are immature RBCs. A **reticulocyte count (retic count)** is often reported as the percentage of reticulocytes in the blood and indicates if the bone marrow is producing an adequate number of RBCs.

PRODUCTION RATES AND NORMAL VALUES

Dependencies

Production rates and normal values depend on age, sex, and clinical conditions/factors.

The Fetus

In the fetus, the RBC count triples from 12 weeks of gestation to term. MCV decreases from 180 fL at 12 weeks to 108 fL at term (which is still macrocytic compared to older children). Retic counts in term infants average ~ 5%, and it is common for nucleated RBCs to circulate freely for several days after birth.

The Newborn

In the first few days after birth, hemoglobin levels are much higher in capillaries than in venous blood due to a loss of plasma from the capillaries. Also, venous hemoglobin, hematocrit, and RBC counts increase between birth and the first 3 days of life due to a postnatal decrease in plasma volume.

The production of RBCs is regulated by erythropoietin (EPO), which is produced by the liver in the fetus. Production switches from liver to kidney soon after birth. EPO production is regulated by tissue oxygenation. At birth, hemoglobin averages 17 g/dL; this relative polycythemia is due to the low arterial P_aO_2 *in utero* that stimulates EPO production and thus increases erythropoiesis. Arterial P_aO_2 rises acutely at birth, resulting in a decrease in EPO production. Nucleated RBCs disappear from the peripheral blood, and the retic count falls. Red cell lifespan during the first 6–8 weeks of life is around 90 days instead of the usual 120 days. This results in the "physiologic anemia of infancy," which reaches its nadir around 2 months of age, with an average hemoglobin level of 9–11 g/dL. If this is found on laboratory evaluation, no further biochemical follow-up is needed. After 6–8 weeks of life, RBC production resumes and retic counts increase, as does the hemoglobin.

The Preterm Infant

The preterm infant has an even more dramatic fall in hemoglobin concentration than the term newborn. By 2 months of age, hemoglobin falls to 9.5 g/dL in infants with birth weights between 1,500 and 2,000 g—and to 9 g/dL for those infants weighing between 1,000 and 1,500 g at birth. Hemoglobin levels drop further for infants with a very low birth weight. Preterm infants have inappropriately low levels of EPO and thus cannot stimulate production of RBCs.

Older Children and Adolescents

In preschool- and school-age children, erythropoiesis keeps up with growth, and the mean hemoglobin increases. The values for boys and girls diverge at adolescence due to the erythroid-stimulating effects of androgens in adolescent males.

MCV falls during the first 6–12 months of life, during which time it reaches its nadir of 77 fL, and then rises throughout childhood and adolescence.

Retic counts are normally < 2% after 4 months of age, and nucleated RBCs disappear from the circulation after the first week of life.

Blood volume is fairly constant after 6 months of age and remains at 75–77 mL/kg.

HEMOGLOBIN

Hemoglobin (Hb) is a tetramer made up of 2 pairs of globin chains, each attached to an iron-containing porphyrin ring (heme). The globin chain is designated by a Greek letter followed by a subscript that shows the number of chains per molecule. For example, normal adult hemoglobin (HbA) contains 2 pairs of α and β chains and is designated $\alpha_2\beta_2$.

In the embryo, hemoglobin is predominantly Gower-1, Gower-2, and Portland, and they contain ζ and ε chains. By 8–12 weeks of gestation, the Gower and Portland hemoglobins disappear and fetal hemoglobin (HbF) predominates. HbF contains α and γ chains and is known as $\alpha_2\gamma_2$. It accounts for 90% of the circulating hemoglobin in a 6-month-old fetus, after which it begins to be replaced by adult hemoglobin. At birth, however, HbF still makes up 70% of the total hemoglobin. By 4 months of age, HbF is less than 20% of the total; and by 1 year of age, it makes up less than 2% of hemoglobin. In patients with hemoglobinopathies, the amount of HbF remains elevated. HbA$_2$ ($\alpha_2\delta_2$), or minor adult hemoglobin, is produced in late gestation and accounts for about 2–3% of total hemoglobin after the first few months of life. HbA$_2$ is elevated in β-thalassemia trait. See Figure 24-1.

OXYGEN TRANSPORT

Oxygen transport is tied to the intrinsic function of hemoglobin. In the fetus and newborn, the oxygen dissociation curve favors oxygen extraction from the maternal circulation. This limits the proportional release of oxygen to the tissues after birth. The oxygen dissociation curve shifts to the right after birth to allow better release of oxygen to the tissues; this is due mainly to the change from HbF to HbA and the effect of 2,3-diphosphoglycerate (2,3-DPG), which is found in RBCs and is a potent affinity modulator.

HbA: $\alpha_2\beta_2$
HbF: $\alpha_2\gamma_2$
HbA$_2$: β thal!

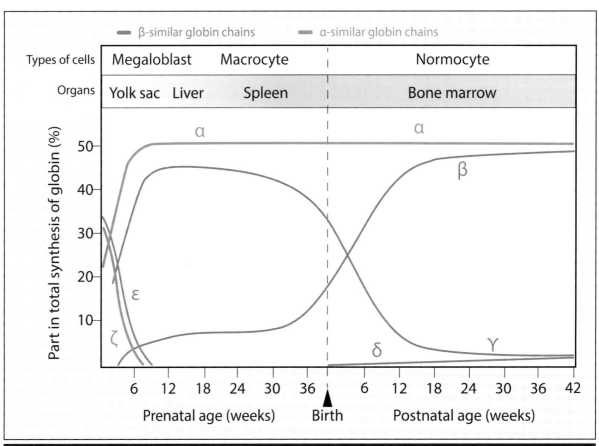

Figure 24-1: Developmental Globin Synthesis

ANEMIA

PREVIEW | REVIEW

- Which tests are recommended in the initial workup of anemia?
- Know Table 24-1.
- Know Table 24-2.
- What is the significance of elevated HbA_2 in the evaluation of microcytic anemia?
- What is hemoglobin Bart? Under what conditions is hemoglobin Bart seen?
- What infection is most commonly responsible for chronic GI blood loss in children worldwide?
- How can you use RDW to differentiate iron deficiency anemia from β-thalassemia minor?
- What is the most common type of hypoproliferative anemia?
- Which animal's milk is low in folate and results in folate deficiency in infants predominantly given this type of milk?
- How do you differentiate between the congenital and juvenile forms of pernicious anemia?
- Which cause of macrocytic anemia can lead to neurologic problems?
- What are the RBC survival defects?
- What is the underlying defect in hereditary spherocytosis?
- How do you diagnose G6PD deficiency? Is testing reliable during a hemolytic crisis?
- What is the genetic defect that results in hemoglobin S?
- What is the average lifespan of a sickle cell?
- How do you diagnose sickle cell disease?
- Which types of bacterial infection result in serious disease in children with sickle cell disease?
- At what age is penicillin prophylaxis started in patients with sickle cell disease?
- What is the most common reason for hospital admission of a patient with sickle cell disease?
- What is the most common first crisis in children with sickle cell disease?
- What is the most common cause of death for adolescents with sickle cell disease?
- Which infection causes aplastic crisis in patients with sickle cell disease?
- What is the acute treatment for a stroke in a patient with sickle cell disease?
- What is priapism? What are the treatment options for priapism with sickle cell disease?
- When are people with sickle cell trait at risk for sickle cell–related complications?
- What is the genetic defect in hemoglobin C?
- What clinical features are found with HbCC and HbC trait?
- How are the direct and indirect Coombs tests performed, and when are they ordered?
- Which pathogens cause cold agglutinin disease in children?

NORMAL ERYTHROPOIESIS

Erythropoietin regulates RBC production. Normal erythropoiesis involves maturation of stem cells: proerythroblasts → erythroblasts of different stages → reticulocytes → mature cells (Figure 24-2). Reticulocytes have lost their nucleus but retain RNA. The mature RBCs in the peripheral blood have lost their RNA. A special stain is used to quantify reticulocytes, but they are easily recognized on a peripheral blood smear (polychromasia).

proerythroblast
↓
basophilic erythroblast
↓
polychromatic erythroblast
↓
pyknotic erythroblast
↓
reticulocyte
↓
mature RBC

Figure 24-2: Erythropoiesis

Mature RBCs have a lifespan of 120 days. The spleen removes old or damaged RBCs, which are then ingested by macrophages, part of the reticuloendothelial system. The hemoglobin is catabolized, and the porphyrin ring of heme is opened, forming unconjugated (indirect) bilirubin. Haptoglobin binds and transports free hemoglobin in serum.

Iron released from heme or absorbed in the intestine from the diet is transported by transferrin to the bone marrow and stored as ferritin. Therefore, ferritin typically reflects iron stores, but remember that it is also an acute phase reactant and does not accurately reflect iron stores if there is ongoing inflammation. (Transferrin saturation and total iron-binding capacity [TIBC] are indirect measures of iron levels as well.)

CLINICAL MANIFESTATIONS OF ANEMIA

Patients are usually asymptomatic, even with significant anemia. Some symptomatic clues are:

- Ice-eating (pagophagia), lethargy: iron deficiency
- Distal paresthesias: B_{12} deficiency
- LUQ abdominal pain: hereditary spherocytosis with splenomegaly
- RUQ pain or intolerance to fatty foods: cholelithiasis from chronic hemolysis
- Constipation and cold intolerance: hypothyroidism

LABORATORY RESULTS (RED CELL INDICES, RETICULOCYTE COUNT, AND PERIPHERAL BLOOD SMEAR)

The initial workup of anemia is often prompted by the clinical presentation, which can include pallor, jaundice, and decreased activity. The evaluation starts with a complete blood count including red cell indices, retic count, and examination of the peripheral blood smear. See Image 24-1 through Image 24-6 for different magnifications of normal peripheral smears and bone marrow aspirates.

One approach to classification of anemias is based on the red cell indices (Figure 24-3). MCV is the average size of RBCs in a specimen, and anemias are characterized as microcytic (low MCV), normocytic (normal MCV), and macrocytic (high MCV). Microcytic anemia results from iron deficiency (Image 24-7), thalassemia, certain hemoglobinopathies, and anemia of chronic disease (ACD; a.k.a. anemia of chronic inflammation). Normocytic anemias result from acute blood loss, certain hemolytic anemias, and ACD. Macrocytic anemias result from B_{12} or folate deficiency (Image 24-8), certain medications (e.g., valproic acid), and inherited bone marrow failure syndromes. Other red cell indices can also give clues to the diagnosis. The RDW is elevated, for example, in patients with iron deficiency. The MCHC is elevated in hereditary spherocytosis.

Retic count is an important test in the evaluation of anemia. Production and maturation defects lead to low retic counts, whereas bleeding, hemolysis, and response to therapy cause a high retic count.

Review of RBC, platelet, and white blood cell (WBC) morphology provides important diagnostic clues. For example, crescent-shaped cells are diagnostic of sickle cell anemia. Spherocytes are seen in autoimmune hemolytic anemia and hereditary spherocytosis. Review the

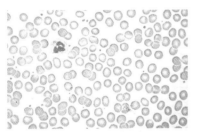

Image 24-1: Normal peripheral smear: low-power view. RBCs, platelets, and segmented neutrophil.

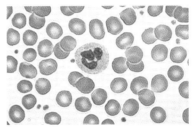

Image 24-2: Normal peripheral smear: low-oil view. Normocytic, normochromic RBCs; platelets; and normal segmented neutrophil.

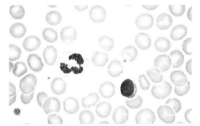

Image 24-3: Normal peripheral smear: high-dry view. RBCs, platelets, normal segmented neutrophil, and normal lymphocyte.

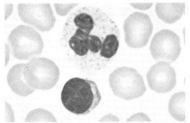

Image 24-4: Normal peripheral smear: high-oil view. Normal RBCs, segmented neutrophil, and lymphocyte. No platelets are visible in this field.

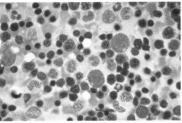

Image 24-5: Normal bone marrow aspirate: low-power view. M:E (myeloid to erythroid) ratio is usually 3:1. This field has more than the normal number of erythroid precursors. Many of the erythroid precursors have dark, condensed nuclei.

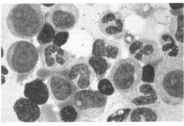

Image 24-6: Normal bone marrow aspirate: low-oil view. 5 erythroid precursors (dark, condensed nuclei). Remaining cells are myeloid precursors/cells—from myoblasts to segmented neutrophils.

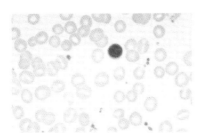

Image 24-7: Iron deficiency. Thrombocytosis, microcytosis, and hypochromia.

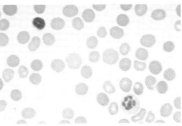

Image 24-8: B_{12} or folate deficiency with pernicious anemia. Low-power view shows hypersegmented neutrophil and macrocytosis.

slide for platelets. Low platelets in association with anemia can indicate Evans syndrome, thrombocytopenic purpura, disseminated intravascular coagulation (DIC), aplastic anemia, or leukemia. Anemia can be a presenting sign of childhood leukemia. Review the WBC morphology for blasts. Table 24-1 on page 24-6 lists specific findings seen on the peripheral blood smear in different types of anemia.

ETIOLOGY OF ANEMIAS

Overview

The etiology of anemia can be classified as either a production defect or a survival defect. Production defects include problems with production of sufficient numbers of RBC precursors in the bone marrow or problems with the maturation of these precursors into fully formed RBCs. Survival defects are problems with the survival of the fully formed RBCs. These can be intrinsic (due to a defect in the construction of the RBCs) or extrinsic (due to a destructive force acting on the normal RBCs). All survival defects result in hemolytic anemia. Table 24-2 on page 24-6 summarizes the production and survival defects that cause anemia.

Production Defects

Overview

Production defects include the following:

- Inherited
  - Thalassemias (also survival defect secondary to hemolysis)
  - Inherited bone marrow failure syndromes (IBMFS; see Stem Cell Disorders on page 24-23)
- Acquired
  - Acquired bone marrow failure
  - Decreased erythropoietin (renal disease)
  - Iron deficiency anemia
  - ACD
  - Folate deficiency
  - B_{12} deficiency (also inherited)
  - Sideroblastic anemia (also inherited)

Inherited Production Defects — Thalassemias

Normal adult hemoglobin has 2 alpha and 2 beta globin chains. Thalassemias are inherited disorders in which there is unbalanced globin chain synthesis due to absent or decreased production of either the beta chain (β-thalassemia) or the alpha chain (α-thalassemia). Each chromosome 16 contains 2 alleles coding for the α-globin chain (4 alleles total), and each chromosome 11 contains 1 allele for the β-globin chain (2 alleles total).

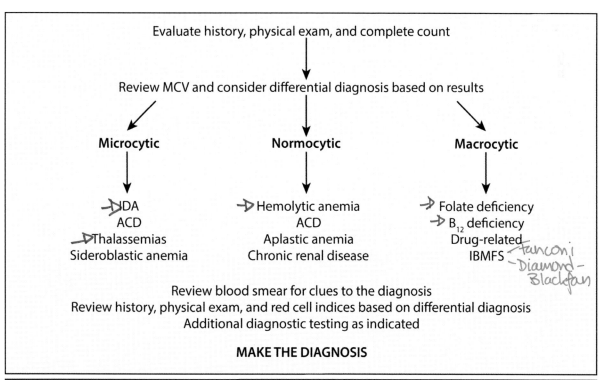

Evaluate history, physical exam, and complete count

Review MCV and consider differential diagnosis based on results

Microcytic

IDA
ACD
Thalassemias
Sideroblastic anemia

Normocytic

Hemolytic anemia
ACD
Aplastic anemia
Chronic renal disease

Macrocytic

Folate deficiency
B_{12} deficiency
Drug-related
IBMFS — Fanconi
— Diamond-Blackfan

Review blood smear for clues to the diagnosis
Review history, physical exam, and red cell indices based on differential diagnosis
Additional diagnostic testing as indicated

MAKE THE DIAGNOSIS

Figure 24-3: Diagnostic Approach to Anemia Based on MCV

Table 24-1: The Peripheral Smear — Significance of Specific Findings

Finding	Meaning
RBC fragments (schistocytes)	Microangiopathic hemolytic anemia (seen in TTP, HUS, HELLP syndrome, DIC, and occasionally vasculitis), severe burns, and valve hemolysis (Image 24-9).
Spherocytes	Autoimmune hemolytic anemia and hereditary spherocytosis (Image 24-10).
Target cells	Significant liver disease, thalassemia syndromes, sickle cell disease Type SC, and homozygous hemoglobin C (Image 24-11).
Teardrop cells (dacrocytes)	Classic for myelofibrosis and other infiltrating bone marrow processes; also seen with thalassemia (Image 24-12).
Burr cells (echinocytes) vs. spur cells (acanthocytes)	Burr cells (Image 24-13 and Image 24-14) are seen in uremic patients. These are distinct and different from spur cells (Image 24-14 and Image 24-15), which are seen in liver diseases.
Hypersegmented PMNs	Megaloblastic anemia (e.g., pernicious anemia/B_{12} deficiency, folate deficiency). See Image 24-8 on page 24-4.
Elliptocytes	Hereditary elliptocytosis (Image 24-16), severe iron deficiency anemia.
Sickle cells (crescent-shaped)	Sickle cell disease (HbSS and HbS β-thalassemia; less common in HbSC; Image 24-17).
Howell-Jolly bodies (nuclear remnants)	Splenectomy or functional asplenia (as seen in sickle cell disease). Howell-Jolly bodies (Image 24-18) are the result of fragmentation of the nucleus (karyorrhexis), causing the formation of small black "pellets." This occurs normally, and the spleen efficiently removes them.
Basophilic stippling (RNA)	Indicates ineffective erythropoiesis; lead poisoning, thalassemia, pyrimidine 5'-nucleotidase deficiency (Image 24-19).
Heinz bodies (denatured hemoglobin)	G6PD deficiency.

Table 24-2: Classification of Anemia — Production and Survival Defects

	Defects	Etiology	Examples
Production Defects	Fewer RBC precursors formed in bone marrow	1) Decreased erythropoietin 2) Bone marrow failure	1) Chronic renal disease 2) Aplastic anemia
	Maturation defects: Cytoplasmic	1) Impaired Hb synthesis 2) Decreased globin synthesis	1) Iron deficiency 2) Thalassemias
		Iron deficiency	Sideroblastic anemia
	Maturation defects: Nuclear	DNA synthesis defects	B_{12}, folate deficiencies
Survival Defects	Intrinsic	1) Membrane cytoskeleton protein 2) Membrane protein deficiency 3) Metabolic enzymes 4) Hemoglobinopathies	1) Spherocytosis, elliptocytosis 2) PNH 3) G6PD deficiency 4) HbSS disease, HbC, HbE
	Extrinsic	1) Immune-mediated hemolytic anemias 2) Drug-induced hemolysis 3) Other causes	1) Autoimmune hemolytic anemia, isoimmune hemolytic anemia of the newborn 2) Penicillin, quinine 3) DIC, mechanical trauma, oxidative injury, hypersplenism

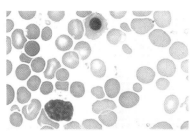

Image 24-9: Burn hemolysis. Hemolytic anemia, nucleated RBC, and spherocytosis. Spherocytes are also seen in immune hemolytic anemia and hereditary spherocytosis.

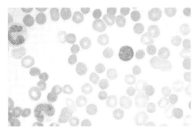

Image 24-10: Hereditary spherocytosis. Note the lack of central pallor. The normal-sized lymphocyte shows that these are microcytic spherocytes.

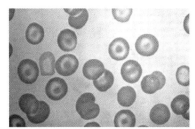

Image 24-11: Target cells: low-oil view.

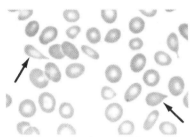

Image 24-12: Teardrop cells (dacrocytes).

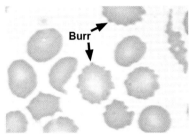

Image 24-13: Echinocytes or Burr cells in uremia. These are RBCs with regular, short, spiny projections. These membrane changes disappear when uremia is corrected.

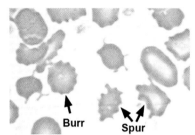

Image 24-14: Hepatorenal failure. Burr cells as seen in uremia, and spur cells as seen in hepatic failure.

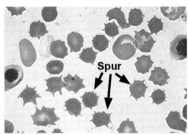

Image 24-15: Acanthocytes (spur cells). Nucleated RBCs. Spur cells are RBCs with multiple irregular projections that vary in length, width, and regularity. Usual cause is hepatic failure.

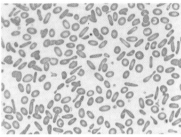

Image 24-16: Hereditary elliptocytosis.

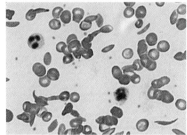

Image 24-17: Sickle cell disease.

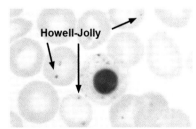

Image 24-18: Postsplenectomy. Howell-Jolly bodies are the dense blue inclusion bodies in the RBCs.

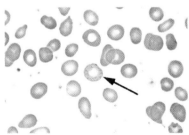

Image 24-19: Basophilic stippling.

There are 3 categories of β-thalassemias (minor, intermedia, and major):

In β-thalassemia, gene variants are classified as β^0 with no beta globin production or β^+ with very reduced beta globin production.

1) **β-thalassemia minor** (heterozygous; i.e., 1 normal beta globin allele (β) and 1 thalassemic allele (β^0 or β^+): mild or no anemia, with a disproportionate degree of microcytosis. These patients are asymptomatic. Hypochromia, microcytosis, target cells, elliptocytes, and basophilic stippling occur. RDW is normal. Finding an $HbA_2 > 3.5\%$ is diagnostic.

2) **β-thalassemia intermedia** (homozygous β^+/β^+): some normal β-globin production and, therefore, milder symptoms compared with β-thalassemia major (below). These patients usually do not require transfusions. Decreased production of β-globin leads to increased delta and gamma chains. Therefore, HbA_2 ($\alpha_2\delta_2$) and HbF ($\alpha_2\gamma_2$) are increased. This is of use diagnostically because quantitative hemoglobin electrophoresis measures the levels of these hemoglobins.

3) **β-thalassemia major** (Cooley anemia; homozygous β^0/β^0 thalassemia or compound heterozygous β^0/β^+ thalassemia): homozygosity for impaired gene synthesis with essentially no β-globin production. The remaining, highly insoluble α-globin precipitates into inclusion bodies (**Heinz bodies**, seen with special staining of the blood smear), causing severe clinical symptoms. Most erythroblasts die in the bone marrow (intramedullary hemolysis), resulting in erythroid hyperplasia in the bone marrow. By 6–12 months of age, most infants show pallor, irritability, growth retardation, hepatosplenomegaly, profound anemia, and jaundice. Expansion of the bone marrow space (due to extramedullary hematopoiesis) in facial bones leads to characteristic changes such as frontal bossing and prominent malar eminences (i.e., "chipmunk facies" in children). Mature RBCs that are produced have a shortened lifespan. On blood smear, RBCs are hypochromatic and microcytic. In addition, the RBCs are abnormally shaped and include target cells, teardrop cells, echinocytes, and fragmented cells. Nucleated red cells are present. Hemoglobin electrophoresis shows almost all HbF. HbA is absent in homozygous β^0/β^0 thalassemia and is present in very small amounts in compound heterozygous β^0/β^+ thalassemia. Patients with β-thalassemia major are transfusion dependent and often develop iron overload, requiring chelation therapy. Iron overload can cause endocrine abnormalities, heart failure, and arrhythmias due to deposition of iron in the organs. Splenectomy is beneficial in some cases, and bone marrow transplant can be curative.

There are 4 categories of α-thalassemias, each of which involves the deletion or dysfunction of 1 or more of the 4 alleles (Table 24-3). The more loci affected, the worse the symptoms:

1) **α-thalassemia trait**: 1 locus, asymptomatic, no hematologic abnormalities (the "silent carrier")

2) **α-thalassemia minor**: 2 loci, asymptomatic, MCV low, little-to-no anemia

3) **HbH disease**: 3 loci, moderate-to-severe hemolysis

4) **Hydrops fetalis**: 4 loci, death *in utero*

Patients with α-thalassemia have differing levels of hemoglobin Bart (a tetramer of gamma chains) on their newborn screen, depending on the number of alleles affected.

Diagnosis of thalassemias on newborn screening (Table 24-3): β-thalassemia major (β^0/β^0) is diagnosed on newborn screening (HbF only). Other β-thalassemias have the normal newborn hemoglobin pattern of fetal hemoglobin and adult hemoglobin A (FA). Alpha thalassemia shows FA with elevated hemoglobin Bart.

Acquired Production Defects

Bone Marrow Failure

Profound endocrine failure due to deficiencies in thyroid hormone, glucocorticoids, testosterone, or growth hormone can lead to anemia. Therefore, hypoproliferative anemia often complicates hypothyroidism, Addison disease, hypogonadism, and/or panhypopituitarism. These are rare in children.

See Stem Cell Disorders on page 24-23.

Decreased Erythropoietin

Patients with renal failure have anemia due to decreased erythropoietin production, and the anemia is usually responsive to recombinant erythropoietin.

Iron Deficiency

The major nutritional deficit of youth is iron deficiency anemia. Iron is essential for the production of hemoglobin. An adult has up to 5 g of body iron, whereas a newborn has as little as 0.25 g. Thus, during childhood and adolescence, a total of 4.75 g of iron must be absorbed. During times of maximal growth, such as infancy or adolescence, the iron requirements exceed the actual iron accrual rate. Only about 5% of dietary iron is absorbed, and most children require 10–15 mg of iron per day to maintain a positive iron balance. During infancy, this requires the use of iron-fortified foods beyond 4 months of age.

Iron deficiency is caused by poor intake, poor absorption, or excess blood loss. Inadequate iron intake is the most common cause of iron deficiency anemia in the pediatric population. In infants and young children, excess intake of cow's milk is a typical factor. In a child with a normal

Table 24-3: Newborn Screening and Hemoglobinopathies

Condition	Hemoglobin Electrophoresis: Newborn*	Hemoglobin Electrophoresis: Children and Adults*
Sickle Cell Disease		
HbSS	FS	S, may have elevated F
HbSC	FSC	SC
HbS β^0 thalassemia	FS	S
HbS β^+ thalassemia	FSA or FS	SA
Sickle cell trait (HbAS)	FAS	AS
Thalassemias		
Beta thalassemia minor	FA	A, elevated HbA$_2$, elevated HbF
Beta thalassemia intermedia	FA or F	A, elevated HbA$_2$, elevated HbF
Beta thalassemia major (β^0/β^0)	F	F
Beta thalassemia major (β^0/β^+)	FA	FA
Alpha thalassemia trait, silent carrier Single alpha gene deletion	FA, may have elevated Hb Bart**	A
Alpha thalassemia minor 2 alpha gene deletions	FA, elevated Hb Bart**	A
Hemoglobin H disease 3 alpha gene deletions	FA, elevated Hb Bart**	A, elevated HbH***
Hydrops fetalis 4 alpha gene deletions	Mainly Hb Bart**	Death *in utero*

* Hemoglobin order is dictated by quantity, high to lower.
** Hb Bart = 4 gamma chains
*** HbH = 4 beta chains

diet, remember to consider bleeding as a cause of iron deficiency. Menstrual loss is an obvious contributor in the adolescent girl. In all age groups, chronic blood loss from the GI tract is a common cause of iron deficiency. GI blood loss results from Meckel diverticulum, *Helicobacter pylori* with gastric ulcer, and inflammatory bowel disease. Children with celiac disease often have concomitant iron deficiency anemia. Worldwide, hookworm infection (*Necator americanus* or *Ancylostoma duodenale*) is the most common cause of chronic GI blood loss. See Infectious Disease, Book 4, for more information. Consider testing all children with iron deficiency anemia for occult GI blood loss.

Most patients with iron deficiency anemia are asymptomatic. Sometimes, there is a history of pica (repeated ingestion of nonnutritive substances). In severe cases, the patient can present with pallor, irritability, poor feeding, tachypnea, or exercise intolerance. In addition to anemia, iron deficiency also causes nonhematologic effects, such as behavior and learning disturbances.

The RBCs in iron deficiency are often microcytic (MCV < 80 fL) and hypochromic (decreased MCHC = Hb/HCT × 100). The retic count is low, as are serum iron and ferritin (iron stores). Remember that ferritin is an acute phase reactant and can be high in the setting of iron deficiency if there is ongoing inflammation. Serum iron-binding capacity is increased because transferrin iron saturation is low.

It is important to distinguish iron deficiency anemia from β- and α-thalassemia trait because microcytosis is present in all of these conditions. To differentiate these traits from iron deficiency, look at the Mentzer index (MCV/RBC). This index is ≥ 13 in iron deficiency and < 13 in thalassemia, which is explained by the fact that the RBC count is generally low in iron deficiency but normal or increased in thalassemia trait. In addition, the RDW is normal in patients with thalassemia trait but is increased in early iron-deficient patients. Ferritin is normal in thalassemia trait and low in iron deficiency. Ferritin is often elevated with β-thalassemia intermedia or major and with hemoglobin H disease (3 alpha gene deletions). Basophilic stippling and target cells can also be seen in thalassemia trait.

It is also important to distinguish iron deficiency anemia from anemia of chronic disease (ACD). ACD is the most common hypoproliferative anemia. It occurs in patients with a chronic malignant, infectious, or inflammatory disorder. Treatment is aimed at management of the underlying disorder.

Understanding the role of hepcidin can be helpful in distinguishing these 2 types of anemia. Hepcidin blocks iron transport. When levels are high, iron absorption is low. In iron deficiency anemia, hepcidin levels decrease in response to low iron stores and iron absorption increases. In contrast, in anemia of chronic disease, iron stores are normal to high, but the cytokine-mediated production of hepcidin inhibits their use and causes anemia. See Table 24-4 for a comparison of lab values in iron deficiency anemia vs. ACD.

Table 24-4: Iron Deficiency vs. ACD		
Lab Parameter	Iron Deficiency	ACD
Iron	Low	Low
TIBC	High	Low
Transferrin saturation	Low	Low to normal
Ferritin	Often low	Normal to high

Iron-refractory iron deficiency anemia (IRIDA) is a rare, inherited condition in which children are unresponsive to oral iron and are only partially responsive to IV iron. This disorder is related to mutations in *TMPRSS6* that increase hepcidin, leading to impaired iron absorption and transport.

Treatment of iron deficiency anemia is aimed at correcting the underlying cause (e.g., limiting cow's milk, looking for GI bleeding). Oral iron therapy is almost always sufficient to correct anemia and replace iron stores. Give oral iron as 3–6 mg/kg of elemental ferrous sulfate per day. Most children can handle the iron without GI upset or constipation (unlike adults). Look for reticulocytosis to begin 3–5 days after beginning therapy and peak at 7–10 days. If the retic count does not rise in response to iron therapy, you must consider patient nonadherence or an alternative diagnosis.

Expect the hemoglobin to increase 1–2 g/dL in the 1st month. It is critical to continue ferrous sulfate therapy, even after the hemoglobin concentration has returned to normal, in order to ensure correction of total body iron deficit. Parenteral iron is rarely indicated. Red cell indices are not accurate in measuring the iron status of patients with α- or β-thalassemia because the MCV is low in patients with thalassemia regardless; serum iron studies are required. Children with α- or β-thalassemia trait do not require iron supplementation unless they have a concomitant iron deficiency.

To prevent iron deficiency, the 2010 AAP recommendations are the following:

• Breast milk is recommended for at least the first 5–6 months of life. Provide elemental iron supplementation of 1 mg/kg/day for infants who are exclusively breastfed beyond 4 months of age. (Premature infants require supplementation by 1–2 months of age.)

• Iron-supplemented formula is recommended for the 1st year of life in infants who are not breastfed.

• Include iron-enriched cereals among the first foods introduced.

• Do not give cow's milk during the 1st year of life to prevent occult GI bleeding. (Iron in cow's milk is poorly absorbed; infants with iron deficiency often have a history of consuming large amounts of cow's milk.)

Folate and Vitamin B$_{12}$ Deficiencies

Folate and B$_{12}$ deficiencies cause slowing of DNA synthesis and delayed maturation of the entire erythrocyte cell line, resulting in large, immature erythrocytes called **megaloblasts**. This, in turn, causes anemia with macrocytosis. Additionally, abnormalities of neutrophils can occur—especially hypersegmentation.

Folate deficiency can result from inadequate dietary intake, increased metabolic demand (e.g., infancy, pregnancy, lactation), malabsorption, or metabolic interference (e.g., methotrexate, sulfonamide). Little folate is stored, so deficiency states can occur quickly. Folic acid supplementation is recommended for sickle cell disease and other hemolytic disorders, but efficacy has not been well established in pediatric patients.

Folic acid taken before and during pregnancy can help prevent neural tube defects in the fetus. All females of childbearing age capable of becoming pregnant need to take folic acid supplementation.

Infants require 3–5 µg/kg/day. Breast milk and cow's milk are sufficient to provide daily allowances. Goat's milk is a poor source of folate and results in megaloblastic anemia in unsupplemented infants if used as the sole food.

Folate deficiency in infancy can follow chronic diarrhea and malabsorptive states. Initially in folate deficiency, homocysteine levels increase, followed by a fall of RBC folate levels to the lower limit of normal. At this point, hypersegmented neutrophils appear, and then RBC folate levels fall below normal. Finally, megaloblastic anemia occurs. In folate-deficient patients, macroovalocytes, large oval RBCs, neutropenia, and thrombocytopenia are common.

Treat with folic acid at a dose of 1–5 mg daily. If the patient has concomitant vitamin B$_{12}$ deficiency, use of high-dose folate can correct RBC problems but worsen neurologic manifestations of B$_{12}$ deficiency. It is, therefore, important to determine if B$_{12}$ deficiency is also present.

Vitamin B$_{12}$ (cyanocobalamin) deficiency in children occurs most commonly because of abnormalities in the absorption of vitamin B$_{12}$. The absorption of vitamin B$_{12}$ is dependent on its forming a complex with intrinsic factor (IF), which is produced by the parietal cells of the stomach. The B$_{12}$-IF complex is then absorbed in the terminal ileum. After absorption, vitamin B$_{12}$ separates from the complex and is released into the circulation. In the plasma, vitamin B$_{12}$ is bound to both the glycoprotein transcobalamin I and to a β-globulin transport protein, transcobalamin II. Cobalamin is metabolized to adenosylcobalamin, which is required for the metabolism of methylmalonic acid (MMA). Risk factors for vitamin B$_{12}$ deficiency are small bowel resection and maternal vegan diet in a child who is exclusively breastfed.

Pernicious anemia is a specific form of B$_{12}$ deficiency. There are 2 types of pernicious anemia in children:

1) **Congenital** pernicious anemia occurs before 3 years of age and is associated with consanguinity with autosomal recessive (AR) inheritance. Gastric histology and acid secretion are normal, but IF is absent. There are no antibodies to IF and no endocrinopathies.

2) **Juvenile** pernicious anemia occurs in older children and is similar to the adult form. This is due to an autoimmune-mediated decrease in gastric IF. In this case, gastric atrophy and decreased secretion of acid and pepsin are commonly found. There are often other autoimmune manifestations, including vitiligo or thyroiditis.

B$_{12}$ deficiency, in contrast to folate deficiency, leads to neurologic symptoms and eventually to irreversible neurologic damage, including bilateral paresthesias, decreased proprioception and vibration sense (dorsolateral column "dropout"), spastic ataxia, central scotomata, and dementia. These neurologic deficits can occur even in the absence of anemia or macrocytosis. B$_{12}$ deficiency can also cause skeletal changes, including osteoporosis and hip/spine fractures.

The diagnostic workup includes measurement of vitamin B$_{12}$ and folate levels. Peripheral smear reveals basophilic stippling of RBCs and Howell-Jolly bodies, macroovalocytosis, anisocytosis, and poikilocytosis. The retic count can be normal or low. Thrombocytopenia is present in half the patients, and often the platelets have bizarre shapes.

Pernicious anemia is commonly diagnosed by assessing the presence of anti-IF antibodies in association with low B$_{12}$ levels and high serum methylmalonic acid (MMA).

Treatment usually requires parenteral vitamin B$_{12}$ for life: monthly subcutaneous injections of 1 mg of cyanocobalamin or hydroxocobalamin.

Inherited and Acquired Production Defects — Sideroblastic Anemias

Sideroblastic anemias are unusual anemias characterized by ringed sideroblasts in the bone marrow; these are normoblasts with iron-laden mitochondria surrounding the nucleus. Normoblasts are normal-sized erythroblasts that are the nucleated immediate precursors to normal erythrocytes.

There are a variety of causes for sideroblastic anemia (both acquired and inherited). The blood smear shows

Pappenheimer bodies, which are often at the periphery of the cell; these are dark blue cytoplasmic inclusions of iron occurring as small single or multiple blue granules.

The peripheral blood smear usually has 2 populations of erythrocytes, including normal-appearing cells along with hypochromic microcytic cells (low MCV; low MCH). This variation in size and shape is reflected in the CBC with a large RBC volume distribution width (RDW). Again, bone marrow shows ringed sideroblasts.

Less common causes can produce normo- to macrocytic erythrocytes.

Survival Defects

Overview

Survival defects can be inherited or acquired. Most inherited survival defects are due to a problem intrinsic to the RBC membrane, hemoglobin, or machinery. Most acquired survival defects are due to external forces acting on the RBCs.

Survival defects include the following:

- Inherited
  ○ Hereditary spherocytosis
  ○ Hereditary elliptocytosis
  ○ Paroxysmal nocturnal hemoglobinuria
  ○ G6PD deficiency
  ○ Sickle cell disease
- Acquired
  ○ Immune-mediated hemolytic anemia

RBC lifespan is shortened, resulting in hemolytic anemia. The body tries to compensate for this by increasing the bone marrow output, resulting in bony changes if the hemolytic process is long-term. The presence of reticulocytosis points to a hemolytic cause. Symptoms include pallor (especially noticeable in the conjunctiva, palm, and nailbeds), scleral icterus, jaundice, and hepatosplenomegaly.

Inherited Survival Defects (Congenital Hemolytic Anemias)

Hereditary Spherocytosis

Hereditary spherocytosis (HS) is the most common congenital hemolytic anemia in populations of northern European origin. The incidence in the U.S. is about 1/5,000 births. A majority of cases are autosomal dominant (AD); however, for 10–25% of patients, no family history is found.

HS is due to a structural or functional abnormality of cytoskeletal proteins, spectrin, ankyrin, and, less commonly, band 3 or protein 4.2. Newly produced RBCs entering the circulation are not spherocytic, but the spherocytic shape gradually occurs due to splenic effects. Spherocytes are more rigid than normal cells and cannot easily pass through pores of the splenic sinusoids. Loss of RBC membrane occurs without a reduction in RBC volume, and the cell becomes more spherical. This cell becomes even less deformable and at greater risk for lysis in the spleen.

Diagnosis is made by finding the presence of anemia (of varying degrees), reticulocytosis, increased MCHC, spherocytes in the peripheral blood smear, and a positive osmotic fragility test.

Some children with HS have a chronic hemolytic anemia, jaundice, reticulocytosis, and splenomegaly. Other children have compensated anemia with few symptoms at baseline. Increasing pallor in a child with HS is a sign of an aplastic crisis, with decreased hemoglobin and retic count typically caused by parvovirus B19 infection. Close monitoring of hemoglobin and retic count is imperative. In contrast, a sudden increase in jaundice is a sign of increasing hemolysis, which also can result in worsening anemia and the need for RBC transfusion. HS can be a life-threatening cause of hyperbilirubinemia/ kernicterus in the neonatal period. Chronic complications include cholelithiasis due to bilirubin stones.

Splenectomy is sometimes required to prolong RBC survival. Prior to splenectomy, administer pneumococcal, *Haemophilus influenzae*, and meningococcal vaccinations to minimize the risk of postsplenectomy sepsis. Postsplenectomy penicillin prophylaxis is also necessary, and urgent medical evaluation is necessary for splenectomized children with fever.

Hereditary Elliptocytosis

Hereditary elliptocytosis (HE) occurs at a rate of 1/2,500 births in the U.S. The most common cause of HE is abnormal spectrin, which is critical for cytoskeletal lateral interactions. There are 2 forms of the disorder, including:

1) **Common HE**, which is asymptomatic and has uniformly elliptical RBCs without other hematologic abnormalities
2) **Hemolytic HE**, which causes splenomegaly with mild-to-moderate anemia and hemolysis and has both spherocytes and elliptocytes

Splenectomy is generally curative.

Paroxysmal Nocturnal Hemoglobinuria

Paroxysmal nocturnal hemoglobinuria (PNH) is a rare, acquired clonal stem cell disorder involving:

• glycophosphatidylinositol (GPI)-linked membrane proteins,
• decay-accelerating factor (DAF, a.k.a. CD55), and
• a homologous restriction factor (HRF, a.k.a. CD59) of the *PIG-A* gene on the X chromosome.

Deficiency of these proteins makes cells more susceptible to complement-mediated lysis. Since it is nonantibody-mediated, the direct Coombs test is negative. (See Table 24-5.)

PNH can appear alone or in association with myelodysplastic syndromes, acute myeloid leukemia (AML), or aplastic anemia. The PNH triad consists of:

1) Hemolytic anemia
2) Pancytopenia
3) Arterial and venous thromboses

Pancytopenia may be the 1st detected laboratory abnormality.

Diagnose with flow cytometry, which detects specific GPI-linked proteins. The direct Coombs test (with complement) is usually normal, because all cells that activate complement are promptly lysed and therefore do not agglutinate in the assay.

Eculizumab (Soliris) is a drug that blocks complement-mediated lysis and has revolutionized treatment for patients with PNH. It has decreased need for transfusions, with 55% achieving transfusion independence in a clinical trial of 11 patients! Bone marrow transplant (BMT) is curative and is indicated for patients with severe refractory pancytopenia or life-threatening thrombosis.

G6PD Deficiency

All 250 variants of X-linked recessive glucose 6-phosphate dehydrogenase (G6PD) deficiency result in decreased amounts of reduced glutathione. The disease is common in African American males, Kurdish Jews, and those living in the lowlands of Greece. Reduced glutathione is an antioxidant required to protect RBCs from

Coombs Test	Description of Test	Positive Test	Possible Indications
Direct	Antibodies against IgG or C3 are prepared in an animal and then mixed with the patient's blood.	Patient's RBCs cells agglutinate—which means there is IgG (or C3) on the surface of the patient's RBCs.	Autoimmune hemolytic anemia Infectious mononucleosis Mycoplasma infection
Indirect	The Rh- and ABO-compatible RBCs are mixed with the patient's serum. (Testing is done to see if the patient's serum contains antibodies that can cause agglutination of other RBCs.)	Patient's RBCs agglutinate.	Incompatible blood match with transfusion Erythroblastosis fetalis

Table 24-5: Coombs Tests

oxidative stress. When an oxidant stress is present (e.g., systemic infection, sulfa drugs, dapsone, primaquine, fava beans), there is an inadequate reserve of reduced glutathione, and RBCs hemolyze. Consider G6PD deficiency as a possible cause for unexplained neonatal jaundice. Symptoms of a hemolytic crisis include sudden onset of pallor, fatigue, and dark urine. Except during an acute hemolytic crisis (when all the affected RBCs have hemolyzed and the remaining RBCs have normal or near-normal G6PD levels), measurement of G6PD level is diagnostic. Peripheral blood stain shows Heinz bodies, which consist of denatured globin. Due to differences in enzyme mutations in African vs. Mediterranean heritage, G6PD disease is typically more significant in those of Mediterranean origin.

Sickle Cell Disease

Sickle cell disease (SCD) is composed of a group of inherited RBC disorders characterized by the presence of hemoglobin S (HbS). HbS is caused by a point mutation in the 6th codon of the β-globin gene, which is located on the short arm of chromosome 11. Adenine is replaced by thymidine, which results in valine being encoded instead of glutamic acid. Upon deoxygenation, HbS polymerizes, leading to sickled RBCs.

4 common types of SCD occur (listed in decreasing order of severity):

- HbSS
- HbSβ⁰ thalassemia (hemoglobin S from one parent and β⁰ thalassemia from the other parent)
- HbSC (hemoglobin S from one parent and hemoglobin C from the other parent)
- HbSβ⁺ thalassemia (hemoglobin S from one parent and β⁺ thalassemia from the other parent)

The type of SCD can be distinguished on the basis of hemoglobin electrophoresis pattern, red cell indices, and genetic testing.

SCD affects 1/375 African American newborns. The disease also affects many other racial groups, including Mediterranean, Middle Eastern, and Asiatic Indian.

HbS forms polymers that damage the RBC and decrease its lifespan. The average lifespan of an RBC in HbSS disease is only 15–50 days (normal = 120 days). Sickled RBCs adhere to and damage endothelial layers of small and large blood vessels, resulting in vaso-occlusion. Vaso-occlusion with ischemia and tissue damage results in acute complications, including pain, acute chest syndrome (ACS), splenic sequestration, priapism, and stroke. Chronic hemolysis results in hyperbilirubinemia and cholelithiasis. Chronic organ damage affects the kidneys, spleen, lungs, and brain. Chronic complications of sickle cell disease include delays in growth and sexual maturation. Median life expectancy for patients with SCD in the U.S. is approximately 50 years.

In the United States, SCD is diagnosed through newborn screening programs (see Table 24-3 on page 24-9).

Prenatal diagnosis is useful when both parents are known to have either SCD or trait. Amniotic fluid, fetal erythrocytes, or chorionic villi can be sampled for testing. At birth, infants have high levels of HbF, which interferes with sickling. Therefore, newborns are not anemic. Symptoms generally occur starting at 6 months of age, as HbF decreases.

Hydroxyurea (Droxia, Hydrea) is the only disease-modifying medication shown to reduce acute and chronic complications. BMT is increasingly utilized as a curative therapy for high-risk patients. Best outcomes are seen with matched related donors.

Risk of infection with encapsulated organisms (*Streptococcus pneumonia, Neisseria meningitidis,* and *H. influenzae*) is high due to functional "asplenia," which is a result of autoinfarction from repeated sickling of RBCs within the spleen. Patients are also at higher risk of infection with *Salmonella,* including bacteremia and osteomyelitis. Prescribe penicillin prophylaxis to infants diagnosed with SCD by newborn screening because it dramatically decreases invasive pneumococcal infections in children < 5 years of age with SCD. Children with SCD require immunizations against encapsulated organisms. Pneumococcal conjugate and polysaccharide vaccines are recommended for all children with SCD.

Pain (vaso-occlusive) crisis is the most common complication of SCD and the most common reason for hospitalization. The first pain crisis in about 1/3 of patients is sickle cell **dactylitis**, a symmetric painful swelling of the hands and feet. As the child ages, the crises usually affect the long bones, vertebrae, sternum, ribs, lower back, and abdomen. Clinically, some children have very few crises, and others have frequent, debilitating crises. Treatment is aimed at relieving pain and providing hydration. IV hydration, NSAIDs, and opioid analgesics are typically used for hospitalized children.

Splenic sequestration is a life-threatening condition that occurs most often in young children with SCD. Children with splenic sequestration of sickled RBCs have massively enlarged and engorged spleens, resulting in abdominal pain, hypovolemia, severe anemia, and shock. Splenomegaly and thrombocytopenia suggest the diagnosis of acute splenic sequestration. IV hydration and RBC transfusion decrease sequestration in the spleen and alleviate symptoms. Splenic sequestration often recurs; children with life-threatening splenic sequestration or recurrent events undergo splenectomy.

Acute chest syndrome (ACS) is defined as the development of a new pulmonary infiltrate with fever, chest pain, tachypnea, and/or hypoxia. Etiology of ACS includes infection, infarction, atelectasis, and/or fat embolism from the bone marrow. ACS can progress rapidly to respiratory failure. ACS is the leading cause of death in adolescents and adults with SCD. Treatment includes respiratory support, hydration (if necessary), and antibiotics that cover pneumococcus, *Mycoplasma,* and *Chlamydia.* Exchange transfusions are administered to patients with significant hypoxia and respiratory distress and to those who do not improve with appropriate respiratory support, hydration, and antibiotic therapy. Exchange transfusion can rapidly decrease HbS and improve symptoms.

Aplastic crisis (red cell aplasia) occurs because of infection with parvovirus B19. Parvovirus B19 destroys early red cell precursors in the bone marrow and causes an abrupt cessation of RBC production. In the patient with SCD, in which RBC lifespan is only 15–50 days and maintaining RBC numbers is predicated on rapid bone marrow production, parvovirus B19 infection can quickly cause a life-threatening anemia. Presenting symptoms can vary and include fever, fatigue, pallor, coryza, and headache. The aplastic crisis is characterized by a falling hemoglobin (over 1–3 days) and reticulocytopenia. The low retic count differentiates aplastic crisis from other causes of worsening anemia. Diagnosis of parvovirus B19 is made using parvovirus DNA polymerase chain reaction (PCR) and/or serology. Elevated IgM indicates acute infection. The acute red cell aplasia is typically short and self-limited, and rapid production of IgM antibodies against parvovirus B19 quickly curbs the infection. Usually, reticulocytosis returns in 1–2 weeks. During this time, periodic transfusions are frequently required.

Stroke risk is high for children with sickle cell anemia (HbSS and HbSβ⁰ thalassemia). The peak incidence occurs in children between 5 and 10 years of age. Children are more likely to have infarctive stroke secondary to occlusion of the large intracerebral blood vessels. Symptoms include weakness, changes in speech, headache, and seizures. If a stroke is suspected or confirmed on physical examination, imaging with CT and/or MRI is done to evaluate for areas of ischemia and vasculopathy. Acute treatment is emergent exchange transfusion, which should be done even before an MRI in patients with sickle cell who are diagnosed with a stroke on the basis of the physical examination. In addition, patients with SCD who have had a stroke require chronic RBC transfusion therapy to keep the HbS < 30% to reduce the risk of recurrence.

Use transcranial Doppler ultrasound (TCD) to screen children with HbSS and HbSβ⁰ thalassemia, starting at 2 years of age. To prevent strokes, chronic RBC transfusions are recommended for children with abnormally high TCD velocities.

Cerebral vasculopathy is a risk factor for stroke. **Moyamoya** disease occurs in some patients with SCD and is the collateral formation of vessels due to vascular occlusion. "Moyamoya" is a Japanese word meaning "puff of smoke"; the vessels on angiography appear to be a cluster of vessels with a smoky appearance. More information about Moyamoya syndrome is found in Neurology, Book 2.

Priapism is a prolonged, painful erection, and it occurs in up to 10% of older boys and adolescents with SCD. It requires rapid intervention to prevent damage to the penis. Consult hematology and urology. Management includes hydration and pain control. In many cases, aspiration of the corpora cavernosa and irrigation with a dilute solution of epinephrine rapidly alleviates the condition. Rarely, surgical intervention (i.e., glans-cavernosum shunt) is indicated.

Other Hemoglobinopathies

Sickle cell trait (HbAS): People with sickle cell trait have normal hemoglobin, peripheral blood smears, and red cell indices. Their life expectancy is normal. It is unusual for a person with sickle cell trait to have any sickle cell–related complications, except in cases of extreme physical exertion or low oxygen tension (e.g., unpressurized aircraft, high altitude). Hyposthenuria (inability to concentrate urine) and renal papillary necrosis with gross hematuria are the most common complications. The incidence of renal medullary carcinoma, a rare kidney tumor, is higher in patients with sickle cell trait. Screening is not necessary due to the rarity of this tumor.

Hemoglobin SC disease (HbSC): Patients with HbSC are usually less anemic and have less severe hemolysis than those with HbSS. These patients have equal amounts of HbS and hemoglobin C (HbC), and there is no HbA. HbC occurs because of the substitution of a lysine for the glutamic acid residue in the 6th position of the β-globin chain. Peripheral smears show microcytosis and target cells but not irreversibly sickled cells. Splenomegaly remains throughout adolescence and adulthood. Adolescents are at risk for retinal disease and avascular necrosis of the hips.

Hemoglobin C disease (HbCC): Homozygotes for HbC have a mild hemolytic anemia and splenomegaly but do not have vaso-occlusive problems. RBCs are microcytic with a large number of target cells on peripheral smear. Heterozygotes (HbAC) have no symptoms and only a large number of target cells as the hematologic manifestation.

Hemoglobin E disease (HbEE): Patients homozygous for HbE have mild hemolytic anemia with significant microcytosis, hypochromia, and target cells. Heterozygotes have minimal findings.

HbEE is very common in the populations of south and southeast Asia (~ 30%) and in northeast India (up to 60%!). It is thought that this is because RBCs with HbEE are resistant to infection by *Plasmodium falciparum*, the protozoan that causes malaria in humans.

Acquired Survival Defects

Immune-Mediated Hemolytic Anemias

The most common form of acquired hemolytic anemia is immune-mediated destruction of RBCs by antibodies. Symptoms include pallor, fatigue, jaundice, and dark urine.

There are 2 broad groups of immune-mediated hemolytic anemias: **autoimmune hemolytic anemia** (AIHA;

warm, cold, or paroxysmal) and **isoimmune hemolytic disease of the newborn** (HDN; a.k.a. alloimmune hemolytic disease of the newborn).

In **warm AIHA**, IgG antibodies specific for the Rh group of RBC antigens can bind to these antigens at body temperature. Macrophages and monocytes are attracted to these IgG-coated cells and start attacking them, converting them to spherocytes and causing them to hemolyze. IgG-coated RBCs and spherocytes are sequestered by the spleen. AIHA is either primary or secondary. Secondary AIHA is seen with infection, certain medications (e.g., penicillins, cephalosporins, NSAIDs), and lymphoproliferative and collagen vascular disorders (e.g., systemic lupus erythematosus [SLE]). Clinical history includes acute onset of pallor, jaundice, and sometimes dark urine. Investigate the patient's history for a new medication or recent febrile illness. Physical exam findings are significant for pallor, jaundice, and splenomegaly.

The direct Coombs test is a necessary part of the evaluation of the child with acute onset of anemia and is positive in AIHA. (See Table 24-5 on page 24-12 for an explanation of the Coombs tests.) Briefly, the direct Coombs test reveals what components (IgG or C3) are "directly" attached to the patient's RBCs, suggesting an autoimmune reaction. The indirect Coombs test reveals antibodies in the patient's serum that have the potential to bind to RBCs.

AIHA can be life-threatening. Treat warm autoimmune hemolytic anemia with corticosteroids. If necessary, transfuse the most compatible RBCs. Splenectomy or immunosuppressive agents are used in refractory cases.

Cold agglutinin disease can occur with *Mycoplasma* and Epstein-Barr virus. IgM-RBC complexes lyse complement and cause intravascular hemolysis. IgM disease is Coombs negative.

Paroxysmal cold hemoglobinuria (PCH) is caused by a cold-reacting IgG (Donath-Landsteiner antibody). This antibody binds at cold temperatures and causes RBC lysis at warm temperatures. PCH is common after viral illness, and treatment is supportive. Keep the patient warm and use a blood warmer for transfusions. Consider plasmapheresis for severe disease. Steroids are less helpful than with warm AIHA.

Isoimmune hemolytic disease of the newborn is a distinctive form of immune hemolytic anemia that presents in infancy due to maternal production of antibodies against fetal RBC antigens that cross the placenta during pregnancy. This can be due to ABO antibodies (ABO incompatibility) or to Rh antibodies (**Rh hemolytic disease of the newborn**). Classification as Rh positive or negative is based upon whether or not the major D antigen is expressed on erythrocytes. The direct Coombs test is positive, as with most AIHAs. Classically, Rh hemolytic disease of the newborn does not occur with the first pregnancy. In contrast, ABO hemolysis can occur with the first pregnancy due to the natural production

of isohemagglutinins. Anemia and hyperbilirubinemia resolve as maternal antibodies are cleared.

See Neonatology, Book 1, for more information on hemolytic disease of the fetus and newborn. Methemoglobinemia is discussed in Emergency Medicine & Maltreatment Syndromes, Book 2.

Drug-Induced Hemolysis

Many drugs cause hemolysis. Penicillin bound to RBCs elicits an antibody that can cause hemolysis. Quinine, methyldopa, and certain cephalosporin antibiotics are also known culprits.

The other causes of extrinsic survival defects:

- DIC
- Mechanical trauma to RBCs
- Oxidative injury
- Hypersplenism

WHITE BLOOD CELL DISORDERS

PREVIEW | REVIEW

- Define severe neutropenia.
- Why should patients with severe neutropenia be evaluated immediately for any fever?
- Differentiate chronic benign neutropenia from cyclic neutropenia.
- What is Kostmann syndrome?
- What is Shwachman-Diamond syndrome?
- Describe neonatal isoimmune neutropenia.
- If an infant presents with delayed separation of the umbilical cord, what diagnosis should be considered?
- What is hyperimmunoglobulin E syndrome?
- Which virus induces an accelerated phase in children with Chédiak-Higashi syndrome?
- What is the defect in chronic granulomatous disease? How do you test for this disease?
- What is the most common neutrophil disorder?
- What is mastocytosis?

NEUTROPENIA

Overview

Severe neutropenia is generally defined as having an absolute neutrophil count (ANC) of < 500 cells/µL. (The ANC is obtained by multiplying the total WBC count by the percentage of neutrophils + band forms.) Moderate neutropenia is generally considered between 500 and 1,000 cells/µL, whereas mild neutropenia is defined by neutrophil counts between 1,000 and 1,500 cells/µL. Patients with severe neutropenia are at marked risk for developing serious bacterial infections. Those with less severe neutropenia frequently develop skin infections, otitis media, or stomatitis. Recurrent bacterial infection is a manifestation of all WBC disorders (neutropenia, as well as qualitative defects). Children with severe neutropenia are often infected with their own skin and bowel flora. Children are at risk for overwhelming bacterial infection; febrile and ill-appearing children with neutropenia require immediate evaluation, blood cultures, and parenteral broad-spectrum antibiotics.

Neutropenias include the following:

- Inherited
  - Cyclic neutropenia
  - Severe congenital neutropenia (Kostmann syndrome)
  - Shwachman-Diamond syndrome
  - Cartilage-hair hypoplasia
- Acquired
  - Neonatal isoimmune neutropenia
  - Chronic benign neutropenia (autoimmune)
  - Virus- or drug-induced neutropenia

Inherited Neutropenias

Cyclic Neutropenia

In cyclic neutropenia, neutropenia occurs at a regular interval of every 21 +/– 3 days. It is characterized by defective maturation of uncommitted stem cells. During 3- to 5-day periods of neutropenia, which usually have an ANC < 200 cells/μL, the patient often presents with fever, aphthous stomatitis, cervical lymphadenitis, and/or rectal and vaginal ulcers. In ~ 10% of cases, infections can be severe or even fatal. Patients with cyclic neutropenia are at particular risk of sepsis caused by *Clostridium septicum*. In about 1/3 of patients, the disorder is inherited in an AD pattern. Mutations involve the *ELA2* gene. Management includes granulocyte colony-stimulating factor (G-CSF) and antibiotics for infections. Oral hygiene is important.

Severe Congenital Neutropenia (Kostmann Syndrome)

Kostmann syndrome is a rare AR disorder. Mutations can involve multiple genes, including *ELA2* and *HAX1*. The ANC is typically < 200 cells/μL. There is also monocytosis and eosinophilia. Children are at risk for severe bacterial infections and early death. Management includes G-CSF (often at high dose). BMT is curative. There is a national registry for patients. Note that some patients acquire a mutation in the G-CSF receptor, followed by a transformation to myelodysplasia and acute myelogenous leukemia; however, malignancy is not attributed to G-CSF therapy.

Shwachman-Diamond Syndrome

Shwachman-Diamond syndrome is an AR disorder resulting from mutations in the *SBDS* gene. Children present with features similar to those of children with cystic fibrosis, including failure to thrive, steatorrhea due to pancreatic exocrine insufficiency, and recurrent infections. Unique features of Shwachman-Diamond syndrome include neutropenia and metaphyseal dysostoses.

A sweat test will be normal. Diagnostic evaluation includes complete blood count, bone marrow aspirate and biopsy, serum isoamylase, serum pancreatic trypsinogen, and fecal elastase levels. Genetic testing is available for *SBDS* gene analysis.

Treatment options include supportive care with pancreatic enzyme replacement and, depending on frequency and severity of infections, G-CSF administration or BMT. Patients are predisposed to myelodysplastic syndrome and AML.

Cartilage-Hair Hypoplasia

Cartilage-hair hypoplasia is an AR form of short-limb dysostosis. It occurs mainly in children of Amish descent and is characterized by sparse or fine hair. Neutropenia occurs in about 25% of cases and is often accompanied by defects in cell-mediated immunity. Varicella zoster infection is particularly troublesome. Patients are at high risk for autoimmune diseases such as immune (idiopathic) thrombocytopenic purpura (ITP) or AIHA. BMT is the treatment of choice for those with recurrent severe infections.

Acquired Neutropenias

Neonatal Isoimmune Neutropenia

Neonatal isoimmune neutropenia (NIN) is a self-limited disease that occurs in about 1/1,000 newborns. NIN is similar to Rh disease except, with NIN, maternal antibodies result from maternal sensitization to neutrophil antigens that are shared by the fetus and the father but are absent from the mother's neutrophils. Maternal IgG antineutrophil antibodies cross the placenta and result in destruction of fetal neutrophils, with a resultant neutropenia. The infant's neutrophil count recovers in 6–12 weeks. Any infection requires quick, appropriate antibiotic therapy. Subsequent siblings are at risk for the same condition.

Chronic Benign Neutropenia

Chronic benign neutropenia is characterized by a persistently low ANC of < 1,000 cells/μL (patients usually have an ANC of 0–500 cells/μL), which is caused by autoantibodies to granulocytes. It is also called autoimmune neutropenia (AIN). It is the most common cause of neutropenia in "healthy" children and must be differentiated from more serious forms of neutropenia. It can be AD or sporadic. Chronic benign neutropenia has a median age of diagnosis of 8–11 months and typically lasts about 2 years.

The disease is mild and usually does not required treatment. G-CSF is given for severe infections.

Virus- or Drug-Induced Immune-Related Neutropenia

The most common etiology of neutropenia in children is viral infection resulting in transient bone marrow suppression. Viral infection can also induce immune-mediated neutropenia. In this case, an anti-viral antibody cross-reacts with a neutrophil or a drug attaches to the neutrophil and acts as a hapten to stimulate antibody production. Viral-induced neutropenia is very common and does not require specific treatment.

Drugs that can cause neutropenia include anticonvulsants, antithyroids, NSAIDs, antihistamines, sulfas, and synthetic penicillins. The neutrophil count is usually not in the severely low range, and significant secondary infections are unusual. If a drug is the suspected cause of neutropenia, then discontinue the drug if possible. Chemotherapeutic agents induce neutropenia (often severe). A table of chemotherapeutic agents is included in Oncology, Book 5.

DISORDERS OF NEUTROPHIL FUNCTION

Overview

Neutrophil function disorders are inherited conditions that frequently present with recurrent infections and a normal neutrophil count. Symptoms include aphthous ulcers, stomatitis, otitis media, cervical lymphadenopathy, and skin abscesses in the first few months of life. Initial workup includes neutrophil count, neutrophil morphology, and either a test for respiratory burst (usually a nitroblue tetrazolium [NBT] dye test if chronic granulomatous disease is a concern) or flow cytometry for other disorders, such as LAD1. See Figure 24-4 for a diagram of normal granulocyte production.

Leukocyte Adhesion Deficiency Type 1

Leukocyte adhesion deficiency Type 1 (LAD1) is a rare AR disorder that particularly affects the adherence-related functions of neutrophils (but also of monocytes and lymphocytes.) The defect is a mutation in the gene that encodes CD18, located on chromosome 21, and results in a lack of formation of adhesion molecules. The neutrophils can properly kill intracellular organisms, but they cannot attach to the infected cells or properly mobilize to the site of infection. Children with LAD1 deficiency have neutrophilia, but the neutrophils do not accumulate at the site of infection. Delayed separation of the umbilical cord and omphalitis are frequently the 1st signs of this disorder. These children have recurrent skin infections, severe periodontitis/gingivitis, and recurrent pneumonias due to bacteria and fungi.

Diagnosis is made using the Rebuck skin window technique and flow cytometry of activated neutrophils. A positive test shows decreased accumulation of tissue neutrophils. BMT is the treatment of choice. Life expectancy without BMT is typically < 2 years.

Hyperimmunoglobulin E Syndrome (Job Syndrome)

Hyperimmunoglobulin E syndrome (hyper-IgE, a.k.a. Job syndrome) presents with at least a 10-fold increase in the serum IgE level, defective chemotaxis, skin disorders, and recurrent infections. Abscesses are common but are "cold": without redness, heat, or pain.

Staphylococcus aureus is the main organism responsible for the skin abscesses. Antibiotics are used for skin infections. Use of trimethoprim/sulfamethoxazole for prophylaxis is indicated. Some recommend treatment with cyclosporine A, recombinant interferon γ, or IV immunoglobulin (IVIG).

See Allergy & Immunology, Book 4, for more information.

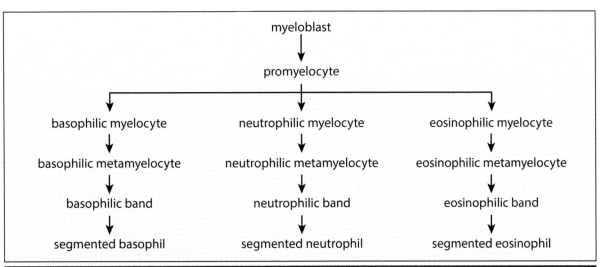

Figure 24-4: Normal Granulopoiesis

Chédiak-Higashi Syndrome

Chédiak-Higashi syndrome is an AR disease that results from a defect in the gene responsible for vesicle trafficking regulatory proteins and causes altered lysosomes and granules within the cells. It presents with partial oculocutaneous albinism with silvery hair, giant lysosomes in all granule-containing cells, neutropenia, bleeding tendency, natural killer cell dysfunction, progressive neurologic decline, and frequent bacterial infections. Infection with Epstein-Barr virus in these patients frequently induces an accelerated phase, typically in the 2nd decade of life. This results in hepatosplenomegaly, lymphadenopathy, and pancytopenia, followed by death. Giant granules in neutrophils and eosinophils on the peripheral smear are pathognomonic for Chédiak-Higashi syndrome.

Treatment during the stable phase is antibiotics for infections. Treatment options for the accelerated phase include steroids and either VP16 or vincristine or a BMT.

Chronic Granulomatous Disease

Chronic granulomatous disease (CGD) is a disorder of neutrophil function in which there is a defect in the respiratory burst, which, under normal circumstances, results in the killing of bacteria. In patients with CGD, the neutrophils can ingest bacteria, but the processes that lead to superoxide anion formation, hydrogen peroxide production, and eventual bacterial killing are impaired. Serious infections occur with those organisms that produce catalase, which include *Staphylococcus aureus*, *Nocardia*, *Aspergillus*, *Burkholderia cepacia*, *Serratia marcescens*, and *Salmonella*. Most cases are X-linked, but 1/3 are AR.

Infants present with recurrent infections with the organisms mentioned above. Skin and perirectal infections are very common. Liver abscesses and osteomyelitis are also frequently seen.

The NBT dye test quantitates reduction of NBT to the insoluble blue compound formazan by NADPH oxidase. A newer flow cytometry–based test (i.e., dihydrorhodamine oxidation) is also available to measure superoxide production. To confirm the diagnosis, look for failure to induce an oxidative metabolic burst during phagocytosis, and/or look for the demonstration of a defect in leukocyte microbicidal activity against catalase-producing organisms. The molecular basis confirms the mode of transmission: Absent proteins p22-phox, p47-phox, or p67-phox are AR, whereas absent glycoprotein GP91-phox is X-linked.

Treatment options include early use of prophylactic trimethoprim/sulfamethoxazole, itraconazole, and interferon-γ to decrease the number of serious infections or, alternatively, BMT.

See Allergy & Immunology, Book 4, for more information.

Myeloperoxidase Deficiency

Myeloperoxidase deficiency is inherited as an AR disorder with a frequency of 1/2,000 births. The absence of myeloperoxidase from azurophilic granules in neutrophils is the most common neutrophil disorder. The disease can present with recurrent mild infections but usually is completely asymptomatic due to variable expression of the defect. Diagnosis is confirmed by finding the absence of neutrophil myeloperoxidase.

DISORDERS OF EOSINOPHILS

Occurrence

In the U.S. and other developed countries, eosinophilia is most commonly caused by allergens; worldwide, the most common cause is parasites. Also, eosinophilia can be seen in Hodgkin disease, leukemias, dermatitis, and GI disorders.

Hypereosinophilic Syndrome

Hypereosinophilic syndrome is an acquired, chronic syndrome whereby an overabundance of eosinophils creates tissue damage. It has no known etiology and is distinct from eosinophilic leukemia, a subtype of AML. **Löffler syndrome** is characterized by hypereosinophilia, endocardial fibrosis, and mural thrombi. Treat with corticosteroids, vinca alkaloids, hydroxyurea, and, if necessary, BMT.

DISORDERS OF BASOPHILS

Basophils are the least numerous WBCs and normally are < 1% of the total circulating WBC pool. Basophils contain histamine and heparin and are the bloodborne equivalent of tissue-bound mast cells. Excess numbers of basophils occur in chronic myelogenous leukemia, ulcerative colitis, and myxedema.

Mastocytosis is a skin condition in which mast cells infiltrate the skin. **Darier sign**, the presence of urticaria caused by rubbing the skin, is seen on physical exam. Diagnosis is confirmed by biopsy. There is a systemic form of mastocytosis that involves infiltration of the bone marrow, liver, spleen, and GI tract. These patients do very poorly.

PLATELET DISORDERS

PREVIEW | REVIEW

- What is the normal platelet lifespan?
- What is Wiskott-Aldrich syndrome?
- What is TAR syndrome?
- What is the next diagnostic step if a patient has an unexpectedly very low platelet count after previously having normal counts?

- What preceding medical history is commonly reported in children diagnosed with ITP?
- Describe the peripheral blood smear findings in ITP. What diagnosis should be considered in a child with giant platelets (the size of RBCs)?
- What are the typical blood counts in children with acute ITP?
- What is the role of bone marrow aspiration and biopsy in the evaluation of a child with thrombocytopenia? What bone marrow findings are consistent with a diagnosis of ITP?
- How soon do platelet counts normalize in children with ITP?
- What are the laboratory and clinical indications for treatment of ITP? What is the typical platelet count trigger for treatment of ITP?
- What are the 1st line treatments for ITP?
- Describe the clinical presentation and management of infants of women with ITP.
- What are the clinical features of vWD?
- What tests are included in the laboratory evaluation of vWD?
- What are the treatment options for children with vWD?
- Giant, abnormal platelets and decreased platelet aggregation in response to ristocetin are seen in which inherited platelet disorder?
- Normal platelet count with decreased platelet aggregation in response to collagen, epinephrine, and ADP are seen in which inherited platelet disorder?
- What does aspirin do to platelets? How long does it last?
- What treatment does reactive thrombocytosis require?

NORMAL PRODUCTION

Platelets normally live 7–10 days in the blood. Megakaryocytes in the bone marrow undergo cytoplasmic fragmentation to form platelets. The production and maturation of megakaryocytes is regulated by thrombopoietin.

Platelets are involved in primary hemostasis, which is the forming of a platelet plug. See Primary Hemostasis — Platelet Plug Formation on page 24-26 for a detailed review of the mechanisms involved with platelet adhesion and aggregation during primary hemostasis.

THROMBOCYTOPENIA

Overview

Thrombocytopenia can be caused by ITP, DIC, thrombotic thrombocytopenic purpura (TTP), hemolytic uremic syndrome (HUS), **HELLP** syndrome (hemolytic anemia, **e**levated **l**iver function tests, **l**ow **p**latelets), dilution, transfusion, or amniotic fluid embolism (during childbirth). Medications/drugs causing thrombocytopenia include heparin, quinine, quinidine, phenytoin, gold salts, and alcohol. Beware that pseudothrombocytopenia may occur due to platelet clumping; see more on page 24-20.

Children with thrombocytopenia have symptoms that include bruising, petechiae, and mucosal bleeding. Severity of bruising and bleeding depends on degree of thrombocytopenia and etiology of thrombocytopenia.

We'll cover a few causes of thrombocytopenia:

- Inherited
  - Wiskott-Aldrich syndrome
  - Myosin heavy chain 9 gene (*MYH9*)–related disorders
  - Amegakaryocytic thrombocytopenia with absent radii (TAR syndrome)
- Acquired
  - Pseudothrombocytopenia
  - Immune (idiopathic) thrombocytopenic purpura (ITP)
  - Thrombotic thrombocytopenic purpura
  - Maternal autoimmune neonatal thrombocytopenia
  - Kasabach-Merritt phenomenon

Inherited Thrombocytopenia

Overview

Thrombocytopenia may be inherited. Consider inherited thrombocytopenia if it occurs at a very young age and is chronic or if the patient has family history of thrombocytopenia. Inherited thrombocytopenia can be mistaken for ITP; consider it if the patient does not respond to ITP therapy. Look at the blood smear.

4 inherited platelet disorders cause abnormal platelet morphology:

1) Bernard-Soulier syndrome (large platelets)
2) Wiskott-Aldrich syndrome (small platelets)
3) *MYH9*-related disorders, including May-Hegglin anomaly (large platelets; white cell inclusions called Döhle bodies)
4) Gray platelet syndrome (pale platelets)

Wiskott-Aldrich Syndrome

WATER

Wiskott-Aldrich syndrome is an extremely rare X-linked disorder characterized by severe thrombocytopenia and small-sized platelets (in contrast to ITP, in which platelets are large) that can present in the neonatal period. Affected boys develop eczema and immunodeficiency. Individuals are at risk for lymphoma later in life. See Allergy & Immunology, Book 4, for more information.

MYH9-Related Disorders

This group of myosin heavy chain 9–related disorders is characterized by AD mutations in the gene for non-muscle myosin heavy chain IIA. This defect leads to defective megakaryocyte maturation. Characteristics on the blood smear include macrothrombocytes and Döhle bodies in WBCs. Clinical characteristics include bleeding tendency and renal failure, sensorineural hearing loss, and/or cataracts.

Amegakaryocytic Thrombocytopenia with Absent Radii (TAR Syndrome)

TAR syndrome is an inherited disorder that presents with bleeding in the neonatal period. Thrombocytopenia is severe, and there is an increased risk of death during the neonatal period and early infancy as a result of intracranial bleeds associated with platelet counts of < 30,000. Half of all affected infants are symptomatic in the 1st week of life, and 90% are symptomatic by 4 months of age. Thrombocytopenic episodes are most frequent during the first 2 years of life and then decrease in frequency. Thrombocytopenia can fluctuate, and levels can even be normal at certain times. Infection and dietary factors, especially cow's milk allergy, sometimes precipitate episodes. Leukocytosis can occur. There are no megakaryocytes in the bone marrow.

These patients also have no radii (Image 24-20), but their thumbs are normal (as opposed to Fanconi anemia and trisomy 18, in which thumbs are abnormal).

In addition to absent radii, upper extremity abnormalities include hypoplastic carpals and phalanges, syndactyly, clinodactyly, and phocomelia. Lower extremity abnormalities are also common and can include hip dysplasia, femoral and/or tibial torsion, and deformities of the knees and/or feet. Dysmorphic features of the face include micrognathia; hypertelorism with a broad forehead; and low-set, posteriorly rotated ears. Congenital heart disease (most often atrial septal defect, isolated ventricular septal defect, or tetralogy of Fallot) occurs in 30–35% of patients with TAR syndrome.

Most survive, and the platelet counts improve spontaneously over time. Treatment, if necessary for clinically significant bleeding, is best accomplished with platelet transfusion.

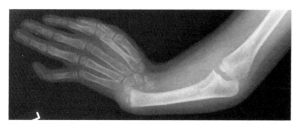

Image 24-20: X-ray demonstrating missing radius in a child with TAR syndrome

Acquired Thrombocytopenia

Overview

Thrombocytopenia is most often an acquired condition and is caused by 1 or more of the following processes:

- Decreased production of platelets (e.g., leukemia, aplastic anemia, viral infection, medications)
- Increased destruction of platelets (e.g., immune thrombocytopenic purpura, medications, DIC)
- Sequestration (pooling) of platelets in an enlarged spleen

If there are normal or increased numbers of megakaryocytes in the bone marrow, you do not have a production problem!

Know:

- Many children with sepsis have thrombocytopenia due to DIC.
- Neonates with CMV present with thrombocytopenia, microcephaly, and/or other congenital anomalies.
- Always review the medication history when evaluating a child with thrombocytopenia.

Pseudothrombocytopenia

If a patient has unexpected thrombocytopenia, then review the blood smear. In some cases, platelet clumping results in a factitiously low platelet count on the automated reader. Platelet clumping results from naturally occurring antibodies that interact with EDTA (ethylenediaminetetraacetic acid) in the blood collection tube. Platelets do not clump in a light blue-top tube (sodium citrate). Redraw the sample in this type of tube.

Immune (Idiopathic) Thrombocytopenic Purpura (ITP)

ITP is a common cause of true thrombocytopenia in children. There are between 1 and 6 cases per 100,000 children per year in the U.S. In this condition, thrombocytopenia results from an immune-mediated destruction of circulating platelets. It is usually acute in onset and self-limited, but it can become chronic or recurrent. ITP is a diagnosis of exclusion, so other causes must be ruled out.

Acute ITP affects boys and girls equally and has a peak between 2 and 5 years of age. Chronic ITP more commonly occurs in adolescents or adults. A history of recent (in the preceding 1–6 weeks) viral infection or immunization is found in a large percentage of those affected. Acute bruising, petechiae, or bleeding is usually the 1st sign.

Petechiae and purpuric lesions occur spontaneously or with minor trauma. No hepatosplenomegaly is noted. In menstruating girls, a platelet count < 10,000 can result in severe blood loss. Intracranial hemorrhage occurs in < 1% of children with ITP and is fatal in 1/3 of these cases.

The major laboratory finding is a low platelet count of varying severity. The few platelets seen on the smear are megathrombocytes—large but not as large as red blood cells. The predominance of giant platelets indicates an inherited platelet disorder (e.g., Bernard-Soulier syndrome). The platelets, recently released in response to the low numbers (which, remember, is due to destruction and not to a production problem), are "reticulated"; that is, they still contain RNA. Bottom line: The bone marrow is cranking out the platelets as fast as it can, but the destructive process is eliminating them just as fast. Unless significant bleeding has occurred, hemoglobin is usually normal in ITP, which helps differentiate it from TTP, HUS, and DIC. In ITP, the WBC is also usually normal.

Note: **Evans syndrome** is when ITP is found in association with AIHA. Some patients with Evans syndrome additionally have autoimmune neutropenia. In this syndrome, autoantibodies are directed at specific, distinctly different antigens on each of the affected blood cell lines.

A bone marrow study is necessary in patients with ITP if:

• features are not classic for ITP and/or
• the platelet count does not increase with initial therapy.

If performed, the bone marrow study shows normal-to-increased megakaryocytes.

Platelet counts normalize in nearly 80% of children with ITP within 12 months of diagnosis. Risk factors for chronic ITP are > 10 years of age, female gender, and insidious onset of original symptoms. In rare instances, ITP is recurrent.

Decision to treat depends on bleeding symptoms and sometimes platelet count. Treatment is not indicated if the platelet count is > 10,000–20,000 and there are no substantial bleeding symptoms. If there is significant skin or mucosal bleeding, initiate treatment; some clinicians start treatment if platelet count falls below 10,000–20,000 even in the absence of significant bleeding symptoms. In all patients, NSAIDs, aspirin, and antihistamines are contraindicated because these interfere with platelet function.

There are 3 main treatments available for acute ITP:

1) IVIG, the 1st line treatment, blocks the Fc receptors of the reticuloendothelial phagocytes and prevents them from binding and destroying the IgG antibody–coated platelets.

2) Corticosteroids have a rapid action that reduces reticuloendothelial destruction of antibody-coated platelets and also slows down antibody production. Various treatment regimens have been used. Note: Corticosteroids can mask a diagnosis of acute leukemia. Consider evaluation for leukemia if clinical presentation includes lymphadenopathy, bone pain, or weight loss and/or if anemia or neutropenia are present.

3) Anti-Rh (D) immunoglobulin causes a mild hemolytic anemia that saturates the Fc receptors of the reticuloendothelial phagocytes and results in increased survival of antibody-coated platelets. There is a black box warning about renal failure due to severe hemolysis, and close monitoring is required. Note: Anti-Rh can be used only in Rh+ patients who are Coombs negative and not splenectomized.

IVIG yields a response rate of 94–97%, followed by anti-Rh (D) immunoglobulin (82–90%) and corticosteroids (79%). Duration of response is variable. Some patients with acute ITP require multiple treatments until thrombocytopenia and bleeding symptoms resolve. Platelet transfusions are not generally recommended because they are destroyed by the same antibodies as the native platelets. In the case of intracranial bleeding, platelets are given with IVIG, high-dose IV steroids, and, rarely, splenectomy.

If ITP becomes chronic, splenectomy, immunosuppressive agents, or thrombopoietin mimetics are treatment options. Splenectomy can be "curative" by eliminating the site of destruction of platelets, but the antibody can remain.

Thrombotic Thrombocytopenic Purpura

Thrombotic thrombocytopenic purpura (TTP) is a thrombotic microangiopathic hemolytic anemia typically caused by antibodies against ADAMTS13, a protease that breaks down ultra-large von Willebrand factor (vWF) multimers. In addition to the anemia, previously healthy patients present with thrombocytopenia. Characteristic lab findings include an elevated LDH, hyperbilirubinemia, and azotemia. The condition is life-threatening because of the risk of thrombosis in small arteries supplying the heart and CNS. The treatment of TTP includes emergent plasma pheresis and corticosteroids.

Maternal Autoimmune Neonatal Thrombocytopenia

Gestational thrombocytopenia (a.k.a. incidental thrombocytopenia of pregnancy) is a fairly common disorder of pregnant women (about 5%). The condition is neither immunologic nor severe. The infants of these mothers are not affected. However, infants whose mothers have ITP may develop thrombocytopenia. This occurs because of the transplacental passage of maternal IgG antiplatelet antibodies. The condition lasts about 1–2 months after birth.

IVIG is given during the 3rd trimester to mothers who have ITP, especially if there is maternal bleeding. IVIG is also given to the newborn with a platelet count < 20,000. If the newborn also has intracranial hemorrhage (< 1% risk), give steroids and platelet transfusions as well.

Kasabach-Merritt Phenomenon

This syndrome is due to the destruction of platelets in certain vascular tumors of the skin, liver, or spleen. These tumors include tufted angiomas and kaposiform hemangioendotheliomas. The syndrome usually presents early in life. Some patients have evidence of a consumptive coagulopathy with low fibrinogen and elevated D-dimers with microangiopathic hemolytic anemia. Management includes medications (steroids, vincristine, propranolol, and interferon-α) and supportive care. The tumors often cannot be surgically excised or embolized if they are too large or inaccessible.

PLATELET FUNCTION ABNORMALITIES

Overview

Etiology of platelet function abnormalities includes:

- Inherited:
  - von Willebrand disease
  - Bernard-Soulier syndrome
  - Glanzmann thrombasthenia
- Acquired:
  - Drug-induced
  - Uremia

Children with platelet function abnormalities most often have normal or near-normal platelet counts with reduced platelet function. Symptoms include bruising, petechiae, and mucosal bleeding.

Inherited

von Willebrand Disease (vWD)

von Willebrand factor (vWF) helps platelets stick to exposed subendothelium and to other platelets; it is also the carrier protein for Factor 8.

vWF multimers in the bloodstream have little affinity for platelets. Affinity increases dramatically when vWF attaches to an altered vascular surface, increasing the aggregation of the platelets at that spot. vWF multimers in the bloodstream are various sizes, ranging from small to ultralarge. The larger the multimer, the more hemostatic potential.

von Willebrand disease (vWD) is usually AD and affects up to 1% of the population. Expression is variable—patients have mild symptoms (bleeding with dental extractions and lifelong easy bruising) to more severe symptoms (frequent recurrent bleeding: nasal, oral, GI, and GU, including recurrent menorrhagia). A frequent 1st manifestation of vWD in girls is heavy menstrual bleeding.

PTT is usually normal but is prolonged in severe subtypes (due to decreased Factor 8), whereas PT is always normal. Bleeding time and platelet function analysis (PFA) test are typically prolonged.

normal PT/PTT
prolonged bleeding time

Individuals with type O blood normally have lower vWF levels. Levels increase during pregnancy and with estrogen therapy.

There are 3 types of vWD:

- **Type 1 vWD** is the most common (90%) and is due to a decrease in the amount of vWF (i.e., is a quantitative problem).
- **Type 2 vWD** results from a qualitative problem with vWF. All cause increased bleeding.
  - Type 2A—decreased binding of vWF to platelets.
  - Type 2B—increased binding of vWF to platelets, but it is a bleeding disorder. This seems counterintuitive but what is thought to happen is that the largest vWF multimers bind to platelets while still in the plasma, making these multimers unavailable to be used in the hemostatic process. The largest multimers have the most hemostatic potential, so the result is a bleeding disorder.
  - Type 2M—decreased binding of vWF to platelets.
  - Type 2N—decreased binding of vWF to Factor 8.
- **Type 3 vWD** is rare (1/1,000,000 in the general population). Patients have undetectable vWF levels and low Factor 8 levels. The bleeding symptoms are similar to those seen in severe hemophilia.

When decreased activity is tied to decreased amount of vWF, it is always a quantity problem—never a binding problem! Hence, **diagnosis of Type 1 vWD** is confirmed with the combination of all of the following:

- Decreased vWF antigen
- Proportional decrease in Factor 8 activity (vWF protein is a cofactor of Factor 8)
- Proportional decrease in biologic activity, as measured by the ristocetin cofactor (rCoF) assay

Diagnosis of Type 2 vWD (A, B, M, and N) requires specialized testing.

Diagnosis of Type 3 vWD is based on finding absent vWF antigen and activity and very low Factor 8 activity.

Diagnostic testing is complicated by increased vWF with stress, such as can occur at the time of blood draw. Delayed processing results in falsely low levels.

Desmopressin (DDAVP) causes a release of stored vWF and Factor 8 from endothelial cells. DDAVP may be used to treat and prevent bleeding in most patients with Type 1 vWD and some patients with Type 2A vWD. Patients with these types of vWD who do not respond to DDAVP or have major bleeding or surgery are treated with vWF/Factor 8 concentrates. Treatment with vWF/Factor 8 concentrates is required for patients with Type 2B vWD, Type 2N vWD, and Type 3 vWD. Cryoprecipitate contains vWF and Factor 8, but it has been replaced by the concentrates that have less risk of viral contamination. These concentrates are preferred over cryoprecipitate because cryoprecipitate contains fibrinogen, Factor 8, vWF, and Factor 13 (which has a higher risk of viral contamination).

The antifibrinolytic agents, ε-aminocaproic acid and tranexamic acid, are useful for minor mucosal bleeding and can be given as an oral rinse to prevent local fibrinolysis.

Menorrhagia is a common symptom of vWD. Treatment options include ε-aminocaproic acid, tranexamic acid, and oral contraceptives.

Bernard-Soulier Syndrome

Bernard-Soulier syndrome is an AR disorder with mild thrombocytopenia and giant, abnormal platelets that do not aggregate in response to ristocetin but do aggregate in response to ADP, epinephrine, or collagen. There is a prolonged bleeding time and PFA test with this disorder. The abnormality is a deficiency of platelet glycoprotein 1b (GP1b) in the platelet membrane, which results in the inability of the platelets to aggregate properly. There is severe mucocutaneous bleeding starting in infancy.

Glanzmann Thrombasthenia

Glanzmann thrombasthenia is another AR disorder with normal platelet counts and poor platelet aggregation in response to ADP, epinephrine, and collagen. It is due to an abnormality in the genes encoding the αIIb-β3 integrin fibrinogen receptor. This results in the inability of platelets to bind fibrinogen and aggregate. There is severe mucocutaneous bleeding starting in infancy.

Acquired

Drug-Induced Platelet Dysfunction

Drug-induced platelet dysfunction can be irreversible or reversible. Aspirin irreversibly inactivates platelet cyclooxygenase and alters platelet function for the entire lifespan of the platelet. In contrast, NSAIDs reversibly inhibit platelet function. Serotonin reuptake inhibitors also inhibit platelet function by depleting platelet serotonin and thus inhibiting serotonin-induced platelet aggregation amplification.

Uremic Platelet Dysfunction

The major cause of bleeding in patients with renal disease is platelet dysfunction that results from impaired platelet adhesiveness and decreased platelet aggregation.

Most commonly, this condition manifests as GI bleeding, but it can also involve the skin, mucous membranes, urinary tract, and respiratory system.

Treatment of platelet dysfunction is needed in symptomatic patients or in those about to undergo a surgical procedure. Options include correction of anemia, desmopressin, dialysis, or administration of conjugated estrogens.

THROMBOCYTOSIS (EXCESS PLATELETS)

Overview

Thrombocytosis is defined as > 500,000 platelets. Platelets are an acute phase reactant. Thrombocytosis in children is usually due to a reaction to some secondary cause: acute or chronic infection, iron deficiency anemia, inflammatory disorders, or acute blood loss. It is a benign condition and does not require specific therapy. Thrombocytosis is also common in mucocutaneous lymph node syndrome (Kawasaki syndrome) and in patients who are hyposplenic or asplenic.

Essential Thrombocythemia

Essential thrombocythemia is a rare myeloproliferative disorder with persistent platelet counts > 1,000,000. Thrombosis and bleeding commonly occur because platelet function is abnormal. Patients who are not bleeding are treated with a platelet aggregation inhibitor, such as aspirin. In addition, a platelet-lowering drug, such as hydroxyurea or anagrelide, is prescribed.

STEM CELL DISORDERS

PREVIEW | REVIEW

- What are the treatment options for children with aplastic anemia?
- Why should blood products be leukoreduced and irradiated in patients with aplastic anemia?
- Describe congenital anomalies seen in children with Fanconi anemia.
- Children with Fanconi anemia are at risk for which malignancies?
- Which virus infects RBCs and results in aplastic crisis in children with congenital hemolytic anemias?
- How do you differentiate among the 3 most common causes of red cell aplasia?

APLASTIC ANEMIA

Aplastic anemia is a condition in which there are a reduced number of RBCs, WBCs, and platelets due to bone marrow aplasia/hypoplasia. Aplastic anemia is a stem cell disorder with the clinical presentation of pancytopenia, rather than anemia, and therefore is a misnomer. Aplastic anemia involves all cell lines, whereas aplastic crisis involves the red cell line only.

The cause is unknown in > 50% of cases, with the remainder due to certain drugs, toxins, infections, or radiation exposure. The dose-related causes include benzene and radiation. Idiosyncratic causes are sulfa drugs, gold, chloramphenicol, and insecticides. Include hepatitis, CMV, Epstein-Barr virus (EBV), HIV, and parvovirus testing in the initial evaluation of aplastic anemia. In addition, evaluate children with aplastic anemia for inherited bone marrow failure syndromes (IBMFS). About 20% of patients with PNH (paroxysmal nocturnal hemoglobinuria) eventually develop aplastic anemia. (See more about PNH on page 24-12.) Other causes of pancytopenia include fibrosis or infiltration with neoplastic cells, such as in neuroblastoma, B_{12} or folic acid deficiency, primary hematologic malignancies, and hemophagocytic lymphohistiocytosis.

The combination of bruising and pallor suggests a marrow disorder affecting > 1 cell line. Typically, these patients present with recurrent infections, mucosal bleeding, and increased menstrual flow in premenopausal females. They can also present with fatigue and petechiae.

Bone marrow examination is necessary in evaluation of any child with pancytopenia. Patients with aplastic anemia have a hypocellular or acellular bone marrow.

Treatment of aplastic anemia:

- Immunosuppressive therapy with antithymocyte globulin (ATG), cyclosporine, and prednisone offers a complete response rate of 65%, although relapses are common.
- Matched BMT, if available, has a 10-year survival rate of > 80%!

A patient treated medically is at risk for a secondary malignancy if the patient has an underlying IBMFS.

To prevent pretransplant alloimmunization, minimize the number of transfusions if possible. If transfusions are required before transplant:

- Do not use family members as donors.
- Use leukocyte-filtered, irradiated blood components.
- Use single-donor platelets.

FANCONI ANEMIA   8-9 yr old w/ pancytopenia

Fanconi anemia is an AR disorder involving poor DNA repair mechanisms. It presents with pancytopenia and occurs at a mean age of 8–9 years. Note: The anemia can begin at birth or be delayed to as late as 48 years of age. Only 3% are diagnosed before 1 year of age and only 10% after 16 years of age, so the majority fall close to the mean age of 8–9 years.

Classically, patients present with short stature, absent or abnormal thumbs, abnormal radii, microcephaly, café-au-lait spots, dark pigmentation, and renal anomalies, although congenital anomalies are not required for the diagnosis. There are at least 15 different mutations, and *FANCA* and *FANCC* are the 2 most commonly affected genes.

Fanconi anemia can present in children as macrocytic anemia with or without other cytopenias. The diagnostic test of choice is the identification of DNA repair abnormalities in cultured peripheral blood lymphocytes, including a high number of metaphases with breaks,

gaps, rearrangements, and other abnormalities. A test is done with diepoxybutane (DEB) or mitomycin C (MMC), which induces chromosomal damage.

On average, patients with Fanconi anemia live into their mid-30s. Most deaths are due to infection (neutropenia) or bleeding (thrombocytopenia), but aerodigestive cancers are common.

Patients with Fanconi anemia have a 15% risk of developing acute myelogenous leukemia. BMT is the only known cure for the aplasia, but it does not decrease risks of other cancers. Because the defect is in DNA repair, use of chemotherapy requires dose reductions. Hepatic malignancy and squamous cell carcinoma are also more common in patients with Fanconi anemia than in the general population. Do not confuse this with Fanconi syndrome, which is a renal condition characterized by generalized proximal tubular dysfunction.

RED CELL APLASIA

Overview

Red cell (RBC) aplasia is defined by anemia in the setting of reticulocytopenia. The most common known causes of RBC aplasia in the pediatric population are parvovirus B19–associated RBC aplasia, transient erythroblastopenia of childhood (TEC), and congenital hypoplastic anemia (Diamond-Blackfan anemia).

Red cell aplasia can also be idiopathic or secondary to drugs (phenytoin and chloramphenicol in particular) or immune disorders (e.g., thymoma, SLE, chronic lymphocytic leukemia).

Parvovirus B19

Parvovirus B19 can infect erythroid progenitors and cause an acute or chronic red cell aplasia. In an otherwise healthy patient, this is a transient phenomenon and is often asymptomatic. However, chronic infection with red cell aplasia can be seen in the immunocompromised.

Remember: In patients with hemolytic anemias such as sickle cell disease, parvovirus B19 infection can cause an aplastic crisis. (See more on aplastic crisis in sickle cell disease on page 24-14.)

Suspect this in patients presenting with red cell aplasia in the setting of fever, rash, and/or arthropathy. The rash can have the "slapped cheek" presentation of erythema infectiosum, one of the presentations of parvovirus B19 seen in otherwise healthy children.

Diagnose by finding parvovirus B19 DNA in serum, blood, or bone marrow cells. Viral studies for CMV, parvovirus B19, and EBV are usually done during workup for any case of red cell aplasia. Lab confirmation is typically not needed if the signs and symptoms are characteristic. Treatment is supportive. IVIG is prescribed for complicated cases in immunosuppressed patients.

Short no thumbs cafe au lait

Transient Erythroblastopenia of Childhood

1-3yr old

Transient erythroblastopenia of childhood (TEC) is an acquired, self-limited condition seen in previously healthy children between 1 and 3 years of age. Affected children exhibit pallor and decreased activity. There is no organomegaly or petechiae on exam.

Laboratory evaluation shows normocytic anemia with reticulocytopenia but without other cytopenias. Parvovirus is not responsible.

Treatment includes supportive care with transfusion for symptomatic anemia. In most cases, the anemia resolves in 1–2 months without transfusions. Children with TEC are not at increased risk of developing additional hematologic problems.

Congenital Hypoplastic Anemia (Diamond-Blackfan Anemia)

macrocytic anemia
< 1yr gage

Diamond-Blackfan anemia (DBA) presents in infancy with macrocytic anemia and reticulocytopenia without other cytopenias. Most children are diagnosed at < 1 year of age. About 1/3 of patients have various congenital deformities, including thumb anomalies; short stature; glaucoma; renal anomalies; hypogonadism; short, webbed necks; congenital heart disease; and intellectual disability.

TEF

Manage these children with transfusions until 6–12 months of age; then try corticosteroids. Because corticosteroids affect bone growth, many wait until 12 months of age. The anemia responds to corticosteroids in up to 80% of patients. Spontaneous remission occurs in about 25% of cases. Chronic RBC transfusions are indicated for those who are steroid refractory or steroid dependent. Consider BMT for patients requiring chronic red cell transfusion therapy.

Differentiating Among the Red Cell Aplasias

If a child comes in with anemia and low reticulocytes, especially consider the aforementioned disorders: parvovirus B19, TEC, and congenital hypoplastic anemia (Diamond-Blackfan anemia). During the history and physical exam, still keep in mind that you are ruling out drugs and autoimmune disorders as causes.

Differentiating the above 3 disorders:

- Parvovirus B19 usually occurs in school-aged children and has associated fever, rash, and arthropathy.
- TEC typically occurs in children between 1 and 4 years of age and has normocytic RBCs and no rash, fever, or arthropathy.
- DBA is most often diagnosed in children < 1 year of age and has macrocytic RBCs. Patients also often have congenital deformities.

HEMOSTASIS

PREVIEW | REVIEW

- Describe primary hemostasis.
- At the bedside, how can you differentiate between a primary hemostatic problem and a coagulation problem?
- Which 5 tests are commonly done in the initial evaluation of a bleeding disorder?
- What does the thrombin time measure?
- What does it mean if the PT is prolonged but the PTT is normal?
- What does it mean if the PTT is prolonged but the PT is normal?
- What does a mixing study show?
- Which clotting factor is low in children with hemophilia A? What will the PT and PTT be in hemophilia A?
- Which clotting factor deficiencies have X-linked inheritance? Which have autosomal inheritance?
- What medication can you give to a child with mild hemophilia A (> 5% Factor 8) before a tooth extraction? Which test should be done prior to relying on this medication for treatment?
- What is hemophilia B? How is it treated?
- Which clotting factor deficiency does not result in bleeding?
- What can cause DIC?
- What are the lab abnormalities seen in DIC?
- Name the vitamin K–dependent coagulation factors.
- Why are individuals with protein C deficiency at risk for warfarin-related skin necrosis?
- Which congenital thrombophilias result in neonatal purpura fulminans in infancy?

HEMOSTATIC PROCESS

Clotting after a vascular injury must be quick to initiate, localized to the area of injury, and durable enough for the healing process to occur.

The entire hemostatic process occurs in 4 overlapping phases:

1) **Primary hemostasis**—local vasoconstriction and formation of a loose platelet plug.

2) **Secondary hemostasis**—circulating coagulation factors, via the clotting cascade, form fibrin that stabilizes the platelet plug.

3) **Clot limitation**

4) **Clot dissolution** (fibrinolysis)

The green-colored text in the following description of the clotting sequence is done to highlight certain key elements in the process.

NORMAL CLOTTING SEQUENCE

Primary Hemostasis — Platelet Plug Formation

Primary hemostasis consists mainly of platelet plug formation, although vasoconstriction and capillary endothelial adhesion (where capillaries collapse and stick closed when empty) also play a part. The fix from the loose platelet plug is temporary and lasts only 12–24 hours, which is why hemophiliacs often do not have a deep bleed until 12–24 hours after trauma. Glycoprotein (GP), either singly or in complexes, are receptors on the platelet surface. Consult Figure 24-5 (**Steps A–G**) as you read through the following descriptions.

Platelet plug formation has 4 processes:

1) **Adhesion** of platelets to subendothelium (**Step A**)— Platelets bind immediately to exposed collagen with GP1a/2a platelet surface receptors. Platelet binding is further reinforced by vWF, a constituent of the subendothelial matrix, which binds platelet surface receptors GP1b/9/5 and GP2b/3a.

2) **Activation**—As the platelets bind to the collagen, the collagen is then able to bind to the platelet GP6 signaling receptor (**Step B**), which initiates a signaling cascade (**Step C**) that results in platelet activation (**Step D**) with the following results.

   • Dramatic flattening and spreading out of the platelet, with pseudopod formation allowing better coverage and more collagen-receptor interaction.

   • Secretion of a host of products by the platelets, including ADP, ATP, vWF, and fibrinogen (**Step E**).

   • Configurational change to GP2b/3a receptors on the platelet surface, allowing binding to fibrinogen—which will result in

platelet-to-platelet aggregation. Remember there are about 50,000 GP2b/3a receptors on the surface of each platelet!

   • Arachidonic acid (AA) is converted by cyclooxygenase (COX) into other precursors of thromboxane A$_2$ (TxA2). TxA2 strongly induces more platelet activation and more thrombogenesis. TxA2 is also a potent vasoconstrictor (**Steps F and G**).

   • ADP has a similar effect as TxA2 on activating platelets (**Steps F and G**).

3) **Aggregation** by platelet-to-platelet cohesion occurs when circulating fibrinogen binds to the newly exposed GP2b/3a receptors on adjacent platelets.

4) **Thrombin**, produced in secondary hemostasis (below), causes a spiraling increase in platelet activation and coagulation (**Steps F and G**).

Primary hemostasis—clinical correlations:

• Bernard-Soulier syndrome is due to a deficiency of GP1b. Platelets bind poorly to vWF. Patients have bleeding gums and significant bleeding with small injuries; women have profuse bleeding with menses.

• Deficiency in the GP2b/3a complex is termed Glanzmann thrombasthenia. Patients are unable to aggregate platelets.

• Clopidogrel blocks the ADP effects on the platelets.

• TxA2 has vasoconstrictive properties and is the presumed cause of Prinzmetal angina.

• Aspirin (acetylsalicylic acid [ASA]) irreversibly acetylates COX and thereby decreases platelet aggregation by preventing the conversion of AA to TxA2. Most other NSAIDs bind reversibly with cyclooxygenase. Chronic ASA use of as little as 40 mg/day causes suppression of 95% of the TxA2.

Secondary Hemostasis — Coagulation

Follow along in Figure 24-6 as you review secondary hemostasis. Most of the inactivated coagulation factors float freely in the plasma—basically waiting for an injury to occur. While the platelets are aggregating (step 3 under Primary Hemostasis — Platelet Plug Formation), the clotting pathway is activated. Factors **12**, **11**, **9**, and **8** form the intrinsic pathway, and the **7a-tissue factor complex** comprises the extrinsic pathway. Both pathways converge to activate **Factor 10.** The final common pathway consists of converting prothrombin to thrombin.

Stop for a minute to look at Figure 24-6 again and appreciate what an important substance thrombin is. Thrombin is critical in both the conversion of fibrinogen to fibrin in the platelet plug (that was formed in primary hemostasis) and in activating Factor 13; the resulting Factor 13a interacts with the fibrin to make a covalently bonded, stabilized, cross-linked fibrin clot. Thrombin is an important platelet activator and also stimulates self-regeneration by activating Factors 5, 8, and 11.

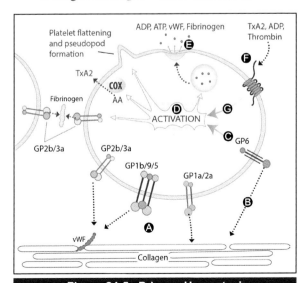

Figure 24-5: Primary Hemostasis

Additionally, thrombin activates platelets in primary hemostasis (see Figure 24-5).

See Disorders of Secondary Hemostasis (Coagulation Factor Disorders) on page 24-28.

CLOT LIMITATION AND DISSOLUTION

Clot size **limitation** occurs because thrombin also modulates its own production by combining with an endothelial cell surface protein, thrombomodulin, to activate protein C. Activated protein C, combined with protein S, deactivates Factors 5a and 8a, thereby limiting thrombin production.

Clot **dissolution** (fibrinolysis) is initiated by tissue plasminogen activator (**tPA**) released from endothelial cells. tPA is an enzyme that catalyzes the conversion of plasminogen to plasmin, which breaks down fibrin and fibrinogen and dissolves the clot.

Protein C also blocks the inhibitor of tPA (platelet activating factor [PAF]).

Clinical correlations quick review:

- Protein C or protein S deficiency cause a thrombogenic tendency. If mild, either deficiency predisposes the patient to deep vein thrombosis (DVT).

- tPA, as a drug, is used for thrombolysis in acute ischemic conditions (e.g., cardiac, limb, pulmonary, stroke).

CLINICAL EVALUATION OF BLEEDING DISORDERS

At the bedside, you can use family history, patient history, and physical examination to establish a differential diagnosis for a patient with a suspected bleeding disorder:

- **Primary hemostatic** problems (90% involve low platelets or platelet dysfunction) result in multiple, tiny, superficial hemorrhages. Patients present with petechiae, ecchymosis, and mucocutaneous bleeding. Remember that vasculitic disorders are a cause of bruising or palpable purpura in a child with a normal platelet count.

- Patients with a **coagulation disorder**, such as hemophilia, develop deep tissue bleeding, including hematomas or hemarthroses.

LAB TESTS IN BLEEDING DISORDERS

Know these 5 tests, which are usually done to quickly assess coagulation and platelet status:

1) Prothrombin time (PT) measures the function of extrinsic and common pathways. (Think Factor 7.)

2) Activated partial thromboplastin time (PTT; a.k.a. aPTT) measures the function of the intrinsic and the common pathways.

[handwritten annotations: "PT=7: extrinsic", "PTT: intrinsic"]

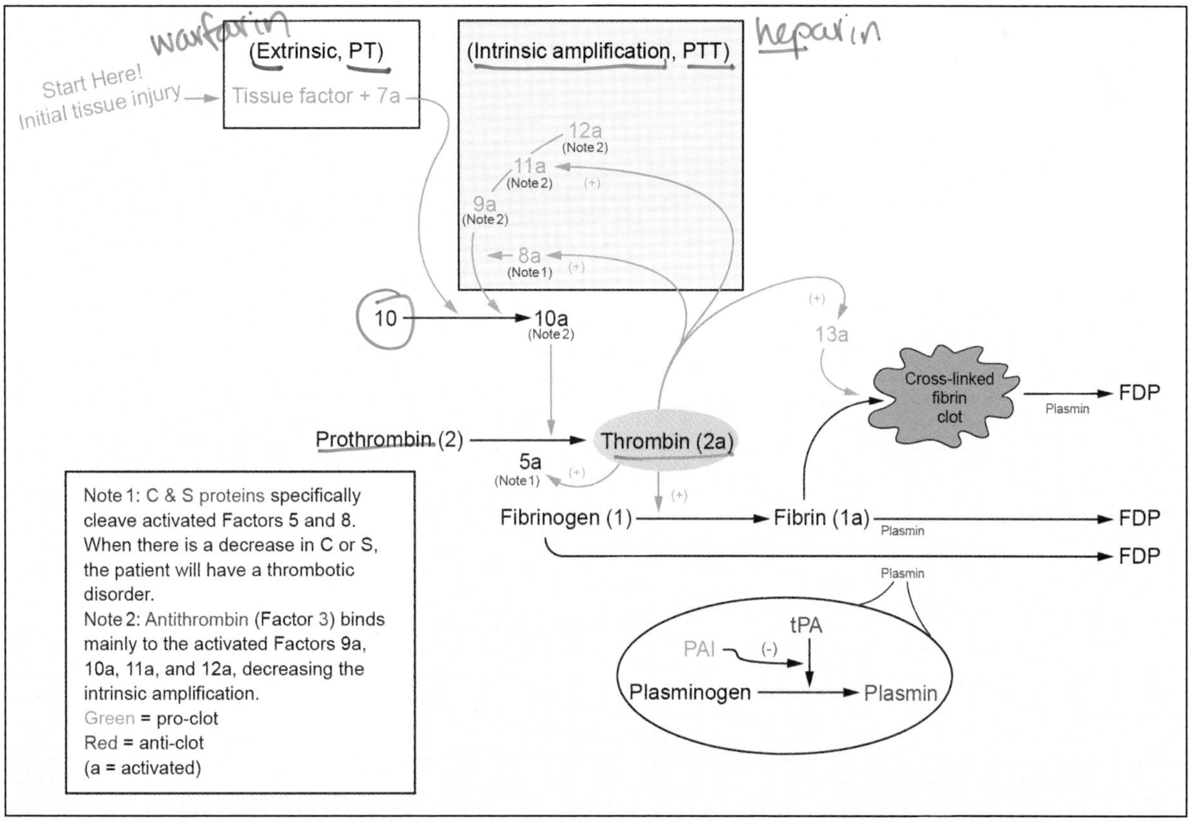

[handwritten annotations on figure: "warfarin", "heparin"]

Start Here! Initial tissue injury → Tissue factor + 7a

(Extrinsic, PT)

(Intrinsic amplification, PTT)

12a (Note 2)
11a (Note 2) (+)
9a (Note 2)
8a (Note 1) (+)

10 → 10a (Note 2)

13a (+)

Cross-linked fibrin clot → FDP (Plasmin)

Prothrombin (2) → Thrombin (2a)

5a (Note 1) (+)

Fibrinogen (1) → (+) → Fibrin (1a) → FDP (Plasmin)

→ FDP

Note 1: C & S proteins specifically cleave activated Factors 5 and 8. When there is a decrease in C or S, the patient will have a thrombotic disorder.
Note 2: Antithrombin (Factor 3) binds mainly to the activated Factors 9a, 10a, 11a, and 12a, decreasing the intrinsic amplification.
Green = pro-clot
Red = anti-clot
(a = activated)

tPA
PAI ⌐ (-)
Plasminogen → Plasmin

Figure 24-6: Coagulation Pathways

3) The thrombin time measures the time of conversion of fibrinogen to fibrin; it is abnormal only if there is a problem with this process. An increased thrombin time reflects decreased or defective fibrinogen, elevated fibrin degradation products (FDPs), or the presence of heparin or heparin-like anticoagulants.

4) Platelet count.

5) Bleeding time (< 10 minutes is normal) reflects the effectiveness of platelet aggregation. In other words, it is a measure of both adequate platelet number and adequate platelet function. Because this test is technically difficult, it is not often used. Instead, rapid platelet function analysis (PFA) is performed.

Review Figure 24-7 and Table 24-6 for an approach to diagnosis based on the PT and PTT and mixing studies.

Know: If there is a greatly increased PTT with a normal PT and normal platelet count, check to see if the PTT normalizes when the patient's plasma is mixed 1:1 with normal plasma (a "mixing study"). If it does correct, the patient has a clotting factor deficiency; if it does not correct, the patient has developed an inhibitor to a clotting factor protein, usually a lupus anticoagulant or Factor 8 inhibitor. When there are Factor 8–specific antibodies, the PTT may initially correct; however, after incubation with normal plasma for 2 hours, it remains prolonged. Factor 8 inhibitors occur in some patients with congenital hemophilia A in response to clotting factor or in older patients with acquired hemophilia A.

DISORDERS OF PRIMARY HEMOSTASIS

Most disorders of primary hemostasis are due to abnormal platelet count or abnormal platelet function. These were discussed on page 24-19 under Platelet Disorders.

DISORDERS OF SECONDARY HEMOSTASIS (COAGULATION FACTOR DISORDERS)

Factor 8 Deficiency (Hemophilia A)

PTT (intrinsic) normal PT (ex)

Overview

Hemophilia A is due to a deficiency of Factor 8. In the intrinsic pathway, activated Factor 8 accelerates by 1,000-fold the cleavage of Factor 10 by activated Factor 9. With either Factor 8 or 9 deficiency, the PTT is increased and the PT is normal.

Factor 8 deficiency is X-linked recessive; i.e., the patient is virtually always male, and the family history might be positive for bleeding in males on the maternal side of the family. Female carriers have one normal Factor 8 gene, but may still have lower Factor 8 levels due to skewed X-inactivation and bleeding symptoms.

There are a few additional facts to know about inheritance of hemophilia:

- A female carrier of hemophilia has:
  ◦ a 50% chance that a male offspring will inherit that bleeding disorder, and
  ◦ a 50% chance that a female offspring will also be a carrier.
- Test children born to the daughters of patients with hemophilia for the relevant bleeding disorder (e.g., Factor 8 or 9 deficiency).
- Approximately 30–50% of children with hemophilia have a negative family history.
- Both Factor 8 and 9 deficiencies can be diagnosed prenatally.

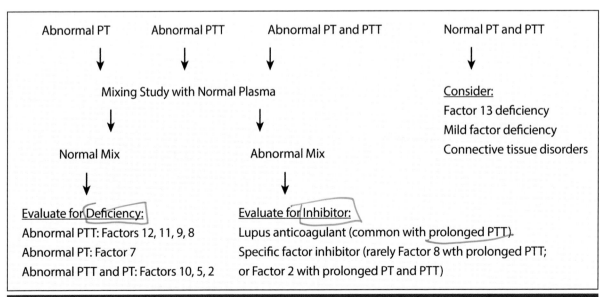

Figure 24-7: Diagnostic Approach to Bleeding Disorders Based on PT, PTT, and Mixing Study

Clinical Presentation

Clinical presentation is similar in Factor 8 and 9 deficiencies, with easy bruising, muscle and joint hemorrhages, and prolonged hemorrhage after surgery or trauma—but typically no mucosal bleeding or excessive bleeding after minor cuts.

Excessive bleeding following neonatal elective circumcision is a classic presentation of hemophilia. Infants can also present with bleeding from heel stick, intramuscular hematoma from hepatitis B immunization, or caput succedaneum with traumatic delivery. In ambulatory patients, hemarthrosis is the most common site for bleeding and presents with pain and reduced mobility. See Table 24-6 for a summary of test results in the factor deficiencies.

With Factor 8 deficiency, the risk of bleeding correlates with the plasma levels of Factor 8. Patients with < 1% of normal have severe disease. Patients with 1–5% activity have moderate disease, and patients with 6–40% Factor 8 activity have mild disease.

It is important to know when to suspect intracranial hemorrhage and how to manage it. A new or worsening headache in a patient with hemophilia is very concerning for a possible intracranial bleed. Symptoms of intracranial bleeding in infants include lethargy and poor feeding. Start factor therapy immediately for hemophilia patients with serious head trauma, even in the absence of loss of consciousness or an abnormal neurologic exam. Consider emergent CT of the head without contrast after factor is administered.

It is important to recognize and aggressively treat bleeding into the forearm. Bleeding in the forearm of a person with hemophilia is an emergency because of the risk of compartment syndrome and nerve damage and long-term risk of contractures. This type of bleeding requires aggressive factor replacement and frequent neurovascular assessment. Patients with compartment syndrome require urgent surgical intervention.

Treatment

DDAVP is a treatment option for some patients with mild Factor 8 deficiency. DDAVP causes a release of vWF and Factor 8 stores from endothelial cells. A DDAVP challenge is done to prove response. If a patient has an adequate response to DDAVP, it can be used as treatment for an acute bleed and prophylactically for a tooth extraction in patients with mild disease (i.e., Factor 8 levels > 5%). DDAVP is not effective in patients with moderate or severe hemophilia.

Patients with moderate or severe Factor 8 deficiency who have acute bleeding are treated with Factor 8 concentrate.

Table 24-6: Lab Results of Inherited and Acquired Bleeding Disorders	
Lab Results	**Etiology**
1) Elevated PT and PTT	Congenital Factor 1, 2, 5, or 10 deficiency Acquired deficiency of vitamin K–dependent Factors 2, 7, 9, and 10 Liver disease DIC Vitamin K deficiency Warfarin, supratherapeutic Antiprothrombin antibody (rare)
2) Elevated PT, normal PTT	Congenital Factor 7 deficiency Acquired Factor 7 deficiency Mild liver disease Mild vitamin K deficiency Warfarin, therapeutic
3) Elevated PTT, normal PT—corrected by addition of normal plasma	Factor deficiency (e.g., Factor 8, 9, 11, or 12* deficiency, vWD with low Factor 8)
4) Elevated PTT, normal PT—not corrected by addition of plasma	Circulating factor inhibitor (e.g., lupus anticoagulant [does not cause bleeding], acquired Factor 8 inhibitor [does cause bleeding], heparin contamination)
5) Normal PT and PTT	vWD Thrombocytopenia Platelet function disorder Dense granule deficiency; storage pool defect Bernard-Soulier (giant platelet) syndrome (absent GP1b) Glanzmann thrombasthenia (absent GP2b/3a)

*Factor 12 deficiency does not cause bleeding.

The most serious side effect of current factor products is development of a **neutralizing inhibitor**, an antibody that inactivates or causes increased clearance of the "foreign" product. This occurs in ~ 25% of patients with severe hemophilia A. If a patient does not respond to clotting factor replacement, suspect the presence of an inhibitor. The presence of an inhibitor can be confirmed with a Factor 8 inhibitor assay. If positive, bypassing agents (i.e., rVIIa and FEIBA) must be used to treat bleeding. Immune tolerance induction (frequent, high doses of Factor 8) is done to provide immune tolerance and eradicate the inhibitor.

It is important to begin the treatment of a bleeding episode with the onset of symptoms and not wait until it is clinically established. Early treatment delays or prevents the hemophilic arthropathy and subsequent severe joint deformity. Prophylactic use of Factor 8 reduces arthropathy.

Factor 9 Deficiency

Factor 9 deficiency is called hemophilia B or "Christmas disease" and is X-linked recessive. It is one-tenth as common as hemophilia A. Presentation is similar to Factor 8 deficiency and is dependent on severity. Treat an acute bleed with a Factor 9 concentrate.

Inhibitors are much less common in hemophilia B. Factor 9 inhibitors can present with anaphylaxis and nephrotic syndrome.

Factor 11 Deficiency (Hemophilia C)

Factor 11 deficiency is autosomal recessive; it is found equally in men and women. It is most common in certain ethnic groups, especially Ashkenazi Jews (up to 8%). Bleeding problems are less common than in those with Factor 8 or 9 deficiency, and these patients usually do not get hemarthroses. The risk of bleeding does not correlate with the level of Factor 11! For some reason, these patients tend to have more mucosal bleeding, such as epistaxis and menorrhagia. Tranexamic acid and ε-aminocaproic acid are useful for mucosal bleeding. For severe bleeding episodes, use fresh frozen plasma.

Factors 5, 7, and 10 Deficiencies

Factors 5, 7, and 10 deficiencies are rare AR bleeding disorders. Know that acquired Factor 10 deficiency can be seen in patients with amyloidosis.

Factor 12 Deficiency

Factor 12 deficiency is an AR disorder. Patients with a decreased Factor 12 (Hageman factor) have a normal PT and a very prolonged PTT (as with Factor 8, 9, or 11 deficiencies), but they do not have a clinical bleeding disorder and can even undergo surgery without worry of bleeding.

Factor 13 Deficiency

Factor 13 deficiency is a rare AR disorder. Ask about consanguinity because offspring of consanguineous parents are at higher risk for rare disorders. These patients can have severe bleeding problems and severe scarring with superficial wounds and yet have a normal PT and PTT. The screening test is the urea solubility assay. Factor 13 activity assays are also available. Prophylactic Factor 13 replacement is often required to prevent severe bleeding. Purified Factor 13 concentrates are preferred over cryoprecipitate.

What bleeding disorders appear with a normal platelet count, PT, PTT, and bleeding time? The major disorders to consider are:

- Mild vWD
- Mild hemophilia
- Factor 13 deficiency (rare)

Table 24-6 on page 24-29 summarizes typical lab results of many of the bleeding disorders.

DIC

Disseminated intravascular coagulation (DIC) is the most common acquired coagulopathy. It is always a secondary condition, so the underlying disease must be treated for the DIC to resolve. DIC occurs in diseases that promote tissue-factor release. These include:

- Massive direct tissue trauma
- Production of tumor necrosis factor (especially seen in solid tumors)
- Sepsis
- Endotoxin production in certain infections
- Placental tissue substances in obstetric patients with placental abruption, dead fetus, or amniotic fluid embolism
- Acute promyelocytic leukemia
- Rattlesnake or viper envenomation

In DIC, large amounts of released tissue factor interact with Factor 7 and initiate coagulation. There is excessive thrombin and plasmin produced, resulting in both increased clot formation (via thrombin cleaving fibrinogen to fibrin) and clot breakdown (via plasmin degradation of fibrin clots). The plasmin breaks down fibrinogen and fibrin into fibrinogen/fibrin degradation products (FDPs; a.k.a. fibrin split products [FSPs]).

Lab results in DIC reflect the above abnormalities with:

- Prolonged PT and PTT.
- Thrombocytopenia.
- Decreased fibrinogen.
- Elevated D-dimer. (This is an FDP specifically produced by the action of plasmin on fibrin.)
- Increased thrombin time (due to both decreased fibrinogen and increased FDPs).
- RBC fragments (i.e., schistocytes, characteristic of microangiopathic hemolytic anemia) seen in

the peripheral smear in up to 50% of patients. The fibrin strands span the small blood vessels and shear the RBCs.

The massive depletion of coagulation factors and platelets and the increased fibrin split products result in bleeding. Symptoms in DIC result from bleeding or microvascular thrombosis as well as the underlying disorder. Some symptoms can include petechiae, ecchymosis, hemorrhage, hypotension, tachycardia, altered consciousness, and GI bleeding.

Treatment of DIC: Treat the underlying disorder! With severe bleeding, give fresh frozen plasma and platelets. Give cryoprecipitate if fibrinogen is low.

Vitamin K Deficiency   1972

Vitamin K deficiency results in decreased production of Factors 2, 7, 9, and 10 and of proteins C and S. Causes of vitamin K deficiency are low stores (e.g., neonates), liver disease, decreased dietary absorption (e.g., no dietary intake of leafy greens, malabsorption, or taking broad-spectrum antibiotics), and antagonists (e.g., warfarin).

Newborn infants are functionally vitamin K deficient and require vitamin K supplements soon after birth. Newborns who don't receive vitamin K at birth are at risk for **vitamin K deficiency bleeding** (**VKDB**), previously known as hemorrhagic disease of the newborn. Other risk factors for VKDB include antibiotics, gastrointestinal malabsorption, and a breastfeeding mother treated with vitamin K antagonists (warfarin, hydantoins, and phenobarbital). Infants can present with bruising, gastrointestinal hemorrhage, or intracranial hemorrhage. See Neonatology, Book 1, for more on VKDB.

Because the vitamin K–dependent coagulation factors are synthesized in the liver, severe liver disease can result in deficiency of these factors.

Vitamin K is a fat-soluble vitamin, so any condition that causes fat malabsorption can result in vitamin K deficiency. Some of these conditions include cystic fibrosis, biliary cholangitis, inflammatory bowel disease, and short bowel syndrome.

Warfarin causes an effective vitamin K deficiency. When warfarin treatment is initiated, if the patient has increased thrombosis (e.g., DVT, pulmonary embolism [PE]), it is due to the negative effect of warfarin on protein C, which has anticoagulant effects. Initially, warfarin therapy causes a prothrombotic effect, which outweighs its antithrombotic effect on Factor 7. This is especially likely to happen if the patient is protein C deficient (patients should be on heparin or low-molecular-weight heparin until a therapeutic dose of warfarin is achieved). 1/3 of patients who develop warfarin-related skin necrosis have a protein C deficiency!

Administer vitamin K to patients with vitamin K deficiency if the patient is bleeding; fresh frozen plasma or nonactivated prothrombin complex concentrate can be used while waiting for the vitamin K to take effect (8 hours). Likewise, the effect of warfarin can be reversed with vitamin K. However, if a patient on warfarin has significant bleeding, give fresh frozen plasma or nonactivated prothrombin complex concentrate for immediate factor replacement.

Lupus Anticoagulants

Lupus anticoagulants (LACs) result in a prolonged PTT. (int) In most cases, a patient with LAC does not present with bleeding. It is associated with thrombosis.

LACs are common in young children in the setting of viral infection. They are not pathogenic and resolve spontaneously.

Use a PTT mixing study to differentiate a congenital factor deficiency from an LAC. The patient's plasma is mixed with an equal amount of pooled normal plasma, and the clotting test is repeated immediately after an established incubation period.

Because only ~ 30–40% of an individual factor is necessary to yield a normal PTT, a patient with a deficiency of a clotting factor corrects completely when mixed with normal plasma (i.e., with normal factor levels). On the other hand, the PTT of patients with inhibitors remains abnormally prolonged after the mix. In these cases, a 1:1 dilution of the patient's plasma is not sufficient to eliminate the full effect of the inhibitor on the PTT.

THROMBOTIC DISORDERS

Thrombotic disorders are rare in infants and children, but they are extremely important clinically. **Venous thrombosis** is more common than arterial thrombosis. Venous thrombosis can occur in upper and lower extremity veins, presenting with extremity pain, swelling, and color change. **Cerebral sinovenous thrombosis** presents with seizures, altered mental status, stroke, and/or headache. **Portal vein thrombosis** occurs in newborns with umbilical vein catheters.

Infants with a history of birth asphyxia, shock, and/or sepsis are at increased risk of developing endothelial cell injury leading to **renal vein thrombus** formation. It is also more common in infants of diabetic mothers and in those with congenital hypercoagulable states. This disorder presents with the sudden onset of gross hematuria and a unilateral or bilateral flank mass. On ultrasound, many infants are found to have a thrombus that extends into the inferior vena cava. Doppler flow studies of the inferior vena cava and renal veins confirm the diagnosis. Microangiopathic hemolytic anemia and adrenal hemorrhage can also occur. Although all 3 signs are not present in every patient with renal vein thrombosis, almost all patients have at least 1 of the following: gross hematuria, unilateral or bilateral flank mass, and/or thrombocytopenia.

Most children with thrombosis have multiple risk factors. The most common cause of DVT in children is a central venous catheter. Other acquired risk factors include trauma, immobilization, smoking, and estrogen-based oral contraceptives. LAC and antiphospholipid antibodies (anticardiolipin and anti-β_2 glycoprotein 1) are acquired risk factors for thrombosis and are associated with higher risk for recurrence.

A strong family history of PE or DVT suggests a congenital hypercoagulable disorder. Antithrombin and proteins C and S are naturally occurring anticoagulants. These proteins help to oppose thrombin's procoagulant activity. Activated protein C, in conjunction with its cofactor, protein S, cleaves activated Factors 5 and 8, rendering them inactive. Recall that activated Factors 5 and 8 are necessary cofactors in the clotting cascade, helping to promote clotting. Antithrombin inhibits thrombin. (Heparin functions as an anticoagulant by accentuating the effect of antithrombin.)

Deficiencies of natural anticoagulants are either acquired (e.g., nephrotic syndrome, asparaginase treatment) or inherited in an AD fashion. Infants who are homozygous for protein S or C deficiency have **neonatal purpura fulminans** with life-threatening thrombosis.

Other inherited thrombophilias include **Factor 5 Leiden** (**activated protein C [APC] resistance**) and prothrombin gene mutations. 5% of the Caucasian population is heterozygous for the *Factor 5 Leiden* gene, which increases the risk of venous thrombosis by 5- to 8-fold. 1% of the Caucasian population is heterozygous for prothrombin gene mutation, which increases the risk of venous thrombosis by 3- to 6-fold. The absolute risk of thrombosis depends on the baseline risk of an individual. Screening for acquired and inherited thrombophilia may be considered for all young patients with thrombosis.

See also Neurology, Book 2, for more information on prothrombotic disorders.

ANTICOAGULATION TREATMENT

The most common anticoagulants used in children are unfractionated heparin, low-molecular-weight heparin, and warfarin. Thrombolytic therapy such as tPA is usually reserved for children with life- or limb-threatening arterial or venous thrombosis. tPA increases the conversion of plasminogen to plasmin in the presence of fibrin, so most of the plasmin made is localized to the fibrin clot. However, tPA also results in systemic lysis and therefore can cause serious bleeding.

TRANSFUSION TREATMENT

RBC transfusions: Packed RBCs are the primary product used; whole blood is rarely used. Exceptions include major hemorrhage from trauma and pediatric cardiac surgery. A donated unit of whole blood is usually separated into packed RBCs, platelets, and plasma. Packed red blood cells (PRBCs) are the product of choice and are ordered according to blood type. A unit is typically a total volume of 250–350 mL of PRBCs reconstituted in plasma. A transfusion of 10 mL/kg typically raises the hemoglobin by 2.5–3 g/dL. Complications of RBC transfusions include hemolytic reaction (life-threatening with fever, chills, flank pain, and oozing from IV sites), febrile nonhemolytic reaction (fever and chills only), or urticarial reaction (hives without other allergic symptoms). A unit of PRBCs has 250 mg of elemental iron. Chronic transfusions result in iron overload.

Platelet transfusions: Alloimmunization can be a problem in patients who receive multiple transfusions. Transfusions can be ordered as random-donor or single-donor (pheresis) products. 1 unit of random-donor platelets/kg raises the platelet count by $\sim 50 \times 10^9$/L. 1 single donor unit is the equivalent of 6–8 random donor units, but this is variable.

The actual platelet transfusion thresholds can be quite low in patients without bleeding who are undergoing chemotherapy. This is a pretty controversial area because all recommendations are from expert consensus statements as virtually all studies have been done only in adults.

Patients with ITP are an exception because these patients almost never require platelet transfusions—even with very low platelet counts (their platelets seem to work better); also, transfusion of platelets is usually ineffective due to destruction. Platelet transfusion in TTP is usually avoided.

WBC transfusions are only rarely done. G-CSF or granulocyte-macrophage colony-stimulating factor (GM-CSF) is used in select circumstances to increase WBCs, most commonly in patients receiving myelosuppressive chemotherapy with active, life-threatening infections or in children with severe congenital neutropenia.

HEMATOLOGIC MALIGNANCIES

PREVIEW | REVIEW

- What is the single most common childhood malignancy?

- Which disorders correlate with increased risk of ALL?

- What diagnosis should you consider in a child with pallor and a limp?

- True or false? Splenomegaly is common in ALL.

- Which cytopenias are seen in children with ALL?

- What test is required to diagnose ALL? What must it show to be diagnostic for ALL?

- What is the most important predictive factor for achieving a 2nd remission in ALL?

- What disorders correlate with an increased risk of AML?

- What can an orbital chloroma signify?
- What procedure is required for the diagnosis of AML?
- What peripheral blood cell finding is pathognomonic for AML?
- Know how to identify an Auer rod associated with AML. (See Image 24-24 on page 24-36.)
- Which leukemia is commonly associated with the Philadelphia chromosome? What is the Philadelphia chromosome?
- Does JMML usually present with a small or enlarged spleen?

LEUKEMIA

Overview

Leukemia is the most common cancer in childhood, accounting for approximately 1/3 of all pediatric cancers. Leukemia is cancer of the WBCs resulting in abnormally functioning cells that crowd out other healthy cells in the bone marrow. The type of leukemia that develops depends on the type of blood cell affected and the stage of development during which the cell becomes malignant. The stem cell differentiates into either lymphoid cells that mature into B- or T-lymphocytes or myeloid cells that mature into granulocytes (see Image 24-21). There are 3 main types of leukemia in children:

1) **Acute lymphoblastic leukemia**—cancer that develops in the lymphoid precursor cells

2) **Acute myeloid leukemia**—cancer that develops in the myeloid precursor cells

3) **Chronic myeloid leukemia**—cancer that develops in the stem cells

Symptoms of leukemia include anemia, fatigue, bruising, bleeding, bone pain, lymphadenopathy, and recurrent infections. Complete blood count is the initial test if leukemia is suspected. If abnormal, a bone marrow biopsy

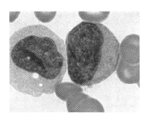
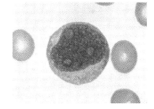
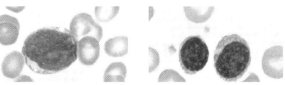

Image 24-21: Myeloblast vs. lymphoblast. UL: Monoblast and myeloblast. UR: Myeloblast. LL: Lymphoblast. LR: Normal lymphocytes are smaller than myeloblasts. Few cytoplasmic granules. Several nucleoli.

is performed as well as a lumbar puncture to determine if the central nervous system is affected. Treatment depends on the type of leukemia.

Acute Lymphoblastic Leukemia

Occurrence   2-5yrolds

Acute lymphoblastic leukemia (ALL) is the single most common childhood malignancy and one of the most curable cancers today. Its incidence peaks between 2 and 5 years of age. Annual incidence is ~ 3/100,000. ALL accounts for about 75% of all pediatric leukemia cases.

Although most patients do not have any known risk factors, there are a few accepted risk factors for ALL. These include the following:

- Prenatal radiation exposure
- Postnatal exposure to high doses of radiation
- Down syndrome
- Ataxia-telangiectasia
- Bloom syndrome
- Fanconi anemia
- Neurofibromatosis

Clinical Findings in ALL

The most common presentation is known as the "4 **P**s": **p**allor, **p**yrexia, **p**urpura, and **p**ain. Fatigue and anorexia are common in the weeks to months before the diagnosis is made. Be aware of the limping 2- to 5-year-old with pallor! The presence of bone pain can distinguish the pancytopenia of leukemia from the pancytopenia of aplastic anemia. Many children with leukemia present with bone pain. Also, watch for the child with persistent oral candidiasis or infiltrated gums.

In addition to fever, bleeding, and bone pain, lymphadenopathy is typical. Generalized lymphadenopathy and hepatosplenomegaly are seen in > 50% of patients.

The lymph nodes, liver, and spleen are the most commonly affected organs, followed by the CNS, testes, and kidneys. Involvement of the CNS or testes is known as extramedullary disease. CNS disease occurs in < 5% of patients and frequently is asymptomatic. If symptoms do occur in CNS disease, they most commonly are headache, nausea, vomiting, lethargy, and/or irritability. Nuchal rigidity and papilledema also can be found but are uncommon. Cranial nerve involvement is rare but has a poor prognosis. Kidney enlargement is common at diagnosis but is not a prognostic indicator.

Laboratory Findings in ALL

Almost 90% of patients with ALL have an abnormal CBC at the time of diagnosis. Normocytic normochromic anemia and reticulocytopenia occur frequently. The WBC count can be very low to very high. Most have an elevated WBC count: 50% have a count > 10,000/μL, and 20% have a count > 50,000/μL. However, it is important to remember that the WBC count can be normal.

Despite relatively high WBC counts at presentation, a majority of patients have severe neutropenia, putting them at an increased risk for infection. Thrombocytopenia is also very common (~ 50% have < 100,000 platelets/μL); thus, many patients have petechiae and purpura. Electrolyte abnormalities are common, and uric acid, phosphorous, potassium, and LDH levels can be high. Renal dysfunction can occur in those with hyperuricemia secondary to tumor lysis.

Definitive diagnosis requires a bone marrow evaluation. The marrow is classically hypercellular and infiltrated with leukemic lymphoblasts (Image 24-22). For the diagnosis of acute leukemia to be made, at least 25% of the marrow must be involved. The absence of blasts in the peripheral blood of a patient with pancytopenia does not rule out the diagnosis of leukemia. A lumbar puncture is performed to evaluate for CNS leukemia, which is diagnosed by the presence of leukemic cells in the cerebrospinal fluid (CSF) or evidence of cranial nerve involvement.

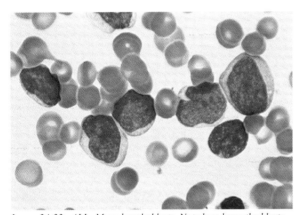

Image 24-22: ALL: Many lymphoblasts. Note how large the blasts are compared to RBCs.

Almost 85% of ALL cases develop from monoclonal proliferation of B-cell precursors; 14% have T-cell lineage; the remaining 1% are mature B-cell ALL.

Good prognostic indicators for ALL:

• Rapid response to treatment
• Hyperdiploidy (> 50 chromosomes or DNA index > 1.16)
• Trisomies of chromosomes 4 and 10
• t(12;21) translocation (*TEL-AML*)
• Female gender

Poorer prognostic indicators for ALL:

• Age < 1 year or > 10 years at diagnosis
• Presence of the Philadelphia chromosome t(9;22)
• Abnormalities of the *MLL* gene; i.e., t(4;11)
• WBC count > 50,000 cells/μL on presentation
• Mature B-cell leukemia
• T-cell leukemia
• African American or Hispanic ethnicity

Treatment of ALL

Treatment regimens for ALL are divided into 4 general categories:

1) Induction therapy
2) Consolidation therapy
3) Maintenance therapy
4) CNS preventive therapy

Most children receive 30–36 months of therapy, depending on prognosis and risk factors. The overall approach to therapy is one of risk stratification, which offers more intensive therapy for the highest risk groups and less therapy and potentially less toxicity for the lowest risk groups.

Induction therapy is the 1st phase of treatment, and its purpose is remission (to destroy the majority of the cancer cells in the blood and bone marrow and restore blood cell production). This includes the use of:

• Vincristine
• Glucocorticoid (dexamethasone or prednisone)
• Asparaginase
• Anthracycline (doxorubicin or daunorubicin) for patients who are higher risk at diagnosis

More than 95% of patients with standard-risk ALL enter remission following induction therapy. The rapidity of clearance of leukemic blasts during the induction month is an important predictor of overall outcome. Mortality rates during induction therapy are 3%, often due to infectious complications.

Every patient with ALL receives **CNS chemoprophylaxis or preventive therapy**, regardless of the initial CNS findings. Usually, a series of lumbar punctures with single-agent intrathecal methotrexate or triple-agent intrathecal therapy is given, reducing the occurrence of CNS leukemia to < 5–10%. CNS preventive therapy begins during the induction phase and continues throughout the treatment program. Children with overt, or at high risk for, CNS leukemia can receive CNS radiation in combination with intensive systemic and intrathecal therapies.

Consolidation therapy is a period of intensified treatment for 6–12 months that begins after induction therapy. This introduces different drugs and combinations that have synergistic effects to reduce the chance for drug resistance. CNS therapy is also intensified. Modern treatment regimens include periods of rest and "re-intensification" in this phase. Cytarabine, anthracyclines, methotrexate, cyclophosphamide, and etoposide (VP-16) are most commonly used.

Maintenance therapy then continues for an additional 18–24 months. Most treatment protocols use daily oral 6-mercaptopurine (6-MP) and weekly methotrexate with intermittent pulses of vincristine and glucocorticoids during the maintenance period.

Outcomes of ALL

Overall cure rates for pediatric ALL are close to 85% and are dependent upon risk stratification.

Expected 5-year event-free survival:

• > 95% for patients with low-risk disease
• 90–95% for patients with standard-risk disease
• 75–90% for patients with high-risk disease
• < 75% for patients with very high-risk disease

For patients who experience relapse, the main site of relapse is the bone marrow. The most important predictive factor for achieving a 2nd remission is the length of time the 1st remission lasted (i.e., the longer the 1st remission lasted, the better the survival rate). Salvage therapies to induce another remission can be very intense. BMT has become standard for treatment of the 1st relapse if it occurs early in the course (< 36 months from initial diagnosis), whereas patients with a late relapse may be salvageable with chemotherapy alone. Isolated CNS and testicular relapses are much less common, each accounting for < 10% of relapses. These extramedullary relapses can potentially be cured by treatment with chemotherapy and radiation therapy.

Long-Term Effects of Therapy

Early and late **CNS toxicity** have been noted in those receiving intrathecal and radiation therapy. Seizures occur in 5–15% of children with standard CNS therapy. Cerebral atrophy, necrotizing encephalopathy, and microangiopathy can occur over time in survivors. Cranial radiation results in neurodevelopmental and neuroendocrine abnormalities (including growth hormone deficiency), and spinal radiation can cause growth retardation. Osteoporosis is an increasingly recognized secondary effect of corticosteroids.

Hepatotoxicity occurs with antimetabolite therapy (e.g., methotrexate, 6-MP). **Cardiomyopathy** is seen with anthracyclines (doxorubicin and daunorubicin). **Infertility** is also an issue for those undergoing chemotherapy during or after puberty. Epipodophyllotoxins (most notably VP-16) have recently been reported to increase the risk of secondary malignancies, specifically **acute myeloid leukemia**. (See Oncology, Book 5, for a list of common therapeutic agents.)

Acute Myeloid Leukemia

Overview

Acute myeloid leukemia (AML) accounts for about 20% of leukemia in children but makes up > 80% in adults. AML survival rates are much lower than those for ALL and are only about 60–70% with current chemotherapy and transplant regimens.

Some conditions predispose to AML:

• Trisomy 21
• Diamond-Blackfan anemia
• Fanconi anemia
• Bloom syndrome
• Kostmann syndrome
• Paroxysmal nocturnal hemoglobinuria
• Neurofibromatosis

Previous exposure to VP-16 and ionizing radiation also predisposes to AML.

Clinical Manifestations of AML

AML frequently presents with signs and symptoms related to the different cytopenias encountered: fatigue and pallor due to anemia; bruising, petechiae, epistaxis, or gum bleeding due to thrombocytopenia; and infection due to neutropenia. Fever is also typical at presentation. Anemia and thrombocytopenia are nearly universal. The median hemoglobin at presentation is 7 g/dL. The WBC count can vary from low to extremely high. Hepatosplenomegaly can occur, as can leukemic infiltration of the skin (**leukemia cutis**), which can be seen with M4/M5 subtypes (Table 24-7). **Chloromas** are a localized mass of leukemia cells and are often present at the time of diagnosis. For example, an orbital or epidural chloroma can be the 1st clue to the diagnosis.

Subtype	Name	Chromosome	Manifestations
M1	Acute myeloblastic leukemia without maturation		
M2	Acute myeloblastic leukemia with maturation	t(8;21)	
M3	Acute promyelocytic leukemia	t(15;17)	DIC
M4	Acute myelomonocytic leukemia	Inversion 16	CNS disease, gingival hyperplasia
M5	Acute monocytic leukemia	11q23 abnormality	CNS disease, gingival hyperplasia
M6	Acute erythroleukemia		
M7	Acute megakaryoblastic leukemia		Common in patients with Down syndrome < 2 years of age

Table 24-7: FAB Classification of AML

Diagnosis of AML

Oncologists use bone marrow evaluation to diagnose AML. Bone marrow morphology, flow cytometry, and cytogenetics are used to classify AML. Finding Auer rods inside peripheral blood blast cells is pathognomonic for AML (Image 24-23 and Image 24-24). With AML, the French-American-British (FAB) classification system is used to differentiate the 7 subtypes (Table 24-7 on page 24-35). Specific karyotypes are associated with some of these subtypes. For example, t(15;17) is found in most cases of **acute promyelocytic leukemia** (APML). Children with APML present with DIC.

Treatment of AML

AML induction therapy usually includes anthracyclines, etoposide, and cytosine arabinoside (Ara-C), which can produce a remission in about 85% of patients. However, induction therapy is quite intense, and it can take 6 weeks or longer for the bone marrow to recover. Most patients are seriously ill during the induction phase, and there is a significant risk of opportunistic infection.

Although the incidence of CNS disease is low, CNS prophylaxis is necessary for AML.

After initial remission, patients with AML are stratified into risk groups based on cytogenetic and molecular features, as well as rapidity of response to therapy. Most **low-risk** patients have good outcomes with chemotherapy alone. **Intermediate-risk** patients with an appropriate HLA-matched sibling donor may benefit from stem cell transplantation; however, outcomes for chemotherapy alone are improving. **High-risk** patients require bone marrow transplantation from the best available donor to have the best chance for long-term disease control. Children with acute promyelocytic leukemia (APL; M3 subtype) represent a unique subset of AML patients who have excellent cure rates. These children receive retinoic acid in addition to chemotherapy—and do not undergo transplant. Also, children with Down syndrome do very well with chemotherapy alone but are at higher risk for side effects.

For those who respond rapidly to initial therapy, the prognosis is better. For those who do not respond or who have a relapse, the prognosis is very poor.

Chronic Myeloid Leukemia (CML) and Juvenile Myelomonocytic Leukemia (JMML)

Chronic leukemia makes up about 2–4% of all cases of leukemia in children. This includes the adult type of Philadelphia chromosome–positive CML and a very rare hematopoietic disease called juvenile myelomonocytic leukemia.

Philadelphia chromosome–positive CML is a disorder of the pluripotent stem cell defined by the t(9;22) translocation (Philadelphia chromosome). This results in the juxtaposition of the *BCR* gene on chromosome 22 with the *ABL* gene on chromosome 9, causing a fusion gene that encodes for a BCR-ABL abnormal protein tyrosine kinase that drives oncogenesis. CML is characterized by an initial chronic phase (2–4 years) of splenomegaly and extreme leukocytosis with complete granulocytic maturation. This chronic phase can evolve into an acute blast crisis that behaves as an aggressive acute leukemia.

Historically, allogeneic BMT during the 1st year of the chronic phase was the preferred treatment for CML, resulting in cure rates as high as 80–90%, though transplant-related morbidity was high.

Most patients presenting in the chronic phase are treated initially with tyrosine kinase inhibitors (TKIs) such as imatinib or dasatinib. TKIs directly inhibit the BCR-ABL oncogenic protein and can induce complete cytogenetic remission in newly diagnosed patients with CML with a favorable side-effect profile. TKIs have not yet proven to be curative, however, so lifelong therapy is recommended.

Juvenile myelomonocytic leukemia (JMML) usually manifests before the age of 2 years. Children with neurofibromatosis Type 1 are at increased risk for JMML. Children present with a markedly enlarged spleen, modest leukocytosis, thrombocytopenia, and elevated

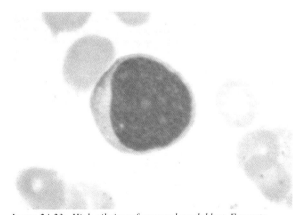

Image 24-23: High-oil view of a normal myeloblast. Few cytoplasmic granules. Several nucleoli.

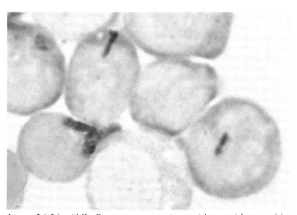

Image 24-24: AML: Bone marrow aspirate with peroxidase-positive blasts and 2 peroxidase-positive Auer rods.

fetal hemoglobin. Skin rashes, including xanthoma, café-au-lait spots, and eczema are common. Monosomy 7 occurs in 30% of patients; there is no Philadelphia chromosome present. Even though there is no blast crisis with JMML, the 5-year survival rate without BMT is < 10%. Allogeneic BMT, with or without pretransplant splenectomy, is the treatment of choice for JMML.

LYMPHOMA

OVERVIEW

Lymphoma refers to cancer of the lymphatic system, which includes lymph nodes, spleen, thymus, and bone marrow. Lymphomas are divided into 2 categories, **Hodgkin lymphoma** and **non-Hodgkin lymphoma**, depending on the microscopic appearance and characteristics of the malignant cells. Hodgkin lymphoma is defined by the presence of Reed-Sternberg cells, which are multinucleated large cells that divide rapidly and live longer than normal cells. Non-Hodgkin lymphomas do not have Reed-Sternberg cells and are subdivided into **Burkitt lymphoma**, **lymphoblastic lymphoma**, and **large cell lymphoma**. Common symptoms of lymphoma include lymphadenopathy, fever, fatigue, night sweats,

weight loss, and difficulty breathing (if chest mass). Worrisome features of lymphadenopathy are:

- Systemic symptoms (e.g., fever, night sweats, weight loss)
- Fixed, nontender nodes
- Supraclavicular nodes
- Lymph nodes > 2 cm with no response to a 2-week course of antibiotics

Diagnosis is made by lymph node or mass biopsy. Treatment depends on the type of lymphoma but usually involves chemotherapy.

HODGKIN LYMPHOMA

Occurrence

Lymphoma is the 3rd most common childhood cancer, and 40% of these are Hodgkin lymphoma. The highest incidence is seen in adolescents between 15 and 19 years of age.

Epidemiology

There are 3 typical age ranges for Hodgkin lymphoma:

1) Childhood ($\leq$ 14 years of age)
2) Young adult (15–34 years of age)—most common form
3) Older adult (55–74 years of age)

The childhood form is mainly seen in poorer socioeconomic environments and has a predominant mixed cellularity histologic subtype. The young adult form is predominantly nodular sclerosing histology and is more common in Caucasian adolescents.

Under the age of 10, boys are more commonly affected, but in adolescence, boys and girls are affected equally. Infectious etiologies, including EBV, have been postulated; however, to date, none have been explicitly implicated. Genetic factors seem to come into play, with increased risk noted in twins and 1st degree relatives, but the specific link is unknown.

Pathology

The classic histologic hallmark of Hodgkin lymphoma is the Reed-Sternberg cell, a large cell with multiple or multilobulated nuclei (looks like "owl's eyes"; Image 24-25 on page 24-38). Most are of B-cell lineage, but those of T-cell lineage are occasionally noted.

There are 4 Rye classifications:

1) Lymphocyte predominance (10–15%)
2) Mixed cellularity (30%)
3) Lymphocytic depletion (rare in children; more common in patients with HIV)
4) Nodular sclerosing (most common)

With modern therapy, the significance of this classification has become diminished.

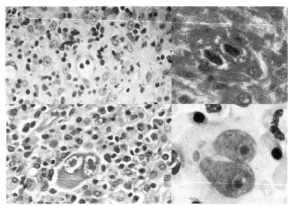

Image 24-25: Hodgkin disease: Views of Reed-Sternberg cell

Clinical Manifestations

The most common presentation for Hodgkin lymphoma is asymptomatic lymphadenopathy, which often involves the cervical or supraclavicular region. Supraclavicular lymphadenopathy is uncommon in inflammatory or infectious conditions and requires further evaluation with chest radiograph to rule out malignancy. 2/3 of patients have mediastinal lymph node involvement, which, on occasion, produces cough or tracheal/bronchial compression. < 10% of children have primary nodal disease below the diaphragm.

1/3 of children have "B" (constitutional) symptoms, which include fever, drenching night sweats, and unexplained weight loss. These B symptoms usually indicate a more advanced disease and a worse prognosis.

Fevers are periodic in character: febrile episodes last several days and are then followed by afebrile periods.

Additionally, cellular immunity is impaired in these patients, so tuberculosis and fungal infections are more common. An especially common infection is varicella zoster.

Itching and alcohol-induced pain (localized to areas involved in the disease; e.g., bones, lymph nodes) are also reported but are not prognostic.

Clinical Diagnosis and Staging

Lab work can show nonspecific findings, but some findings are helpful as prognostic indicators.

Diagnosis of Hodgkin's is confirmed by excisional biopsy of an accessible lymph node. Staging is accomplished by a combination of the radiographic techniques noted below.

Once the histologic diagnosis is made, staging workup includes the following studies:

• CBC
• ESR
• Serum ferritin
• Liver function tests
• CXR (to rapidly evaluate for mediastinal mass)
• Chest/Abdomen/Pelvic CT with contrast
• PET scan
• Bone marrow aspiration and biopsy

The above staging tests help guide treatment and determine prognosis. The following are unfavorable features:

• Albumin < 4 g/dL
• Hemoglobin < 10.5 g/dL
• Male gender
• Stage IV disease (see below)
• WBC count ≥ 15,000 cells/μL
• Absolute lymphocyte count < 600 cells/μL or < 8% of total WBC count

The Ann Arbor staging classification is the international standard for staging of Hodgkin disease (Table 24-8).

Therapy

Hodgkin disease was one of the earliest cancers effectively treated by radiation therapy, chemotherapy, or a combination of both modalities.

Therapy for Hodgkin disease is risk adapted and response based. Patients are assigned to low-, intermediate-, or high-risk groups based on clinical stage and the presence or absence of B symptoms and bulk disease. It has

| Table 24-8: Ann Arbor Staging of Hodgkin Disease ||
Stage	Definition
I	Involvement of a single lymph node region or localized involvement of a single extralymphatic organ or site
II	Involvement of ≥ 2 lymph node regions on the same side of the diaphragm
III	Involvement of lymph node regions on both sides of the diaphragm
IV	Disseminated involvement of ≥ 1 or more extralymphatic organs or tissues

A symptoms = absence of B symptoms
B symptoms = at least 1 of the following:
        Unexplained weight loss of > 10%
        Unexplained recurrent fevers
        Drenching night sweats	

also been shown that rapid responders to therapy have better prognoses than slow responders. Some low- and intermediate-risk patients have good long-term disease control with chemotherapy alone, whereas high-risk patients still receive radiation therapy to maximize the chance of a long-term cure.

Historically, radiation therapy was the mainstay of treatment and was very effective at controlling disease. However, acute and long-term toxicities were substantial. The long-term side effects of radiation therapy, depending on the field of radiation, include growth retardation, thyroid failure, early coronary artery disease, pulmonary fibrosis, and increased risk of secondary malignancies, including breast cancer.

The combination of chemotherapy and radiation was found to improve treatment outcomes compared to radiation alone.

The chemotherapy regimens that are used are multiagent to prevent drug resistance. The first multiagent chemotherapy regimens used to treat Hodgkin disease were:

- **MOPP** (nitrogen **m**ustard, vincristine [i.e., **O**ncovin, Vincasar PFS], **p**rocarbazine, and **p**rednisone) and
- **ABVD** (doxorubicin [**A**driamycin], **b**leomycin, **v**inblastine, and **d**acarbazine).

Treatment-related risks of MOPP are AML and infertility. Treatment-related risks of ABVD are dose-dependent side effects of cardiomyopathy (doxorubicin) and pulmonary toxicity (bleomycin).

Current chemotherapy regimens are based on the initial success with MOPP and ABVD. Risk stratification and response to therapy guide current protocols. Risk stratification allows for reduction, and possible elimination, of the most toxic chemotherapeutic agents in some patients and radiation therapy in select groups of patients.

Prognosis

Hodgkin lymphoma is a very treatable disease with cure rates approaching 90% in patients with early-stage disease and 80–85% in those with late-stage disease. However, treatment-related morbidity can be substantial.

NON-HODGKIN LYMPHOMA

Overview

Non-Hodgkin lymphoma (NHL) is the most common type of lymphoma to occur in pediatrics (NHL 60% vs. Hodgkin lymphoma 40%). There are no distinct age groups for NHL; infants can even be affected. Males outnumber females 3:1.

There is a high rate of NHL in children with:

- Ataxia-telangiectasia
- Wiskott-Aldrich syndrome
- HIV
- Other immunosuppressive diseases

EBV DNA is present in the tumor cells of 95% of endemic cases of Burkitt NHL in equatorial Africa, but it is found in only 15–20% of U.S. cases. NHL can occur from B-cell, T-cell, or indeterminate-cell origin.

Classification

Overview

Most pediatric cases are high-grade, diffuse neoplasms. There are 3 main histologic subtypes:

1) Small, noncleaved cell lymphoma (Burkitt and non-Burkitt subtypes, B-cell origin)
2) Lymphoblastic (80% T-cell origin, 20% early B-cell origin)
3) Large cell (T-cell, B-cell, or indeterminate-cell origin)

The most common form of childhood NHL in the U.S. is the sporadic form of Burkitt lymphoma, which makes up about 50% of pediatric NHLs. This is followed by lymphoblastic lymphoma (30–40%) and large cell lymphoma (15–25%).

Burkitt Lymphoma

Burkitt lymphoma is the most common form of NHL in the U.S., with 90% of Burkitt-type lymphomas originating from relatively mature B cells in Peyer patches within the GI tract, most commonly at the ileocecal junction. Only about 10% of U.S. cases begin in the B lymphocytes within the Waldeyer ring (adenoids/tonsils).

A majority of patients present with an abdominal mass or pain with nausea and vomiting. Jaw involvement is very common in the African form but occurs in only about 15% of U.S. cases. Burkitt lymphoma is the fastest-growing malignant tumor—it can double in 2–3 days! Consequently, **tumor lysis syndrome** is common (more under Supportive Care During Cancer Chemotherapy on page 24-40).

Lymphoblastic Lymphoma

Lymphoblastic lymphoma represents approximately 33% of NHLs. The cells of this tumor are biologically indistinguishable from lymphoblastic leukemia. About 80% are of thymic T-cell origin. Symptoms develop quickly over several weeks. The clinical presentation includes respiratory distress from tracheal and bronchial compression by an anterior mediastinal mass; nontender cervical, supraclavicular, or axillary nodes; and involvement of the liver, spleen, and kidneys. These are typically seen in adolescent males. The other 20% of lymphoblastic lymphomas are of B-cell lineage and present in unusual locations such as skin or bone.

Large Cell Non-Hodgkin Lymphoma

Large cell NHLs contain cells with large nuclei and can manifest anywhere, including abdominal disease like Burkitt's and mediastinal disease like lymphoblastic lymphoma. Large cell lymphomas can also go to unusual sites such as skin, bone, or lung. CNS disease is rare, and bone marrow disease is less likely.

The lymphadenopathy with large cell NHL is usually tender, which separates it from the other lymphomas. Also, constitutional symptoms (e.g., fever, night sweats, weight loss) are much more common in large cell disease. Most large cell lymphomas are of B-cell origin, but T-cell and null-cell types are also seen.

Diagnosis and Staging

Biopsy of an enlarged lymph node is usually required for diagnosis but can be dangerous, depending upon the location of the tumor. If airway obstruction is a problem, then sedated procedures are risky and are avoided.

Staging is generally based on the volume of the tumor. The St. Jude/Murphy staging system is the most widely used. Localized disease makes up Stages I and II. Stage I involves a single tumor or single anatomic node except for the mediastinum or abdomen. Stage II involves ≥ 2 nodal areas on the same side of the diaphragm, 2 extranodal tumors on the same side of the diaphragm, or a resectable primary GI tumor. Stages III and IV represent advanced disease. Stage III has involvement of both sides of the diaphragm, all mediastinal or other intrathoracic tumors, all unresectable abdominal diseases, and all paraspinal or epidural tumors. Stage IV is defined by any CNS or bone marrow involvement; it occurs in < 25% of cases.

Treatment

Treatment of NHL consists mainly of chemotherapy, with a typical regimen being **CHOP** (**c**yclophosphamide, doxorubicin [**h**ydroxydaunorubicin], vincristine [**O**ncovin], and **p**rednisone). Rituximab, an anti-CD20 monoclonal antibody, is a treatment option for tumors that are positive for CD20. Patients with abdominal tumors that are resected at diagnosis have an excellent prognosis with short-course, postoperative chemotherapy. Radiation therapy is usually limited to CNS disease or emergency situations (airway obstruction).

Prognosis

Most pediatric patients have a good prognosis, with > 80% survival rate overall. This varies depending on the type and stage at diagnosis. Long-term sequelae from therapy can include infertility, heart failure, and secondary cancers.

SUPPORTIVE CARE DURING CANCER CHEMOTHERAPY

PREVIEW | REVIEW

- How do you manage fever in a patient on chemotherapy?
- What is tumor lysis syndrome?

Advances in supportive care have improved outcomes. Key among these are prevention and management of infection and tumor lysis syndrome.

Children with fever must be emergently evaluated for bacterial sepsis and other invasive infection. Give broad-spectrum antibiotics as soon as cultures are obtained. Admit patients with severe neutropenia to the hospital for further evaluation and antibiotics. Initial therapy with an antipseudomonal β-lactam (e.g., cefepime or ceftazidime), piperacillin-tazobactam, or carbapenem is used. Vancomycin is used when additional gram-positive coverage is needed. Children are at risk for *Pneumocystis* pneumonia and are prescribed trimethoprim/sulfamethoxazole prophylactically. Some treatment protocols include prophylactic antibiotics and antifungals.

The immune system of a child receiving chemotherapy is impaired, so live viral vaccines during treatment are contraindicated.

Tumor lysis syndrome is a medical emergency and describes the metabolic complications of rapid cell lysis noted with initiation of chemotherapy or with high cellular turnover from certain tumors (e.g., AML with hyperleukocytosis, Burkitt lymphoma, T-cell ALL). Hyperkalemia, hyperphosphatemia, hypocalcemia, and renal insufficiency (due to hyperuricemia) occur. Tumor lysis is expected with initial therapy. Prevention includes hyperhydration with fluids that don't contain potassium. Allopurinol, which prevents formation of uric acid, is 1st line medication for the prevention of tumor lysis syndrome. Urate oxidase, which breaks down uric acid, is prescribed for patients with very high levels of uric acid. Watch for decreased urine output as a sign of kidney damage due to tumor lysis syndrome. Tumor lysis labs include uric acid, electrolytes (especially Ca^{2+}, K^+, and PO_4^-), and renal function.

Children frequently require transfusion support. Blood products must be irradiated in order to prevent life-threatening graft-versus-host disease.

↑K⁺ ↑phos ↑uric acid ↓Ca

THE MEDSTUDY HUB: YOUR GUIDELINES AND REVIEW ARTICLES RESOURCE

For both the review articles and current Pediatrics practice guidelines, visit the MedStudy Hub at

medstudy.com/hub

The Hub contains the only online consolidated list of all Pediatrics guidelines! Guidelines on the Hub are continually updated and linked to the published source. MedStudy maintains the Hub as a free online resource, available to all physicians.

MedStudy®

ONCOLOGY

SECTION EDITOR

Courtney Thornburg, MD
Associate Professor of Pediatrics
University of California—San Diego
La Jolla, CA

MEDICAL EDITOR

Lynn Bullock, MD
Colorado Springs, CO

REVIEWER

Donald W. Coulter, MD
Associate Professor, Pediatrics
University of Nebraska Medical Center
Children's Specialty Physicians
Specialty Pediatric Center
Omaha, NE

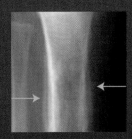

Table of Contents

ONCOLOGY

CANCER INCIDENCE

The overall annual incidence of childhood cancer in the United States is approximately 125/1,000,000 (for children < 15 years of age). The following chart demonstrates the breakdown of the types of cancer by percentage in the 0- to 15-year age range (Table 25-1).

Table 25-1: Types of Cancer in the 0- to 15-Year Age Range	
Type	**% of Total Childhood Cancers**
Leukemias	25
CNS tumors	17
Neuroblastoma	7
Non-Hodgkin lymphoma	6
Wilms tumor	6
Hodgkin disease	5
Rhabdomyosarcoma	3
Retinoblastoma	3
Osteosarcoma	3
Ewing sarcoma	2

LEUKEMIAS

See Hematology, Book 5, for discussion of the leukemias.

TUMORS OF THE CNS

PREVIEW | REVIEW

- Neurofibromatosis Type 1 is associated with which type of CNS tumor?
- Which tumor is characteristically associated with neurofibromatosis Type 2?
- What type of tumor is seen with tuberous sclerosis?
- What type of tumor is seen in von Hippel-Lindau disease?
- Which cranial nerve finding is commonly seen in children with brain tumors?
- What clinical finding is important to look for in an infant you suspect of having a brain tumor?
- What does the "sun-setting" sign refer to?
- Differentiate the presentations between infratentorial and supratentorial lesions.
- Describe Parinaud syndrome.
- What symptoms can occur if a CNS tumor has spread to the leptomeninges?

- What is the mainstay of therapy for most CNS tumors?
- Which age group normally is not treated with CNS radiation therapy due to increased risk of toxicity?
- What are the most common presentations for medulloblastoma?
- If ependymoma tumors involve the 4th ventricle, what complication can occur?
- What is the most common type of primary CNS tumor in children?
- Describe the clinical findings in cerebellar astrocytoma tumors.
- Which type of astrocytoma has the most aggressive clinical behavior?
- How do pineal tumors present?
- Name some of the complications from craniopharyngiomas.
- Meningiomas are more common in which patients?

OCCURRENCE

CNS tumors make up 15–20% of all childhood cancers and are the most common solid neoplasms of childhood. In most parts of the world, an intracranial mass lesion in childhood is likely to be a neoplasm. The incidence of brain tumors in all children is 3/100,000 per year. With current treatments, ~ 65% of children with brain tumors survive into adulthood.

EPIDEMIOLOGY OF BRAIN TUMORS

Occurrence

There is no difference between the sexes in the incidence of brain tumors. Caucasian children have a slightly higher incidence than African American children. Data shows that the incidence of brain tumors is increasing, but some clinical researchers attribute part of this increase to the invention of MRI and the ability to diagnose these tumors more easily.

Risk Factors for Brain Tumors

Neurofibromatosis Type 1 (discussed in Genetics, Book 5) predisposes to CNS tumors, especially optic gliomas. Other tumors include meningiomas, ependymomas, neurosarcomas of the cranial nerves, and spinal cord astrocytomas.

Neurofibromatosis Type 2 characteristically produces bilateral vestibular schwannomas. Other tumors include retinal gliomas, meningiomas, gliomas, and cranial and peripheral nerve schwannomas.

The tumor most commonly seen with tuberous sclerosis is a subependymal giant cell tumor, which arises in the midline. In and of itself, it generally is benign, but it can grow quite large and produce pathology due to impingement on other structures.

Li-Fraumeni syndrome is a familial cancer syndrome that leads to an increased risk of gliomas, ependymomas, and choroid plexus carcinomas.

Turcot syndrome has an increased risk of glioblastoma multiforme and medulloblastoma.

Nevoid basal cell carcinoma syndrome (a.k.a. Gorlin syndrome) is associated with medulloblastomas.

von Hippel-Lindau disease increases the risk of hemangioblastomas in the cerebellum, medulla, and spinal cord.

Animal studies report that *N*-nitroso compounds, including nitrosamines, increase the risk of brain tumors. Pesticides and insecticides also have been implicated. Ionizing radiation is a known risk factor. Prenatal exposure to electromagnetic fields (e.g., electric blankets) and exposure to high-tension power lines also have been implicated.

CLINICAL PRESENTATION

Overview

See Figure 25-1 for common brain tumor locations.

Children with brain tumors can vary in their presentation. Many demonstrate signs and symptoms of increased intracranial pressure, including headache (especially morning), vomiting, and irritability. Diplopia, due to 6th nerve palsy, is also a fairly common sign. Other symptoms include changes in academic performance, fatigue, and personality changes. The "classic" brain tumor headache is a complaint of pain on awakening, which is relieved by vomiting, then lessens during the day. Frequently, though, these classic symptoms do not appear for several months. Signs and symptoms of increased intracranial pressure are a neurosurgical emergency.

Infants pose a specific problem in diagnosis because they obviously do not "complain" of headache and present nonspecific symptoms that can be confused with a common viral illness. Irritability, anorexia, and vomiting

are common symptoms. However, remember: The infant's cranial sutures are not fused, so a helpful diagnostic tool in an infant with these symptoms is to check head circumference or look for a bulging fontanelle.

Developmental delay and motor abnormalities are common in infants with brain tumors. Loss of developmental milestones is a worrisome feature. Impairment of upgaze and downward deviation of the eyes ("sun-setting") can be early signs of increased intracranial pressure.

Infratentorial Lesion Presentations

Infratentorial lesions (generally of the cerebellum and below) arise in the posterior fossa and often cause problems with coordination and cranial nerve dysfunction. Tumors of the 4th ventricle present with signs of increased intracranial pressure, with or without brainstem dysfunction. Cerebellar hemisphere tumors usually present initially with lateralizing signs, such as limb dysmetria (an aspect of ataxia, with impaired ability to control the distance, power, and speed of an act), rather than increased intracranial pressure. Seizures are uncommon with posterior fossa tumors. The inability to move both eyes conjugately or to adduct an eye on attempted lateral gaze implies brainstem pathology.

Supratentorial Lesion Presentations

Supratentorial lesions (in brain structures above the cerebellum) commonly present with headaches, weakness, and seizures. Temporal lobe lesions result in seizures with alterations in sensorium, with or without motor signs. Tumors of the supplementary motor regions can result in seizures presenting as twisting movements, posturing of the limbs, and forced tonic movements of the eyes and head. Some lesions produce generalized seizures without focality. EEG can be helpful, but a normal EEG does not rule out a brain tumor.

Tumors of the "silent area" of the cerebral cortex (the frontal and parietal lobes) rarely cause any symptoms, unless significant growth results in mass effect.

A large number of childhood tumors arise in the midline 3rd ventricle and suprasellar regions and can result in compression of visual pathway structures. It is important to attempt to elicit visual field deficits.

Parinaud syndrome is a triad of impaired upward gaze, dilated pupils with better reactivity to accommodation than to light, and retraction or conversion nystagmus with lid retraction. It is caused by compression or infiltration of the midbrain tectum, particularly with pineal tumors.

Leptomeningeal Tumor Presentations

Dissemination to the leptomeninges occurs in ~ 15% of childhood CNS tumors. Symptoms include intermittent

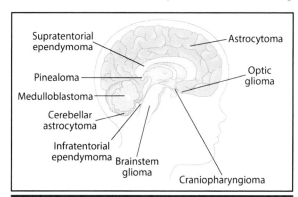

Figure 25-1: Common Brain Tumor Locations

Supratentorial ependymoma
Astrocytoma
Pinealoma
Optic glioma
Medulloblastoma
Cerebellar astrocytoma
Infratentorial ependymoma
Brainstem glioma
Craniopharyngioma

mental status changes; neck, back, or radicular pain; weakness; and bowel and/or bladder dysfunction.

DIAGNOSIS

When available, MRI has replaced CT scan as the modality of choice for diagnosis of brain tumors. Generally, biopsy is required for histologic confirmation and to determine therapy. This is usually done with tumor resection surgery; however, in instances where the tumor cannot be safely removed, stereotactic biopsy may be performed. For gliomas and germ cell tumors, the removed tissue sometimes does not correspond to the most pathologic part of the tumor and can result in a high-grade astrocytoma (worse pathology) misdiagnosed as a low-grade astrocytoma (better pathology). Tumors that cannot be safely biopsied are treated empirically based on the most likely diagnosis, given the location.

TREATMENT

Surgery

Surgical resection is the mainstay of therapy for most tumors of the CNS. If complete resection with negative margins is not possible for a malignant tumor, then a 99% reduction in tumor burden is the goal to increase the effectiveness of radiation and chemotherapy. Preoperative corticosteroids reduce both intracranial pressure and tumor edema; these are tapered slowly after surgery.

Radiation Therapy

Radiation therapy is used to treat most malignant brain tumors and some benign brain tumors. One challenge remains—delivering the maximal effective dose while sparing as much normal brain tissue as possible. Several techniques, such as proton beam radiation, provide a more focused beam with less scatter and are being increasingly used in children. Due to the significant acute and long-term toxicity, radiation therapy is usually avoided in children < 3 years of age. Chemotherapy is often used to delay the use of radiation therapy until patients are older.

Chemotherapy

Pediatric oncologists increasingly use chemotherapy to treat childhood brain tumors. It is standard to use chemotherapy for medulloblastoma and high-grade astrocytoma outside of the brainstem. Agents must cross the blood-brain barrier; commonly used drugs include vincristine, cisplatin, etoposide, and cyclophosphamide. See Table 25-2 starting on page 25-4 for chemotherapy agents and side effects.

PRIMITIVE NEUROECTODERMAL TUMORS

Occurrence

Primitive neuroectodermal tumors (medulloblastomas, pineoblastomas, and central neuroblastomas) occur anywhere in the CNS but are most commonly seen in the posterior fossa, in which case they are known as medulloblastomas. If the primitive neuroectodermal tumors occur in the pineal gland, they are called pineoblastomas. In the cerebral cortex, they are known as central neuroblastomas or supratentorial primitive neuroectodermal tumors. The medulloblastomas have the best prognosis of these 3 tumors.

Medulloblastomas

Primitive neuroectodermal tumors are the most common type of malignant CNS tumor in childhood, and medulloblastomas account for most of these. Medulloblastomas make up ~ 33% of all infratentorial tumors in children. Hydrocephalus is present in ~ 75% of patients at the time of diagnosis. Children with medulloblastoma typically present with morning headache, vomiting, and lethargy. Ataxia is common and involves the trunk or limbs. Most patients are symptomatic for < 3 months before the diagnosis is made. Head-tilt can occur due to 4th cranial nerve dysfunction or impending cerebellar herniation.

Surgical resection at diagnosis often results in all or most of the tumor being removed unless it has infiltrated the 4th ventricle or a cerebellar peduncle, which makes complete resection difficult. Use postoperative gadolinium-enhanced MRI to assess for leptomeningeal involvement and lumbar puncture to look for tumor cells.

Radiation after surgery is a mainstay. Chemotherapy is also frequently used in those with high-risk disease. Prognosis is poor in those with younger age, disseminated disease, brainstem infiltration, larger tumor sizes, and certain histologic and cytogenetic tumor features. For infants who cannot tolerate radiation therapy, high-dose chemotherapy with autologous stem cell support is an alternative in the highest-risk patients.

The other types of primitive neuroectodermal tumors (i.e., pineoblastomas and central neuroblastomas) are much rarer than medulloblastomas. These tumors, especially those of the pineal area, are usually disseminated at the time of diagnosis; survival rates are worse with this lesion than with cerebellar lesions. Cerebral lesions are less likely to disseminate.

EPENDYMOMA

Ependymomas arise from the ependymal lining of the ventricular system: ~ 75% occur in the posterior fossa, with the remainder occurring in supratentorial areas. Ependymomas make up 8–10% of all primary childhood brain tumors and account for 10–15% of the posterior fossa tumors.

Drug	Action	Side Effects	Diseases Treated
Table 25-2: Common Chemotherapeutic Agents			
ANTIMETABOLITES			
Methotrexate	Folic acid antagonist	— Myelosuppression — Renal and hepatic toxicity	ALL Non-Hodgkin lymphoma Osteosarcoma Brain tumors
6-Mercaptopurine (6-MP)	Inhibits purine synthesis	Myelosuppression Hepatotoxicity	ALL
Cytosine arabinoside (ara-C)	Inhibits DNA polymerase	Myelosuppression — Fever Systemic inflammation	ALL AML Hodgkin lymphoma Non-Hodgkin lymphoma
ALKYLATING AGENTS			
Cyclophosphamide	Inhibits DNA synthesis	— Hemorrhagic cystitis Secondary leukemias (e.g., AML) Increased infertility with high doses	ALL Hodgkin lymphoma Non-Hodgkin lymphoma Neuroblastoma Wilms tumor Rhabdomyosarcoma Ewing sarcoma Brain tumors Germ cell tumors
ANTIBIOTICS			
Doxorubicin	Binds to DNA	Cardiomyopathy	ALL Hodgkin lymphoma Non-Hodgkin lymphoma Neuroblastoma Wilms tumor Rhabdomyosarcoma Osteosarcoma Ewing sarcoma Germ cell tumors Hepatoblastoma
Daunorubicin	Binds to DNA	Cardiomyopathy	ALL AML
Bleomycin	Binds to DNA	Pulmonary fibrosis	Hodgkin lymphoma Germ cell tumors
VINCA ALKALOIDS			
Vincristine	Inhibits microtubule formation	— Peripheral neuropathy	ALL Hodgkin lymphoma Non-Hodgkin lymphoma Neuroblastoma Wilms tumor Rhabdomyosarcoma Ewing sarcoma Brain tumors Hepatoblastoma
Vinblastine	Inhibits microtubule formation	Leukopenia	Hodgkin lymphoma

Table 25-2: Common Chemotherapeutic Agents (Continued)			
Drug	**Action**	**Side Effects**	**Diseases Treated**
ENZYMES			
L-asparaginase	Depletes L-asparagine	Pancreatitis Increased glucose Thrombosis	ALL AML
STEROIDS			
Prednisone/Dexamethasone	Unknown	Cushing syndrome Cataracts Diabetes mellitus Hypertension Osteonecrosis	ALL Hodgkin lymphoma Non-Hodgkin lymphoma Hemophagocytic lymphohistiocytosis
OTHER			
Cisplatin	Inhibits DNA synthesis	Nephrotoxicity Ototoxicity Neurotoxicity	Hodgkin lymphoma Neuroblastoma Osteosarcoma Brain tumors Germ cell tumors Hepatoblastoma

Etoposide (VP-16)	Topoisomerase inhibitor	Secondary leukemias
		  (e.g., AML)
			ALL
			AML
			Hodgkin lymphoma
			Non-Hodgkin lymphoma
			Neuroblastoma
			Wilms tumor
			Rhabdomyosarcoma
			Osteosarcoma
			Ewing sarcoma
			Brain tumors
			Germ cell tumors
			Hemophagocytic
			  lymphohistiocytosis

Symptoms depend on where the tumor occurs. If the tumor is in the 4th ventricle, cerebral spinal fluid (CSF) flow is blocked, with accompanying symptoms of nausea, vomiting, and morning headache. Diplopia typically occurs. Most patients have symptoms for 6–9 months before diagnosis. Tumors of the brainstem have more focal deficits and are diagnosed earlier.

MRI is the diagnostic tool of choice. Hydrocephalus is almost always present.

Surgery is the mainstay of therapy, and ease of resection determines chance of cure. Postoperative radiation therapy seems to increase overall survival. Chemotherapy is not beneficial.

GLIOMA

Overview

Gliomas, which can arise anywhere in the CNS, make up 50–60% of brain tumors in children and are the most common primary childhood CNS tumors. These tumors can be astrocytomas or gliomas. Prognosis for gliomas depends on the location and histologic grade.

Cerebellar Astrocytoma

Cerebellar astrocytomas make up 12% of all brain tumors in children and are the most common posterior fossa tumors of childhood. They also have one of the best prognoses (> 90% have 5-year survival). They peak in the 2nd decade. Most occur in the cerebellar hemisphere, but they occasionally involve the vermis.

The most common type is known as the pilocytic juvenile cerebellar astrocytoma.

Symptoms with lateral cerebellar astrocytomas include clumsiness and unsteadiness of the arms and legs. Headaches and vomiting also occur. Diagnose with MRI or CT.

Treatment strategies include surgery, radiation, and chemotherapy. In children with complete resection of the tumor, radiation and chemotherapy may not be required.

Brainstem Glioma

Brainstem gliomas make up 10–20% of CNS tumors in children < 15 years of age. Peak incidence is between 5 and 8 years of age. Diffuse, infiltrating lesions have the

ONCOLOGY

poorest prognosis, and most children die within 2 years of diagnosis. MRI is the best imaging modality and is used to determine the diagnosis without biopsy due to the substantial risk of surgery in this area. Treatment can involve radiation and/or chemotherapy, and outcomes remain very poor.

Diencephalic Glioma

Gliomas of the visual pathway and diencephalon make up 5% of all childhood brain tumors. Most of these tumors that involve the optic nerve occur within the 1st decade. The chiasmal tumors commonly occur in infants or in the 2nd decade. Neurofibromatosis Type 1 is found in ~ 70% of patients with optic pathway tumors. Surgery is generally delayed as long as possible because of the risk of destroying the remaining sight. Radiation is generally the therapy of choice. Chemotherapy may be of benefit in children < 5 years of age with progressive chiasmatic lesions.

High-Grade Astrocytoma

Astrocytomas account for 40% of all childhood brain tumors, and 25% of these are aggressive or high-grade. These tumors have an increased potential for malignancy. Glioblastoma multiforme is the most aggressive of these tumors.

Headache is the earliest and most common symptom. Vomiting, seizures, motor symptoms, and behavioral abnormalities are next most common.

MRI is best for diagnosis.

Treat surgically, but note: High-grade astrocytomas generally infiltrate the brain and cannot be completely excised. Radiation therapy may improve survival. Recently, high-dose chemotherapy and autologous, peripheral blood stem cell rescue have shown promise in adult and pediatric studies, but outcomes remain poor.

GERM CELL TUMORS

Germ cell tumors make up 50% of pineal tumors and 5–10% of parasellar tumors. Germinomas make up ~ 65% of germ cell tumors.

Pineal tumors can present with **Parinaud syndrome**: a triad of impaired upward gaze, dilated pupils with better reactivity to accommodation than to light, and retraction or conversion nystagmus with lid retraction. Suprasellar germinomas produce pituitary and hypothalamic dysfunction, such as growth hormone failure and diabetes insipidus. Teratomas also occur and frequently show calcium deposits.

 Alpha-fetoprotein (AFP) and beta human chorionic gonadotropin (β-hCG) are secreted by mixed germ cell tumors—but not by other pineal tumors.

Surgical resection is difficult because most are in the pineal region. Radiotherapy is the primary mode of therapy, but chemotherapy also is effective for many tumors.

CRANIOPHARYNGIOMA

Craniopharyngiomas are benign tumors that are derived from squamous epithelial cells and arise in the suprasellar region. They make up ~ 10% of all childhood brain tumors. Although benign, they are locally invasive and can affect many structures, including the optic chiasm, carotid arteries, 3rd cranial nerve, and pituitary stalk.

Headaches and vomiting are typical presenting symptoms. > 50% of children with craniopharyngioma have visual changes due to optic involvement. Because of pituitary involvement, endocrinologic signs (such as growth failure, short stature, and polydipsia) often accompany these tumors. Changes in personality or sleep patterns are also common presenting signs.

Diagnostic imaging with CT or MRI identifies the lesion. Calcifications in the suprasellar region are present in most cases. Surgery is recommended for many craniopharyngiomas, but location is frequently a problem. Radiation is usually required. Diabetes insipidus is a common complication of surgery.

CHOROID PLEXUS TUMORS

Choroid plexus tumors are rare. The choroid plexus papilloma is benign and accounts for 66% of such tumors. The tumors can occur in the first few days of life; ~ 80% appear before the 2nd birthday. Most present with signs and symptoms of hydrocephalus because of excess CSF production or because the tumor obstructs CSF flow. Treat with surgical resection.

MENINGIOMA

Meningiomas are rare in children except in those with neurofibromatosis Type 2—in which they can occur as early as 1 year of age. Meningiomas also occur in long-term survivors of other brain tumors who have received radiation therapy.

Treatment is surgical resection. Meningiomas are almost always benign.

NEUROBLASTOMA

PREVIEW | REVIEW

- What is the most common malignancy diagnosed in infancy?
- From where do most neuroblastomas arise?
- What symptoms does VIP cause in neuroblastoma?
- How do you diagnose neuroblastoma?

- At what age of diagnosis do children have the best prognosis in neuroblastoma?
- What is the treatment for the different neuroblastoma risk groups (low, intermediate, and high risk)?

OCCURRENCE

Neuroblastoma makes up 8–10% of all childhood cancers and is the most common malignancy diagnosed during infancy. It is slightly more common in boys than girls. The median age of diagnosis is 22 months, and 97% of such cancers are diagnosed before 10 years of age.

PATHOLOGY

Neuroblastoma is one of the small, round, blue-cell tumors of childhood. The malignant cells derive from neuroblasts of the postganglionic sympathetic nervous system. The amount of neural differentiation varies; therefore, the cells can form ganglioneuromas, ganglioneuroblastomas, and/or neuroblastomas. Molecular and genetic factors that influence diagnosis and prognosis include amplification of the *MYCN* oncogene, tumor cell DNA content (ploidy), and structural genetic changes.

CLINICAL PRESENTATION

40% of neuroblastomas arise in the abdomen within the adrenal medulla and 30% originate in the nonadrenal abdomen, including paravertebral ganglia, pelvic ganglia, and the organ of Zuckerkandl (a small mass of chromaffin cells located along the aorta). About 20% occur in the paravertebral ganglia of the chest or neck. The most common presentation of neuroblastoma is a nontender abdominal mass—typically retroperitoneal. Neuroblastoma in the high thoracic and cervical area can cause Horner syndrome (unilateral ptosis, miosis, and anhydrosis). Involvement of the spinal canal can occur with resulting paralysis or loss of bowel/bladder function in the lower lumbar region.

Most neuroblastomas have metastasized before diagnosis. Metastases can go to distant lymph nodes, bone, bone marrow, liver, and skin (which manifests as subcutaneous bluish nodules). In infants < 1 year of age, it is characteristic to have a small primary tumor with dissemination limited to the liver and skin. This generally has a good prognosis and is referred to as Stage 4S. For children > 1 year of age with metastatic disease, the prognosis is quite poor. Periorbital ecchymosis (raccoon eyes) due to orbital metastases must be distinguished from trauma/child abuse.

Paraneoplastic syndromes can occur but are not that common. Look for intractable secretory diarrhea and abdominal distention due to secretion of vasoactive intestinal peptide (VIP). The **VIP syndrome** occurs with ganglioneuroblastoma or ganglioneuroma and resolves with removal of the tumor.

Opsoclonus-myoclonus-ataxia syndrome (dancing eyes–dancing feet syndrome) occurs in about 5% of newly diagnosed neuroblastoma patients. Rapid and chaotic eye movements, ataxia, and myoclonus characterize it. As a presenting symptom, it warrants a workup for neuroblastoma. These symptoms can resolve with removal of the tumor, but up to 80% of children can have long-term neurologic deficits.

DIAGNOSIS

Diagnosis requires biopsy with histologic evidence of neural origin of the tumor or, in the case of bone marrow diagnosis, compatible "clumps" of cells.

Because neuroblastomas are derived from neural crest cells, they take up and metabolize catecholamines. An increased level of catecholamine metabolites in the urine (homovanillic acid [HVA] and vanillylmandelic acid [VMA]) is often found at diagnosis. Urinary catecholamine excretion in neuroblastoma is useful both in diagnosis and for tumor screening and off-therapy follow-up.

In the workup of neuroblastoma, the following tests are usually done: bilateral bone marrow aspirate and biopsy, plain radiographs, bone scintigraphy, CT, and MRI. Metaiodobenzylguanidine (MIBG) scintigraphy for evaluation of bone and soft tissue involvement is also standard for staging because the majority of neuroblastomas take up the radionuclide.

PROGNOSTIC INDICATORS

Prognosis is determined by multiple clinical and biologic factors.

Better prognosis:

- Child's age at diagnosis—Best prognosis is for < 18 months of age.
- Ploidy of the tumor—Hyperdiploidy confers better outcome in patients < 18 months of age.
- Favorable histology.

Poorer prognosis:

- Extent of tumor—Patients with metastatic disease do very poorly.
- Unfavorable histology.
- *MYCN* oncogene copy number—Increasing number of copies correlates with poorer prognosis.
- Chromosome 1p deletion—Deletion is a poor prognostic sign.

TREATMENT

Overall, therapy is based on risk-group stratification established by the International Neuroblastoma Staging System (INSS). Risk groups are based on a combination of stage and biologic features. The lowest-risk groups are treated with surgery alone. Intermediate-risk groups receive surgery and chemotherapy. Treatment of

ONCOLOGY

high-risk disease includes surgery, standard chemotherapy, high-dose chemotherapy with autologous stem cell rescue, radiation, cis-retinoic acid, and immune-modulating therapy. Even with aggressive therapy, outcomes in high-risk children are poor.

Drugs used in the treatment of neuroblastoma include cyclophosphamide, ifosfamide, cisplatin, carboplatin, doxorubicin, and etoposide.

LYMPHOMA

See Hematology, Book 5, for discussion of lymphoma.

KIDNEY NEOPLASMS

PREVIEW | REVIEW

- What is the most common primary malignancy of the kidney in childhood?
- What congenital disorders and syndromes are associated with Wilms tumor?
- List the conditions in WAGR syndrome.
- What is the most common presentation for Wilms tumor?
- What is the mainstay of therapy for unilateral Wilms tumor?
- True or false? Most unilateral Wilms tumor patients receive chemotherapy.

WILMS TUMOR

Overview

Wilms tumor (nephroblastoma) is the most common primary malignant tumor of the kidney in childhood. It occurs about equally in boys and girls, with no racial differences noted. The mean age of diagnosis is 42–47 months for unilateral tumors and 30–33 months for bilateral tumors.

An important feature to remember is the association of Wilms tumor with other congenital anomalies and syndromes in up to 7% of patients.

Wilms-associated disorders:

- GU anomalies (4.4%, including cryptorchidism and hypospadias)
- Hemihyperplasia (a.k.a. hemihypertrophy; 3%)
- Sporadic aniridia (1%)

Wilms-associated syndromes:

- **WAGR** syndrome:
  - **W**ilms tumor
  - **A**niridia
  - **G**U abnormalities
  - Intellectual disability (mental retardation)
- Beckwith-Wiedemann syndrome (BWS):
  - Organomegaly
  - Macroglossia
  - Omphalocele
  - Hemihyperplasia
  - Wilms tumor
- Denys-Drash syndrome:
  - Wilms tumor
  - Nephropathy
  - Male undervirilization

Infants with BWS or hemihyperplasia are at risk for developing Wilms tumor and other embryonal tumors such as hepatoblastoma. Screening guidelines for Wilms tumor are available.

Wilms tumor can be characterized by a number of genetic factors. The Wilms tumor suppression gene (*WT1*) at chromosome 11p13 and another gene at 11p15.5 have been implicated. Also, familial Wilms tumor genes have been noted.

Pathology and Staging

Classically, Wilms tumor is a solitary growth that can occur in any part of either kidney. It is well demarcated and compresses the normal kidney parenchyma. The tumor usually is triphasic—made up of epithelial, blastemal, and stromal elements—which is favorable histology. Poor histology, or anaplasia, is found in only 10% of cases but accounts for 60% of deaths.

Stage 1 tumors are limited to a single kidney and can be completely excised. Stage 2 disease extends beyond the kidney but can still be completely excised. Patients with Stage 3 disease have residual tumor confined to the abdomen, and patients with Stage 4 disease have hematogenous spread, most frequently to the lung. Stage 5 disease indicates bilateral kidney involvement and occurs in only 5–10% of cases.

Histologic subtype remains the most powerful prognostic factor. Children with favorable histology tumors have better than 90% survival at 2 years regardless of stage. Anaplasia is a predictor of poor outcomes.

Clinical Presentation

The median age of diagnosis of Wilms tumor is about 3 years of age, with the most common sign being an asymptomatic abdominal or flank mass. Only about 50% of patients have nausea, vomiting, or abdominal pain. Many masses are found incidentally on physical examination or by the parents while bathing the child or changing a diaper. Gross hematuria occurs in a small percentage. Also, remember to look for the common associated syndromes and anomalies: aniridia, hemihyperplasia, and genitourinary (GU) abnormalities. Hypertension occurs in about 25% of patients and is due to renal ischemia from tumor impingement of the renal artery. Evaluation includes CXR, CT scan of the abdomen and chest, ultrasound, and echocardiogram.

Treatment

For unilateral disease, nephrectomy with removal of the primary tumor is the mainstay of therapy. Assessment of tumor spread at the time of surgery is important. Most patients then receive postsurgical chemotherapy.

Presurgical chemotherapy is indicated if:

- there is extensive tumor thrombus to the intrahepatic vena cava or
- there is thrombus more proximally to the right atrium or
- the primary tumor is deemed unresectable without significant surgical morbidity.

In bilateral disease (Stage 5), a renal biopsy of each kidney determines the histologic stage and appropriate chemotherapy; and, typically, bilateral parenchymal-sparing resection is performed.

The chemotherapy regimen is routinely based on staging and histologic type. Patients with Stage 1 or 2 favorable histology tumors get vincristine and actinomycin D for 18 weeks; those with Stage 3 or 4 receive combination vincristine, actinomycin D, and doxorubicin for 24 weeks.

Abdominal radiation therapy is not necessary for those with Stage 1 or 2 favorable histology disease. It is useful in Stage 3 and 4 disease. Whole-lung irradiation is a possibility for those with pulmonary metastatic lesions seen on imaging studies.

OTHER KIDNEY NEOPLASMS

Nephroblastomatosis is a term signifying diffuse nephrogenic rests (precursor lesions to Wilms tumor) throughout one or both kidneys. These occur in all bilateral and about 1/3 of unilateral Wilms tumors. The presence of nephroblastomatosis in one kidney leads to careful examination of the other kidney. Careful follow-up with ultrasound or MRI is necessary over time to look for evolution into Wilms tumor.

Mesoblastic nephroma is the most common congenital renal disorder, presenting as a firm, solitary mass of the kidney. It looks like a leiomyoma, is a benign tumor, and resection is curative.

Renal cell carcinoma is very rare in children but occasionally occurs in adolescence. It presents with abdominal pain and hematuria. Complete resection can be curative, but those with residual disease or metastases have a poor prognosis because it does not respond well to therapy.

SOFT TISSUE TUMORS

PREVIEW | REVIEW

- What is the most common soft tissue tumor in childhood?
- What tissue/cell type is affected by rhabdomyosarcoma?
- Which sites are common for the botryoid subtype?
- How does rhabdomyosarcoma present?
- What is the treatment for rhabdomyosarcoma?

RHABDOMYOSARCOMA

Occurrence

Rhabdomyosarcoma is the most common soft tissue tumor of childhood and makes up about 5% of all childhood cancers. Almost 2/3 of cases are diagnosed in children 6 years of age and younger. Although the majority of cases are sporadic, rhabdomyosarcoma can occur with Li-Fraumeni syndrome. Patients with Li-Fraumeni syndrome have a germ line mutation in the *p53* gene and are at risk for soft tissue tumors, adrenocortical carcinoma, and early-onset breast cancer.

Pathology

Rhabdomyosarcoma arises from the same embryonic mesenchyme as striated skeletal muscle.

There are 2 main histologic types:

1) **Embryonal**, found in 60–70% of cases, has a more favorable prognosis. 2 subtypes of embryonal are **botryoid**, which has projections similar to a cluster of grapes (seen most commonly in the vagina, bladder, nasopharynx, and middle ear), and **spindle cell**, which usually presents with limited disease. Both subtypes have an excellent prognosis.

2) **Alveolar**, found in 20–30% of cases, occurs more commonly in the trunk and extremities and has the worst prognosis.

Clinical Presentation

The most common presentation is a mass lesion. The head and neck are the most common sites, and this includes the orbit and parameningeal sites such as the nasopharynx. The next most common site is the GU tract, followed by extremity and truncal tumors. Tumors of the orbits can cause proptosis and ophthalmoplegia. GU tumors present with a pelvic mass causing urinary frequency, urinary obstruction, or constipation. Vaginal bleeding can lead to suspicion of child abuse. In female infants, there can be a protruding polypoid vaginal mass (**sarcoma botryoides**).

Osteosarcoma occurs at a higher rate in people with the following conditions:

- Hereditary retinoblastoma
- Li-Fraumeni syndrome
- Rothmund-Thomson syndrome (i.e., short stature, skin telangiectasias, small hands/feet, hypoplastic or absent thumbs)
- Radiation therapy for Ewing sarcoma or other malignancies

Benign conditions with malignant transformation to osteosarcoma include:

- Paget disease
- Endochondromatosis
- Multiple hereditary exostoses

Pathology

There are 4 pathologic subtypes of osteosarcoma:

1) Osteoblastic (~ 50% of cases)
2) Fibroblastic (~ 22% of cases)
3) Chondroblastic (~ 25% of cases)
4) Telangiectatic (~ 3% of cases)

All show highly malignant and pleomorphic spindle cells in biopsy. Osteosarcoma usually occurs in the metaphyseal region of long bones and invades the medullary cavity; the diaphyseal region is involved in < 10% of cases. These 4 subtypes have no prognostic differences.

Clinical Presentation

Unilateral pain and swelling are the most common presenting findings. The most commonly affected joint is the knee, followed by the shoulder. Frequently, the adolescent thinks this is a sports injury or sprain. Investigate any pain not responding to conservative therapy in a reasonable amount of time. Routine lab work is usually not helpful and is typically normal, although LDH or alkaline phosphatase can be elevated.

Clues:

- Deep bone pain.
- Nighttime awakening.
- Palpable mass.
- X-ray showing a periosteal reaction (sunburst pattern is classic but is neither common nor specific).
- Codman triangle can also be seen on x-ray. It is a reaction seen at the junction of the mass and periosteum caused by the ossification of only the edge of the raised periosteum.

Diagnosis

Biopsy must be performed on any lesion suspected of being a bone tumor. MRI of the lesion and entire bone is done before surgery to evaluate the tumor for its proximity to nerves and blood vessels and to look for skip lesions (i.e., lesions in the bone that are not physically connected).

The most common site for metastasis is the lungs. Therefore, before biopsy, a CT of the chest and a radionuclide bone scan are performed to assess stage of disease. Biopsy should be done by an experienced orthopedic oncologist.

Treatment

With chemotherapy and surgery, the 5-year survival rate in patients with nonmetastatic osteosarcoma is 65–75%. Preoperative chemotherapy is standard, followed by limb salvage operations, when feasible, and further chemotherapy postsurgery. The degree of tumor necrosis at the time of resection is prognostically significant. Chemotherapeutic agents include doxorubicin, cisplatin, and methotrexate. Patients with distant bone metastases and widespread lung metastases have a poor prognosis.

EWING SARCOMA

Pathology

Ewing sarcoma is an undifferentiated sarcoma of bone but can also arise from soft tissue. It is in a group of small, round-cell, undifferentiated tumors of neural crest origin. A majority of patients have a t(11;22) translocation, whereas the rest have a t(21;22).

Clinical Presentation

Clinically, these patients present with pain and swelling, similarly to those with osteosarcoma. Children with Ewing sarcoma are more likely to have systemic findings such as fever and weight loss, and they can be misdiagnosed as having osteomyelitis. Flat bones (e.g. ribs, pelvis) and the diaphyses of the long bones are more commonly affected, as compared to the metaphyseal involvement in osteosarcoma. Paraspinal and vertebral primary tumors are also more common with Ewing's.

Suspect Ewing sarcoma in a patient with pain, swelling, and fever, with an x-ray showing a primary lytic lesion with a lamellated or "onion skin" periosteal reaction (Image 25-2).

Diagnosis

Full workup includes CT of the chest, bone scan, and bone marrow aspirate/biopsy from at least 2 sites. Preoperative MRI is done of the tumor and the entire bone to assess the extent of the lesion. Confirm the diagnosis with a tissue biopsy.

Treatment

Chemotherapy is usually given 1st and includes vincristine, doxorubicin, cyclophosphamide, ifosfamide, and etoposide. Pain relief occurs rapidly with chemotherapy.

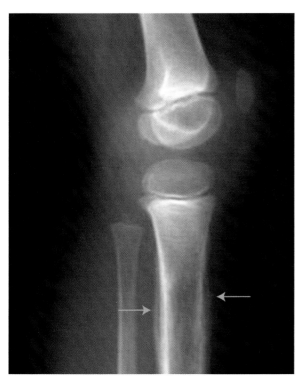

Image 25-2: Ewing sarcoma with "onion skin" periosteal reaction

Local control is accomplished by either complete surgical resection or radiation therapy.

Prognosis is excellent (> 75% cure rate) in those with small, nonmetastatic, distally located extremity tumors. Those with bulky pelvic tumors, metastatic disease at diagnosis, and bone marrow involvement have a poorer prognosis.

OSTEOCHONDROMA

Osteochondroma is a very common benign bone tumor in children. Many cases are asymptomatic and never recognized. Most occur in the metaphysis of long bones, particularly the distal femur, proximal humerus, and proximal tibia. The lesion continues to grow until skeletal maturity.

Most are discovered between 5 and 15 years of age as a bony, nonpainful mass. On x-ray, they appear as stalks or broad-based projections from the surface of the bone. Usually, there is a cartilage "cap," which can be as thick as 1 cm. Transformation to a malignant chondrosarcoma is very rare in children but occurs in about 1% of adults. Typically, they are left alone unless the lesion is large enough to cause symptoms, in which case the lesion is excised.

ENCHONDROMA

Enchondroma is a benign solitary lesion of hyaline cartilage that occurs centrally in the bone. The hands are typically affected. Most patients can just be observed. Enchondroma is listed sometimes as a distractor on

exams, so be aware of it, but realize it is unlikely to be the correct answer.

Ollier disease is a disorder with multiple enchondromas in various locations and results in short stature, limb length inequality, and joint deformity. Malignant transformation is common.

Maffucci syndrome manifests as multiple enchondromas with angiomas of the soft tissue. Malignant transformation is common.

CHONDROBLASTOMA

Chondroblastoma is a rare, benign cartilage-forming lesion of the epiphysis of long bones. Patients present in their early 20s with complaints of mild-to-moderate pain in the hip, shoulder, or knee. Chondroblastomas can be cured if treated with curettage and bone grafting before joint destruction occurs. This is also sometimes listed as a distractor in exam questions.

OSTEOID OSTEOMA

Osteoid osteomas are benign tumors that usually occur in males between 5 and 20 years of age. Clinically, there is a characteristic unremitting and worsening pain (worse at night) that, in contrast to osteosarcoma, is relieved with aspirin or other NSAIDs. The most common bones involved are the proximal femur and tibia. Palpation and range of motion do not worsen the pain. X-rays show a round or oval metaphyseal or diaphyseal lucency surrounded by sclerotic bone. About 25% cannot be seen on plain radiograph but can be seen on CT scan. Treatment is with surgical excision.

OSTEOBLASTOMA

Osteoblastoma is a benign bone-forming tumor that causes local destruction of bone and grows over time. It most commonly affects the vertebrae. Dull, aching pain for months is the usual presenting complaint. Treatment is removal of affected bone and, if necessary, grafting and spinal stabilization.

NASOPHARYNGEAL CARCINOMA

PREVIEW | REVIEW

- What virus increases the risk of nasopharyngeal carcinoma?

Nasopharyngeal carcinomas are rare, making up < 1% of childhood malignancies. More cases are seen in China and occur with Epstein-Barr virus (EBV) infection and prior radiation exposure. Children with nasopharyngeal carcinoma present with paraneoplastic syndromes, including clubbing, fever of unknown origin, and syndrome of inappropriate antidiuretic

ONCOLOGY

hormone secretion (SIADH). Surgery is necessary for staging and diagnosis. Most tumors respond to radiation therapy, and chemotherapy can be beneficial; however, prognosis depends upon whether the tumor has spread to the cervical lymph nodes or beyond.

THYROID CANCER

Consider thyroid cancer in any child with a solitary thyroid nodule. A solitary mass is much more likely to be cancer in children and adolescents than it is in adults. See Endocrinology, Book 3, for more on thyroid cancer.

GONADAL NEOPLASMS

PREVIEW | REVIEW

- True or false? Few gonadal malignancies are germ cell tumors in pediatrics.
- Where are most teratomas located?
- Which patient with a teratoma is particularly predisposed to undergo malignant transformation (i.e., what age and what location)?
- Which germ cell tumors have elevated AFP and/or β-hCG tumor markers?
- What tissue is found in choriocarcinoma?
- With which karyotypes do gonadoblastomas occur?

OCCURRENCE

Almost all gonadal neoplasms are germ cell tumors. They represent 3% of all tumors in children. 2/3 of germ cell tumors in children are extragonadal. The peak ages for occurrence of these tumors are ~ 3 years of age and then again during adolescence. 1/3 of germ cell tumors in children are malignant, but these are mainly in older children and adolescents. Cryptorchidism is a risk factor for developing testicular cancer. Nearly all neonatal germ cell tumors are benign.

CLINICAL PRESENTATION

Presenting symptoms vary depending on the location of the tumor. Ovarian tumors present with a mass, abdominal pain, and distention. Ovarian torsion can occur. Testicular tumors present with a scrotal mass with or without pain.

EVALUATION

If a testicular mass is palpated, order an ultrasound to determine if the mass is solid or not. (If it is, the next step is inguinal orchiectomy.) Never perform a needle biopsy

due to the risk of seeding the biopsy tract. Evaluation of an ovarian mass begins with ultrasonography (add Doppler if ruling out torsion). A solid mass is considered to be cancer until proven otherwise. Order a CT or MRI if diagnosis is unclear from the ultrasound.

Cross-sectional imaging (CT or MRI) is used to detect metastatic disease to the lungs and retroperineum.

TERATOMA

Teratomas can be benign or malignant and represent intermixed tissues that originated from pluripotent stem cells foreign to the anatomic sites in which they occur.

Sacrococcygeal teratomas are the most common congenital germ cell tumor and can be found prenatally on ultrasound or after delivery on examination.

Histologically, teratomas can be mature (composed of well-differentiated adult-type tissues) or immature (composed of embryonic tissues). Malignant elements such as a yolk sac tumor or choriocarcinoma may be present. Teratomas most commonly occur in the sacro-coccyx, ovaries, testes, and anterior mediastinum. Classically, they have components from all 3 embryonic layers (endoderm, mesoderm, and ectoderm), but generally, tumors presenting at a site foreign to the anatomic site are considered teratomas with ≥ 1 embryonic layers. Look for teeth and hair and other "weird stuff" (abnormal tissues) on x-ray!

In an infant with sacrococcygeal teratoma, the risk of malignant transformation increases to 50% once the infant is older than 2 months of age. If malignant elements are discovered, chemotherapy is indicated.

GERMINOMA

Germinoma is a malignant germ cell tumor that can occur in the ovary (dysgerminoma) and the testes (seminoma) as well as extragonadally. The typical extragonadal presentation is intracranial and can present with hydrocephalus, headache, vomiting, or abnormal vision. It responds very well to radiation and chemotherapy. The ovarian and testicular forms respond to surgical resection and chemotherapy. Even though they are malignant, germinomas are often tumor marker negative (AFP and β-hCG).

EMBRYONAL CARCINOMA

Embryonal carcinoma is made up of primitive malignant cells and occurs most commonly in the testes of adolescents. Pure embryonal carcinomas do not typically produce AFP, but can cause an elevation in β-hCG. Surgical resection is sufficient if the disease is confined to the testicle; any tumor markers elevated at diagnosis return to normal postoperatively. Chemotherapy can be given if the tumor is outside the testes or if the tumor markers do not fall after resection.

ENDODERMAL SINUS (YOLK SAC) TUMOR

AAFP

This is the most common malignant childhood germ cell tumor. It most often occurs in the infantile testis, ovary, or sacrococcyx. AFP is a very reliable tumor marker, whereas β-hCG is absent. It can also occur in the intracranial region, and radiation and chemotherapy are required. For testicular or ovarian involvement, surgery is done 1st, followed by chemotherapy.

CHORIOCARCINOMA

β-HCG

Choriocarcinoma is a malignant tumor characterized by the finding of syncytiotrophoblast tissue. It typically occurs mixed with other germ cell tumor histologies. It most commonly occurs in the ovary, anterior mediastinum, and intracranial regions. AFP is absent, but β-hCG is a very reliable tumor marker. Therapy is the same as for endodermal sinus tumor.

GONADOBLASTOMA

Gonadoblastoma occurs in dysgenetic gonads, usually 46,XY or 46,XY/45,XO karyotypes. 80% have female phenotype. Gonadoblastoma is thought of as a carcinoma *in situ* and has low risk for metastases—except that it frequently occurs with germinoma, which commonly metastasizes. Due to the high potential risk of malignant transformation of the gonadoblastoma, the dysgenic gonads are removed.

SEX CORD TUMORS

Sex cord tumors are not germ cell tumors, but they are commonly in the differential for germ cell tumors. They are all very rare in children. These include Leydig cell tumor, Sertoli cell tumor, Sertoli-Leydig cell tumor, granulosa cell tumor (both juvenile and adult types), and mixed sex cord–stromal tumor. Leydig cell tumors produce androgens, and Sertoli cell tumors produce estrogen. Surgery is typically curative.

GI TUMORS

PREVIEW | REVIEW

- What pancreatic tumors are seen in association with autosomal dominant MEN1 syndrome?
- Which tumor is seen in Zollinger-Ellison syndrome?
- What is the cancer risk of having familial adenomatous polyposis?

SALIVARY GLAND TUMORS

Salivary gland masses are of an infectious etiology the majority of the time. The most common neoplasms are benign hemangiomas and lymphangiomas, which typically present in infancy. Hemangiomas usually involute without surgery; if not, they often respond to steroids or propranolol therapy. Lymphangiomas can be removed surgically if the facial nerve can be preserved.

There are several salivary gland tumors that are of epithelial origin, the most common being the benign mixed tumor. This occurs in adolescent girls and is curable by surgery.

Malignant tumors are very rare and include mucoepidermoid carcinoma, acinic cell carcinoma, and adenocarcinoma of the salivary gland. They are excised completely, and radiation therapy can be used if needed. Chemotherapy protocols have not been developed. Prognosis is good, but local recurrence is common.

STOMACH CARCINOMA

Stomach carcinoma is exceedingly rare in children in the U.S. Prognosis is poor, and surgery is the only curative method.

PANCREATIC TUMORS

Pancreatic tumors are rare and can be of either endocrine or nonendocrine origin. Insulinoma and gastrinoma are the most commonly seen (especially on exams) and occur with the autosomal dominant multiple endocrine neoplasia Type 1 (MEN1) syndrome. Insulinoma presents with hypoglycemia with inappropriate insulin and C-peptide levels. Gastrinoma presents with refractory gastric ulcers (Zollinger-Ellison syndrome).

Pancreatoblastomas occur only in childhood and are embryonal tumors that secrete AFP. Resection can be curative, and chemotherapy may be beneficial.

Pancreatic carcinoma of the exocrine pancreas is very rare in children.

COLONIC TUMORS

Colonic tumors are discussed in more detail in Gastroenterology, Book 2, but here are a few key points:

- Isolated colonic polyps in children are seldom premalignant.
- Familial adenomatous polyposis is an autosomal dominant disorder with a 100% risk of colon cancer. Colectomy is recommended.
- Generalized juvenile polyposis is inherited as autosomal dominant and is precancerous.
- Gardner syndrome (multiple intestinal polyps and tumors of the mandible and soft tissue/bone) and Turcot syndrome (primary brain tumor—medulloblastoma and multiple colorectal polyposis) include adenomatous polyps and therefore pose a risk of cancer as well.
- Lynch syndrome is hereditary nonpolyposis colorectal cancer. It is quite rare.

ONCOLOGY

LIVER TUMORS

PREVIEW | REVIEW

- What are the most common liver tumors in children < 3 years of age?
- What tumor marker should be checked in all children with liver tumors?
- What is the most common benign liver tumor?
- What is the most common primary malignant liver tumor?

OVERVIEW

Liver tumors are rare in children. Nearly 70% of liver tumors are malignant, and hepatoblastomas make up the majority of these in children < 3 years of age. Hepatocellular carcinoma increases in frequency in older children and adolescents. Of the benign lesions, hemangioendothelioma is the most common and occurs in children < 2 years of age.

Most liver tumors are painless. However, many can produce jaundice, weight loss, anorexia, and fever.

All children with a hepatic tumor need to have AFP checked.

Diagnosis is confirmed with biopsy unless hemangioendothelioma or cavernous hemangioma is suspected.

HEMANGIOENDOTHELIOMA

Hemangioendothelioma is the most common benign tumor of the liver in childhood. Biopsy is not indicated. Solitary lesions can be resected if necessary. If the lesion is unresectable or a consumption coagulopathy is present, treat with corticosteroids or propranolol; if there is no response, use vincristine. If the patient is without symptoms, no therapy is necessary because these lesions eventually regress.

Other benign tumors include mesenchymal hamartoma, focal nodular hyperplasia, and liver cell adenoma. These can all be surgically resected. Remember that a solitary adenoma is occasionally seen in adolescent females on oral contraceptives.

HEPATOBLASTOMA

Hepatoblastoma is the most common primary malignancy of the liver in childhood. It most commonly occurs in children < 3 years of age, and there is increased risk in premature infants and patients with Beckwith-Wiedemann syndrome. AFP is usually significantly elevated. It typically presents as an asymptomatic abdominal mass. Resection is recommended up front if possible. Treatment with chemotherapy as well as additional surgery and liver transplant depend on risk group. When indicated, chemotherapy includes cisplatin, fluorouracil (5-FU), and vincristine. Liver transplant is necessary if a complete resection is not possible after multiple rounds of chemotherapy.

HEPATOCELLULAR CARCINOMA

Hepatocellular carcinoma is the 2nd most common primary liver malignancy and the most common occurring in children > 3 years of age (usually adolescent age). About 1/2 of patients have elevated AFP, and 1/3 have cirrhosis. Hepatitis B or C infection is a risk factor. Surgical resection is the only curative option, but, unfortunately, only about 1/3 of these tumors are resectable. Chemotherapy is not typically beneficial for these tumors.

CLUES TO DIAGNOSIS

Clues:

- A child < 6 months of age with multiple liver lesions and a normal AFP most likely has **hemangioendothelioma**.
- A 2-year-old ex-premature infant with a liver mass and significantly elevated AFP is likely to have **hepatoblastoma**.
- An 8-year-old with a solitary mass and an elevated AFP most likely has **hepatocellular carcinoma**.
- For an adolescent female on oral contraceptives presenting with a hepatic mass, think **adenoma**.
- In children < 2 years of age with a normal AFP, **hemangioendothelioma** is the most likely diagnosis.
- Metastatic disease to the liver in children < 2 years of age is most likely a **neuroblastoma**; in older children, it can be **lymphoma**, **sarcoma**, or **Wilms tumor**.

CANCER SURVIVORSHIP

PREVIEW | REVIEW

- What are late effects of cancer radiation treatment?
- Nephrotoxicity as a late effect is common after which chemotherapy drug?

With the advances in treatment, more and more patients are surviving cancer. Long-term follow-up is important due to the late sequelae in cancer survivorship.

Late effects of radiation therapy include hormonal dysfunction and second cancers occurring in the affected field. For example, growth hormone deficiency is common after cranial radiation, and infertility is common after gonadal radiation. Cranial radiation causes an increased risk for low-grade (meningioma) and high-grade (glioblastoma) tumors.

Late effects of chemotherapy depend on the specific drugs used for treatment. Secondary acute myeloid leukemia (AML) occurs at a higher rate with etoposide or cyclophosphamide. Nephrotoxicity is common, especially after cisplatin. There is increased infertility after high doses of cyclophosphamide and other alkylators. See Table 25-2 on page 25-4.

General late effects can include increased risk of obesity, liver dysfunction, and second cancers. There is a higher risk of heart disease when anthracyclines are given in conjunction with radiation that covers the heart.

Guidelines for long-term follow-up for survivors of childhood, adolescent, and young adult cancers are available from the Children's Oncology Group.

HISTIOCYTOSIS

PREVIEW | REVIEW

- Which cells are abnormally activated in histiocytic disorders?
- What is the median age for LCH to occur?
- Which organ systems are high-risk in LCH?
- Which endocrine disease can be seen with LCH involving the pituitary gland?
- Distinguish between primary and secondary HLH.
- What are the diagnostic criteria for HLH?

NOTE

The histiocytoses are a heterogeneous group of disorders characterized by abnormal proliferation, activation, and cytokine release by cells involved in phagocytosis and antigen presentation, such as dendritic cells, monocytes, macrophages, and histiocytes.

LANGERHANS CELL HISTIOCYTOSIS

Occurrence

Langerhans cell histiocytosis (LCH) is the most common of the histiocytoses and occurs at an incidence of 4/1,000,000 per year. The median age at presentation is 2½ years, and the male-to-female ratio is close to 1.

Clinical Presentation

Gingival hypertrophy and oral ulcers are early signs of LCH. The most frequent presenting signs are skin rash in the diaper area or scalp (petechiae and brown scaly papules, which can resemble bad cradle cap) or lytic bone lesions, most commonly in the skull, that are often painful. Patients can also present with fever, weight loss, diarrhea, diabetes insipidus (from pituitary involvement), and a history of draining otitis.

Pathology

On skin biopsy, LCH lesions show a large number of pathologic Langerhans cells, which are accompanied by lymphocytes, macrophages, granulocytes, eosinophils, and multinucleated giant cells. Diagnosis is confirmed by finding CD1a or CD207 (langerin) by immunohistochemistry. Birbeck granules are seen on electron microscopy.

Patients are classified as high or low risk based on specific organs involved. High-risk sites include the liver, spleen, lungs, and bone marrow. Low-risk sites consist of skin, bones, lymph nodes, and the pituitary gland. Treatment depends on disease characteristics.

Treatment

Treatment of disease limited to the skin may include topical steroids, surgery, phototherapy, and/or systemic chemotherapy. Indications for systemic chemotherapy, such as oral methotrexate and mercaptopurine, include painful lesions, infected lesions, and other secondary complications. Single bone lesions can undergo curettage and be observed. The recommended treatment of multifocal bone disease or combinations of skin, lymph node, pituitary, and bone lesions is a combination of prednisone and vinblastine for 12 months. Low-risk patients have cure rates of > 90%, and, even if they experience a relapse, most are ultimately cured of their disease. Therapy for high-risk disease adds mercaptopurine to the prednisone/vinblastine regimen.

Patients with high-risk organ involvement can have mortality approaching 50%. The degree of response following 6 weeks of induction therapy is predictive of outcome, with rapid responders doing much better than slow responders. Advanced refractory multisystem risk disease often requires bone marrow transplantation for the best chance of long-term disease control.

HEMOPHAGOCYTIC LYMPHOHISTIOCYTOSIS

Hemophagocytic lymphohistiocytosis (HLH) is due to immune dysregulation.

Primary HLH is a rare autosomal recessive disorder that occurs at a rate of about 1/1,000,000 per year. It usually occurs before 1 year of age, and there is a strong association with consanguinity. Genetic testing is indicated. Secondary HLH occurs later, with EBV and other infections acting as a trigger. Suspect HLH in ill children with cytopenias and hepatosplenomegaly. If you do not think about it, you won't diagnose it.

Other symptoms include fever, lymphadenopathy, and rash. CNS disease presents with seizures and altered mental status. Laboratory evaluation shows pancytopenia, hyperferritinemia, hypertriglyceridemia, and hypofibrinogenemia.

Diagnosis of HLH requires at least 5 of the following criteria:

1) Fever

2) Splenomegaly

3) Peripheral blood cytopenia of ≥ 2 lineages

4) Hypertriglyceridemia and/or hypofibrinogenemia

5) Hemophagocytosis without evidence of malignancy in bone marrow, spleen, or lymph nodes

6) Elevated serum ferritin

7) Low or absent natural killer (NK) cell activity

8) Elevated soluble IL-2 receptor (soluble CD25)

Family history is also helpful in defining primary HLH. Not all patients clearly meet all criteria; however, given the rapidly progressive nature of the disease, if HLH is clinically suspected, begin therapy as soon as possible. 1st line therapy includes dexamethasone and etoposide. Intrathecal methotrexate is given for CNS disease. Bone marrow transplant is indicated for children with primary HLH and children with secondary HLH who are refractory to chemotherapy or relapse.

THE MEDSTUDY HUB:
YOUR GUIDELINES AND
REVIEW ARTICLES RESOURCE

For both the review articles and current Pediatrics practice guidelines, visit the MedStudy Hub at

medstudy.com/hub

The Hub contains the only online consolidated list of all Pediatrics guidelines! Guidelines on the Hub are continually updated and linked to the published source. MedStudy maintains the Hub as a free online resource, available to all physicians.

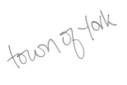